Second Edition

# VISUAL PERCEPTION

**Steven H. Schwartz, OD, PhD**

State College of Optometry
State University of New York
New York, New York

APPLETON & LANGE
Stamford, Connecticut

99 00 01 02 03 / 10 9 8 7 6 5 4 3 2



**Library of Congress Cataloging-in-Publication Data**

Schwartz, Steven H.
Visual perception : a clinical orientation / Steven H. Schwartz.—
2nd ed.
p. cm.
Includes bibliographical references and index.
ISBN 0-8385-9466-2 (case : alk. paper)
1. Visual perception. 2. Vision disorders—Pathophysiology.
I. Title.
[DNLM: 1. Visual Perception. 2. Vision. WW 105 S399v 1999]
QP475.S38 1998
612.8′4—dc21
DNLM/DLC
for Library of Congress 98-20409

Acquisitions Editor: Lin Marshall
Production Editor: Lisa M. Guidone
Art Coordinator: Eve Siegel/Jennsin Services
Art Studio: ElectraGraphics
Designer: Mary Skudlarek

ISBN 0-8385-9466-2
90000
9 780838 594667

PRINTED IN THE UNITED STATES OF AMERICA

# Contents

# Foreword

*If we believed that we must try to find out what is not known, we should be better and braver and less idle than if we believed that what we do not know is impossible to find out and that we need not even try.*

Socrates, *The Meno*

The core of any profession is its basis in scientific knowledge, and for those in the eye and vision care professions, we are indeed fortunate that our core is so rich and deep and broad. Vision science draws its facts and its theories from a wide range of sources—physics, optics, anatomy, physiology, biochemistry, psychology, and cognitive neurosciences. While much of our core knowledge traces back to Leonardo da Vinci, Thomas Young, Helmholtz, Hering, and Wheatstone, vision science is a dynamic field, and our current knowledge also owes a great debt to more recent contributions by such modern workers as Granit, Wald, Hubel and Wiesel, Enroth-Cugell and Robson, and Nathans. Over the more than 20 years since Cornsweet's excellent book on the topic, there has been an explosion in our knowledge and understanding of visual neurophysiology, genetics, development and aging, and many other key aspects of visual function.

While there are many books dealing with aspects of visual science in great depth, there are few books written on the topic with a view to the clinical importance of the topic for those in the eye and vision care professions. In this book, Dr. Steven Schwartz has, I believe, succeeded in covering a broad range of subjects in visual science, and in bringing home the clinical relevance of each section to the reader.

No single volume can address all of visual science; however, this book covers an extraordinarily broad range of clinically important topics, which include color vision and its defects, spatial vision, temporal aspects of vision, psychophysics, physiology, and development and aging. The second edition incorporates new material on extrastriate visual processing, motion perception, and the molecular genetics of color vision—all rapidly developing areas. Dr. Schwartz has a keen understanding of both the fundamental aspects of vision and their clinical implications, and his unique approach, which brings the science and its applications together, will make this book a very popular one in teaching visual science to optometry students.

Dr. Schwartz has a real skill for explaining difficult concepts in very simple (but technically accurate) terms. Moreover, this book goes well beyond the basics, including information from anatomy to perception, and always highlights the clinical implications. Throughout the book, Dr. Schwartz manages to convey much of the excitement of important new developments, while providing the reader with suitable caution as to what aspects of the unfolding stories are still controversial.

Dr. Schwartz displays a real empathy for his readers. For example, in the *Color Vision* chapter, after accurately describing the very difficult concepts related to the CIE system, Dr. Schwartz assures readers by telling them "If you are having difficulty understanding this system, do not feel alone." This is a nice touch, and Dr. Schwartz then goes on to provide helpful suggestions for gaining deeper understanding. The discussion questions (and the "hints") are also likely to be helpful to both teachers of vision science and to the students using the book.

In summary, this book represents a comprehensive text on visual science, providing fundamental concepts in an engaging and interesting style. This information does not exist in any other single volume, and the close links forged between the basic knowledge and the clinical applications make the book particularly appealing for optometric and ophthalmologic students, faculty, and researchers.

Dennis M. Levi, OD, PhD
University of Houston
November, 1998

# Preface

A patient with early cataracts complains of a profound reduction in vision. When we measure the patient's visual acuity, however, we find little or no reduction. How do we explain this apparent lack of consistency between the patient's severe complaint and the near-normal visual acuity? On the basis of our knowledge of visual perception, how do we best treat this patient?

Eye care professionals routinely diagnose and treat conditions that have profound effects on visual perception. But how well do we understand the fundamentals of visual perception and their application to clinical practice? My experience tells me that the rich body of knowledge developed in recent decades regarding visual perception is not fully utilized in routine clinical practice.

Although there are several fine textbooks on visual perception, none are written for the eye care professional. This text is intended to provide those essentials of *monocular* visual perception on which successful clinical practice is predicated.

The text stresses fundamental concepts and models of monocular visual perception. These models are physiologically based. Although a patient may present with a perceptual complaint, the disease or disorder affects the structures of the visual system. Consequently, clinically useful models of visual perception link perception with anatomy and physiology.

In addition to providing a basic science background, each chapter discusses the clinical relevance and application of the material. Clinical information is presented in such a manner that beginning clinicians will benefit from the discussions.

The second edition has been expanded to include certain of the myriad advances in our understanding of visual perception that have occurred in recent years. In particular, new materials on extrastriate visual processing, motion perception, and the molecular genetics of color vision are covered. Virtually all chapters have been substantially updated to include new information. As in the first edition, an effort has been made to present complex and sophisticated concepts in a manner that is concise, comprehensible, and clinically relevant, while maintaining an appropriate degree of scientific rigor.

The concepts presented in each chapter build on those developed in previous chapters. Therefore, if the reader chooses to skip chapters, he or she may need to refer back to preceding chapters for a fuller understanding of the material.

Self-assessment questions are presented at the conclusion of many chapters, with answers given at the end of the book. These questions are intended to develop and reinforce key concepts.

# Acknowledgments

Special thanks go to Mrs. Pat McCollum for transforming my nearly indecipherable scribblings into legible text. Pat's patience in handling the numerous revisions and frequent rewritings was remarkable and is greatly appreciated.

Drs. Michael Barris, Ralph Jensen, David Lee, Dennis Levi, Michael Loop, and Joel Pokorny graciously gave of their time to review portions of the original manuscript. Their insightful and encouraging input made my job considerably easier.

Dr. William Cochran, Dr. Norman Haffner, Ms. Linda Marshall, Ms. Cheryl Mehalik, and Dr. Douglas Poorman demonstrated confidence in this project and provided essential encouragement. For this I am very thankful.

I would also like to thank Drs. Bryan Deck and Jeannie Stone for their thoughtful comments on earlier versions of the manuscript. Their input helped me to maintain the primary focus of the book—teaching visual perception to clinicians.

Below are listed those individuals that generously provided feedback regarding the first edition of the textbook or reviewed portions of the second edition manuscript.

**Michael C. Barris, PhD**
College of Optometry
Nova Southeastern University
Ft. Lauderdale, Florida

**Mike Fendick, OD, PhD**
College of Optometry
Nova Southeastern University
Ft. Lauderdale, Florida

**Peter F. Hitchcock, PhD**
W. K. Kellogg Eye Center
University of Michigan
Ann Arbor, Michigan

**Jeff Hovis, OD, PhD**
School of Optometry
University of Waterloo
Waterloo, Ontario

**Ralph J. Jensen, PhD**
Southern College of Optometry
Memphis, Tennessee

**David Lee, OD, PhD**
Illinois College of Optometry
Chicago, Illinois

**Dennis M. Levi, OD, PhD**
College of Optometry
University of Houston
Houston, Texas

**Michael S. Loop, PhD**
School of Optometry/The Medical Center
University of Alabama at Birmingham
Birmingham, Alabama

**Alan Riezman, OD**
Jerry L. Pettis VA Hospital
Loma Linda, California

**Scott B. Steinman, OD, PhD**
Southern College of Optometry
Memphis, Tennessee

**Dean Yager, PhD**
State College of Optometry
State University of New York
New York, New York

**Robert L. Yolton, OD, PhD**
College of Optometry
Pacific University
Forest Grove, Oregon

# 1

# Experimental Approaches

The neurons that constitute the visual system are organized to analyze and process an enormous amount of information. This information includes color, motion, detail, and depth. The central issues in visual perception concern the manner in which this information is processed.

Three classic experimental approaches are used to study visual perception: **anatomic, neurophysiologic,** and **psychophysical.** To understand the utility of these different experimental strategies, consider an analogy. The visual system can be considered comparable, in some respects, to a complex electronic machine. How would we go about understanding a novel complex electronic device?

One approach is to carefully open up the machine and determine its structure. Diagrams are made that show the locations of the various components of this device and the connections these components make with each other. This methodology is analogous to an anatomic approach. The structure of the apparatus is determined with the expectation that it will provide insight into the function of the apparatus.

A second approach is to determine the functions of the individual components that compose the device. Electronic probes, such as voltmeters, are used to record electrical activity from various components, circuits, and wires within the machine. The flow of information, in terms of electric current, is determined. This approach is analogous to an electrophysiologic methodology. The electronic flow of information within the apparatus is determined with the goal of determining how the apparatus processes information.

A third approach is to determine the operational capabilities of the device. If the device has a keyboard, information is typed into this keyboard and the response of the machine is determined. The various dials and switches on the apparatus are adjusted, and the effect of these manipulations on the machine's function is determined. In essence, the apparatus is treated as a **black box** (Fig. 1–1).

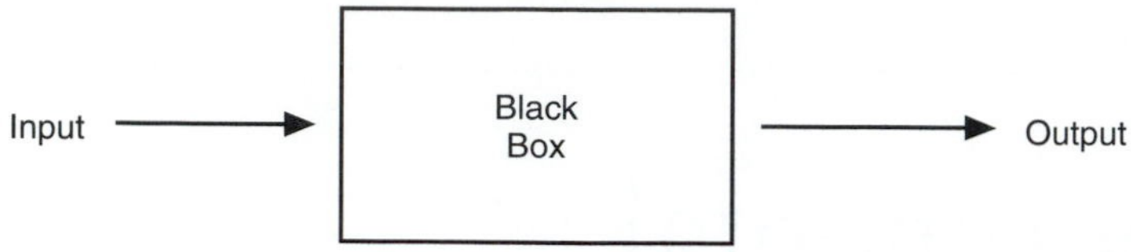


**FIGURE 1–1.** Psychophysical approaches frequently treat the visual system as a black box. A precisely specified input is presented to the system, and the output is determined. From the input–output relationship, the operational characteristics of the system are determined.

Information is fed into the black box and the output is determined. This noninvasive approach—it does not require the apparatus to be dismantled—is psychophysical in nature. By manipulating the input to the apparatus and observing its response, the operational capabilities of the device are determined.

Each of the preceding approaches (anatomic, neurophysiologic, and psychophysical) is essential for full comprehension of the mechanisms that underlie visual perception. The anatomy of the visual system must be elucidated to understand the flow of information within the system. Neurophysiologic investigations are necessary to understand the processing of information at various levels of the visual system. And psychophysical studies are central to an understanding of the capabilities and operating strategies of the visual system.

A new experimental approach, which does not readily lend itself to the machine analogy, is **brain imaging.** In brain imaging studies, the brain's metabolic activity is observed in an alert subject while the subject performs a specified task. For instance, metabolic activity is assessed while a subject views a moving target. The areas of the brain that exhibit the most activity (compared to the baseline activity measured when the subject views a stationary target) are presumably involved in processing motion information. This new research technique is very promising because it allows us to monitor neural activity in alert human subjects.

The data and models presented in this book are derived from these basic experimental approaches. The clinical application of the material, however, rests largely with psychophysical procedures. Psychophysical testing, because it is noninvasive, can be used to assess function on clinical populations. For this reason, the book emphasizes psychophysical experimentation.

# 2

# Introductory Concepts

To study visual perception, it is necessary to be familiar with certain basic aspects of ocular anatomy and physiology and the physics of light. In this chapter, these topics are briefly introduced. Although the discussion is neither detailed nor comprehensive, it provides background material critical to the study of visual perception.

## *VERY BASIC OCULAR ANATOMY*

### *Three Ocular Layers: Sclera, Uvea, and Retina*

Figure 2–1 shows a horizontal cross-section of the human eye. At birth, the average eye has an **axial length** (cornea to retina) of 17 mm, and grows to an average length of 25.4 mm (1 in) in the adult.

The eye can be thought of as consisting of three different layers. The outermost layer is the sclera, the middle layer is the uvea, and the innermost layer is the retina.

The sclera is the white portion of the eye that is apparent on gross observation. This layer consists largely of collagen. It provides support and protection for the internal elements of the eye. The sclera is continuous with the cornea, which is the transparent tissue at the most anterior aspect of the eye.

The uvea is a highly vascularized tissue that, among other functions, plays a large role in providing nutrition to the various elements of the eye. The uvea is divided into three components: the iris, the ciliary body, and the choroid.

The **iris** constricts in response to light and dilates in the absence of light. By controlling the diameter of the pupil, the iris helps to regulate the amount of light that enters the eye.

The **ciliary body** has two primary functions. First, it contains a muscle, the ciliary muscle, that focuses the lens for near vision. This process is referred to

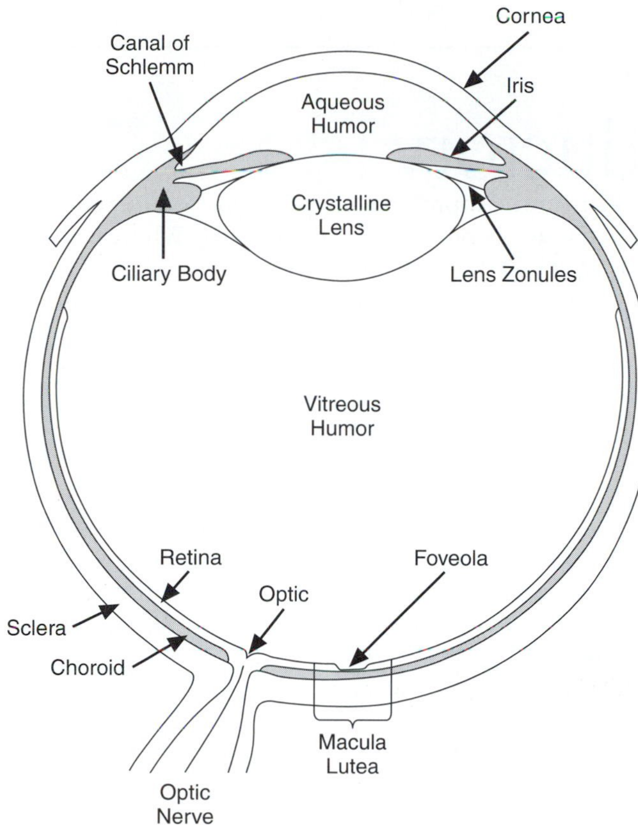


**FIGURE 2–1.** Cross-section of the human eye. (*Adapted from Salzmann M.* The Anatomy and Physiology of the Human Eyeball in the Normal State [*translated by Brown EVC*]. *Chicago: University of Chicago Press; 1912.*)

as **accommodation.** Second, the ciliary body is the source of the **aqueous humor.** The aqueous humor provides nourishment to certain internal eye structures, including the cornea and the lens.

The **choroid** forms the bulk of the uveal tract. The choroid serves the important role of providing blood to the outermost aspects of the retina.

The **retina** is the innermost tissue layer of the eye. It is an exceedingly complex, multilayered neural element that is only 0.2 mm thick. The preceding optical elements focus images on the retina. The retina then begins the complex task of analyzing these images.

### *Ocular Anatomy from Anterior to Posterior*

In the previous section, we considered ocular anatomy in terms of layers going from the outer sclera to the inner retina. In this section, we consider ocular anatomy proceeding from the anterior to posterior aspect of the eye.

The most anterior aspect of the eye is the **cornea.** The cornea is a five-layered transparent structure. Approximately two thirds of the refractive power (focusing power) of the eye is provided by the cornea. Whereas the eye's total refractive power is about 60 diopters, the cornea's power is 40 diopters (Millodot, 1982). Mismatches between the refractive power of the cornea and the axial length of the eye are responsible for most refractive errors.

The aqueous humor is contained within the **anterior** and **posterior chambers** of the eye. (The anterior chamber is bounded by the posterior surface of the cornea and the anterior surfaces of the crystalline lens and iris, while the posterior chamber is bounded by the posterior surface of the iris and the anterior surface of the vitreous humor.) The aqueous is continuously produced by the ciliary body and drained by the **canal of Schlemm.** The canal of Schlemm is located in the angle of the eye, where the iris inserts into the ciliary body. This structure runs circumferentially around the eye.

The aqueous humor exerts a pressure, referred to as the **intraocular pressure (IOP),** of about 16 mm Hg that helps to maintain the structural integrity of the eye. In certain forms of **glaucoma** the IOP is elevated, presumably leading to retinal damage. Elevated IOPs can result from the overproduction of aqueous, poor drainage of aqueous from the eye, or a combination of these factors.

Posterior to the iris is the **crystalline lens.** The lens provides about one third of the dioptric power of the eye. When viewing a distant object, the lens power is approximately 20 diopters. When viewing a near object, the dioptric power of the lens increases, thus allowing near objects to be clearly viewed. As previously mentioned, this process is referred to as accommodation. Accommodation occurs when the ciliary muscle constricts. This releases tension on the **lens zonules** and allows the lens to assume a more "natural" position in which its anterior surface bulges forward (Fig. 2–2). This bulge in the lens anterior surface produces an increase in the dioptric power of the lens and, consequently, the eye itself.

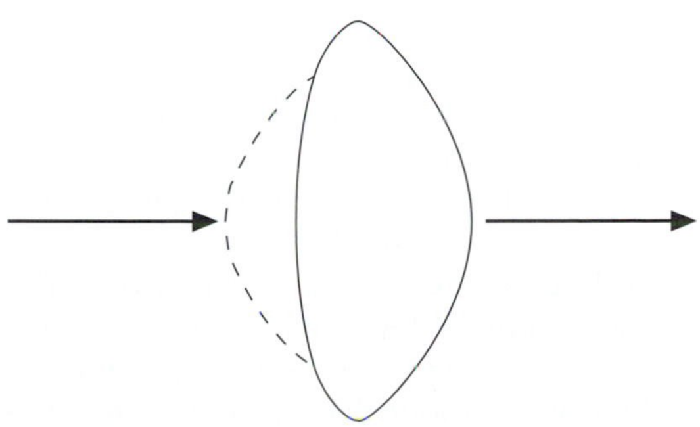

**FIGURE 2–2.** When viewing distant objects, the anterior surface of the lens is relatively flat (solid line). To focus near objects, the anterior surface bulges forward (dashed line). This decreases the radius of curvature of the anterior lens surface, producing an increase in the dioptric power of the lens.

As we age, our ability to accommodate diminishes, apparently due to reduced elasticity of the crystalline lens. By the time most people are in their middle 40s, their ability to accommodate has diminished to the point where they cannot read without plus lenses, a condition referred to as **presbyopia.**

The crystalline lens becomes less transparent with age, apparently due to the destructive oxidative effects of free radicals. If the loss of transparency becomes significant and results in a loss of visual acuity, the patient is said to have a **cataract.** During cataract surgery, one of the most common surgical procedures, the lens is removed and replaced by a synthetic lens.

The **vitreous humor** makes up the bulk of the eye volume. It consists largely of collagen and hyaluronic acid and has a gel-like structure. The vitreous provides structural and nutritive support for the retina in addition to creating a dioptrically critical space.

Posterior to the vitreous humor is the retina. It is on this tissue that the visual world is focused. For our study of visual perception, this is the most important ocular tissue.

## *Basic Retinal Anatomy and Postretinal Pathways*

In some respects, the eye can be considered to be analogous to a camera. Like a camera, the eye focuses the world on a light-sensitive element. In the case of a camera, this element is photographic film; for the eye, it is the retina.

This analogy falls apart when we examine the roles of the film in a camera and the retina in the eye. The film in a camera undergoes a chemical reaction in response to the light that falls on it. This provides the outlines of the photograph. Shades of black and white are dictated by the intensity distribution of the light that falls on the film. Colors are a bit more complex, but follow the same basic principles. The film of a camera acts as a passive receiver of light and simply provides a point-by-point representation of the light distribution falling on it.

The retina behaves very differently from photographic film. The retina is a multilayered neural tissue that begins the process of actively analyzing the image that falls upon it. The retina highlights certain information and disregards other information. In this sense, the retina makes decisions regarding which information is vital to the animal's survival and, consequently, which information will be transmitted to higher visual centers.

Early vision scientists considered the retina to be a passive receiver, much like photographic film. In this simple view, the retina was thought to transmit a point-by-point photographic representation of the focused visual image onto higher visual centers.

This simple view implies that there is an area of the brain that "views" this photographic image. In fact, early scientists envisioned a homunculus, or little person, sitting in the brain and viewing these images. The simplistic nature of this conception becomes apparent when we consider that this theory requires another homunculus to be sitting in the head of the original homunculus. In fact, the natural conclusion of this theory would be an infinite series of progressively smaller homunculi, each viewing the image in the preceding homunculus' brain.

Modern visual science provides abundant empirical evidence that the retina sends a complex neural signal to the brain. Although this signal bears a close resemblance to the image that falls on the retina, it does not represent a point-by-point representation of this image.

This hypothesis is nicely illustrated by studying the visual systems of lower animals. Because lower animals have smaller brains, proportionately more visual processing takes place in the retina than is the case for higher animals. For example, the retina of the frog is capable of detecting a bug and triggering the decision to strike the bug with the frog's tongue (Lettvin et al, 1959). The frog's retina actively analyzes the image that falls upon it, and this analysis serves as a basis for the animal's behavior.

The same is true to a much lesser extent in the mammalian retina. Color, motion, and contrast information are analyzed by the retina and transmitted as a complex signal to higher centers in the brain. Because of the complex neural processing performed by the retina, it typically is assumed to be a part of the brain. The same basic processes that occur in the brain proper also occur in the retina.

Next we discuss basic functional retinal anatomy. In later chapters, we discuss information processing within this complex structure.

### *Retinal Layers*

Figure 2–3 is a schematic flowchart of retinal processing. The photoreceptors (rods and cones) respond to light and transform this radiant energy into electrical activity. This electrical activity is transmitted to retinal bipolar cells and then to retinal ganglion cells. The retinal ganglion cells have long axons which leave the eye and synapse in the dorsal lateral geniculate nucleus (dLGN), a midbrain structure.

This photoreceptor → bipolar cell → ganglion cell arrangement reflects the feed-forward, or **centripetal,** nature of retinal organization. In addition to this feed-forward arrangement, however, there are lateral connections within the retina. These provide for the lateral, or horizontal, transmission of retinal information. As indicated in Figure 2–3, **horizontal** and **amacrine** cells are involved in this lateral integration of retinal information.

In addition to the feed-forward nature of the retina and the lateral interactions, there is also a feedback transmission of information. In this pathway, referred to as the **centrifugal pathway,** information is transmitted from the ganglion cell region back toward the photoreceptors by **interplexiform** cells (Lindberg and Fisher, 1986).

Figures 2–3B, 2–4, and 2–5 show cross-sections of the primate retina. Note

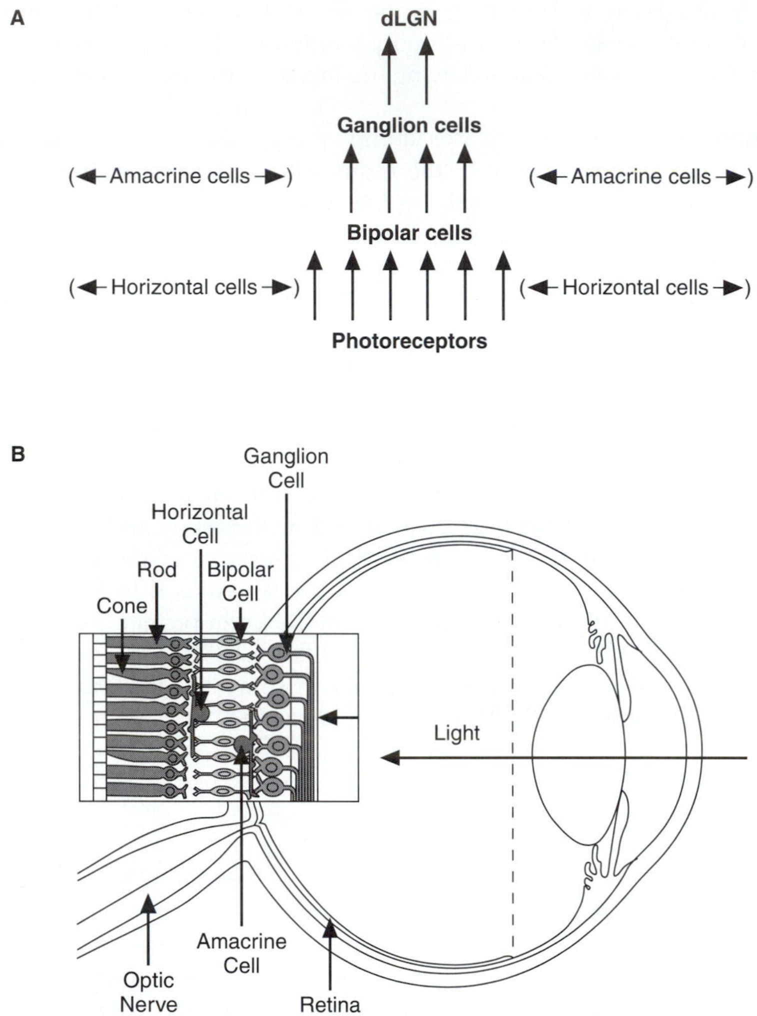


**FIGURE 2–3. A.** Schematic flowchart of retinal processing. A feed-forward pathway consists of the photoreceptors → bipolar cells → ganglion cells. The horizontal and amacrine cells participate in lateral integration within the retina. **B.** Magnified section of the retina that shows that light must pass through the inner retinal layers before it reaches the photoreceptors. The photoreceptors absorb light quanta and convert this radiant energy into electrical activity. (*From Hubel DH.* Eye, Brain, and Vision. *New York: Scientific American Library; 1988. Reprinted with permission of W. H. Freeman and Company.*)

that light passes through the vitreous, through the inner layers of the retina, and then onto the photoreceptors, which are located in the outer retina. The inner retinal elements do little to degrade the retinal image because they are somewhat transparent and, as we will learn, laterally displaced in the region of the retina that is associated with the best vision, the fovea.

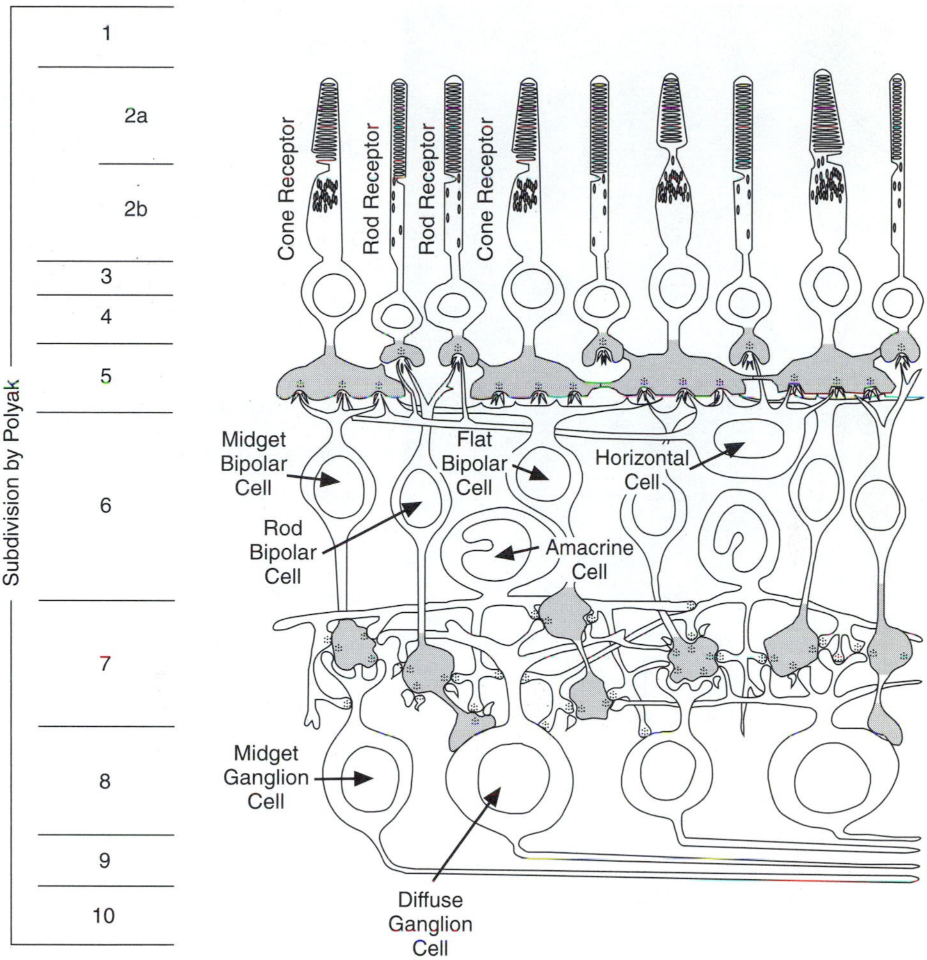


**FIGURE 2–4.** Schematic of retinal organization as proposed by Dowling and Boycott (1966). Beginning at the outer retina, the retinal layers are (1) retinal pigment epithelium, (2a) outer segments of the photoreceptors, (2b) inner segments of the photoreceptors, (3) outer limiting membrane, (4) outer nuclear layer, (5) outer plexiform layer, (6) inner nuclear layer, (7) inner plexiform layer, (8) ganglion cell layer, (9) nerve fiber layer, and (10) internal limiting membrane. Light would come from the bottom of the diagram and pass through the inner retina before reaching the photoreceptors. Subdivisions proposed by Polyak (1941) are given in the margin. (*From Wyszecki G, Stiles WS.* Color Science: Concepts and Methods, Quantitative Data and Formulae. *Copyright 1982. Reprinted by permission of John Wiley & Sons, Inc.*)

In the discussion that follows, we examine retinal anatomy going from the outer layers to the inner layers. The outer retina comprises those elements proximal to the sclera, whereas the inner retina comprises those elements proximal to the vitreous.

The outermost layer of the retina is the **retinal pigment epithelium**

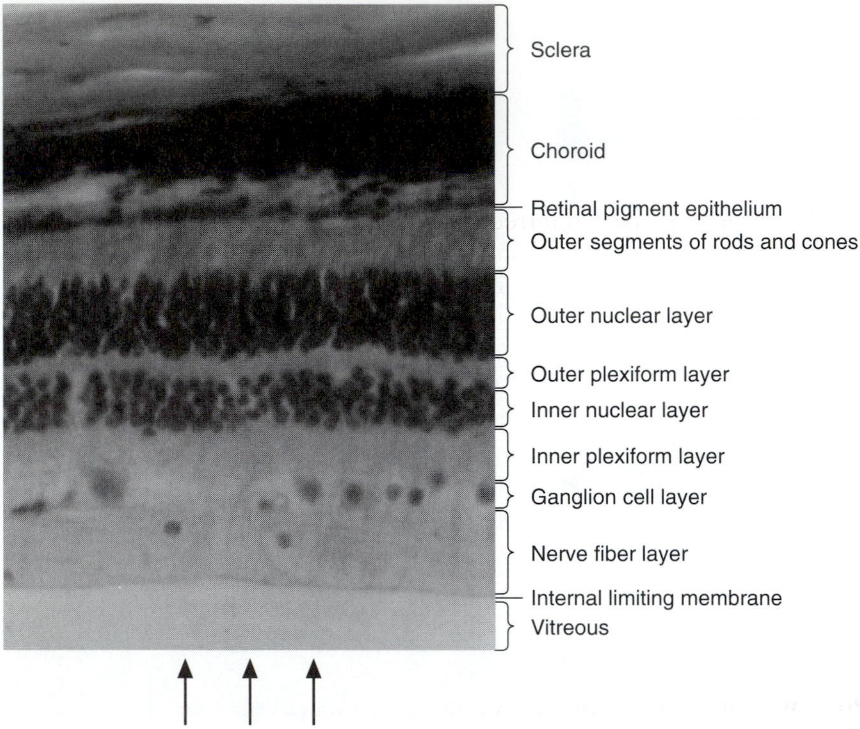


**FIGURE 2–5.** Cross-section of the peripheral monkey retina. Not labeled are the inner segments of the rods and cones and the outer limiting membrane. Note that light must pass through the inner retina prior to reaching the photoreceptors. Also note that the number of photoreceptors greatly exceeds the number of ganglion cells. This illustrates the convergence of information within the retina. (*Photomicrograph courtesy of Dr. Ralph Jensen.*)

**(RPE).** The RPE is not responsive to radiant energy and does not participate in the encoding of visual information. This tissue does, however, play a critical role in providing nutritional support for the photoreceptors. As discussed in Chapter 3, the RPE phagocytizes the continuously produced outer segments of the photoreceptors (Young, 1970, 1971). In addition, the darkly pigmented RPE absorbs light photons that are not absorbed by the photoreceptors and, thereby, reduces light scatter within the eye.

Inner to the RPE are the **photoreceptors.** The photoreceptors manifest a very high level of metabolic activity, among the highest in the body. It is for this reason that they are located in the outer retina close to the choroidal blood supply.

The photoreceptors fall into two categories: **rods** provide nighttime vision and **cones** provide daytime vision. The outermost aspect of a photoreceptor is the **outer segment.** This contains a photopigment that absorbs light and converts this radiant energy into electrical activity. The outer segments form a distinct retinal layer.

The next retinal layer consists of the **inner segments** of the photoreceptors. This layer contains many of the organelles of these cells, excluding their nuclei.

A thin structural layer, referred to as the **outer limiting membrane,** separates the inner segments of the photoreceptors from their nuclei. The photoreceptor nuclei form a distinct layer, which is referred to as the **outer nuclear layer (ONL).**

The first synapses within the retina occur within the **outer plexiform layer (OPL).** This layer consists of the dendrites of the bipolar and horizontal cells and the synapses these cells make with the photoreceptors.

Inner to the OPL is the **inner nuclear layer (INL).** This layer consists of the cell bodies of the bipolar, horizontal, and amacrine cells.

The second stage of synapses within the visual system occurs within the **inner plexiform layer (IPL).** Contained within this layer are the various synapses among the bipolar, amacrine, and ganglion cells.

The innermost cell body layer of the retina is the **ganglion cell layer.** There are two major classes of ganglion cells. The smaller **midget,** or **parvo (P),** cells comprise about 80 percent of the ganglion cells and the larger **parasol,** or **magno (M)** cells about 10 percent of the ganglion cells (Lennie et al, 1990).

The axons of the ganglion cells constitute the next layer, which is referred to as the **nerve fiber layer.** These axons exit the eye and form the **optic nerve,** the second cranial nerve, and synapse in the midbrain. As these axons are not normally myelinated within the eye, they do not significantly interfere with vision. These axons do, however, become myelinated once they leave the eye.

The innermost retinal layer is the **internal limiting membrane.** This membrane acts as an interface between the retina and the vitreous humor.

The preceding description of retinal anatomy is basic and omits many details of both scientific and clinical importance. For example, there are thought to be about 20 different types of amacrine cells. The description does, however, point to the richness and complexity of retinal organization. The many different categories of retinal neurons and their complex synaptic connections, all point to a high degree of information processing within the retina.

A key feature of retinal organization is lateral interaction. Horizontal and amacrine cells integrate information laterally within the retina. These lateral interactions allow for the processing of visual information across space. This important issue is discussed in more detail in Chapters 7 and 13.

There is a significant convergence of information within the retina. A convergence of retinal information is implied by the existence of considerably more photoreceptors than ganglion cells; there are more than 100 million photoreceptors and only 1 million ganglion cells (Østerberg, 1935; Curcio and Allen, 1990). The implication of this reduction in the number of cells as we progress to higher levels of the retina is that visual information is processed as it is transmitted from the photoreceptors to the ganglion cells. Some information is highlighted and encoded, whereas other information is lost.

The diameter of the optic nerve and the number of ganglion cell axons it contains are limited by the structure of the skull. This anatomic limitation makes it necessary for there to be a convergence of information within the retina. Of clinical relevance is the vulnerability of the optic nerve to eye disease. All retinal information is contained within this structure, and any damage to it can have profound effects on vision.

### *Optic Disk and Foveola*

Figure 2–6A is a photograph of the retina. This photograph and the drawing given in Figure 2–6B show the appearance of the normal retina as observed during ophthalmoscopy. The retina and other ocular structures, as seen during ophthalmoscopy, are referred to as the **fundus.**

The **optic nerve head,** or **optic disk,** is a prominent feature of the fundus. This structure represents the bundle of ganglion cell axons as they leave the eye and form the optic nerve. The whitish appearance of the optic nerve head is due to the myelin sheath that covers these axons as they leave the eye. Normally, the ganglion cell axons do not acquire a myelin sheath before they reach the optic nerve head.

There are no photoreceptors in the area of the optic disk. Consequently, this area of the retina provides no vision. The result is a **physiologic blind spot** in each eye, located approximately 15 degrees temporal to the point of fixation. Physiologic blind spots can be demonstrated by observing Figure 2–7.

Temporal to the optic disk is a highly specialized region of the retina referred to as the **fovea** by clinicians. (The term, fovea, has different meanings to clinicians and anatomists as indicated in Table 2–1, which gives the dimensions of these structures.) The fovea is the area of the retina with which you are now reading these words. It subtends a visual angle of about 1.2 degrees, twice the angular subtense of the moon (Pirenne, 1967). It is the area of the retina that provides the best detail-oriented vision (visual resolution).

Observe the E in Figure 2–8. The letter is easily resolvable. Yet, while looking at the E, the surrounding letters are not easily resolvable. This is because the letter E is falling on the fovea, while the other letters fall on more peripheral regions of the retina.

A number of anatomic features distinguish the fovea from other regions of the retina. In the fovea, there are only cones; rods are absent. The packing density of these foveal cones is greater than for any other region of the retina (see Fig. 3–7).

To maximize foveal vision, the neural elements of the inner retina are pushed aside to allow light to fall directly on the photopigment-containing outer segments of cones. This pushing aside of retinal elements produces a pit, referred to as the **foveal pit** (Fig. 2–9).

A

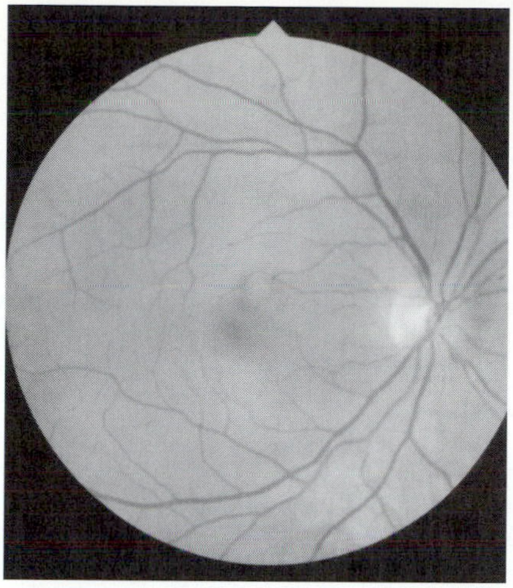

B

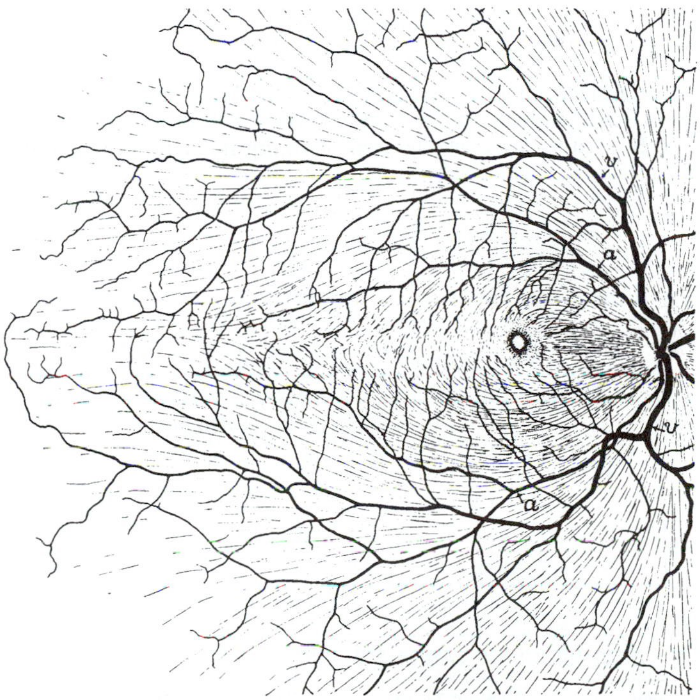


**FIGURE 2–6. A.** Photograph of a normal fundus of a right human eye. Vessels that supply the inner retina emerge from the optic nerve head. The avascular fovea is left (temporal) of the optic nerve head. (*Photograph courtesy of Dr. Mohammad Rafieetary.*) **B.** Sketch of the fundus of a rhesus monkey. Note the avascular fovea which is left (temporal) of the optic disk. The striations show the course of the nerve fiber layer. (*From Polyak SL.* The Retina. *Copyright 1941. Reprinted by permission of the University of Chicago Press.*)

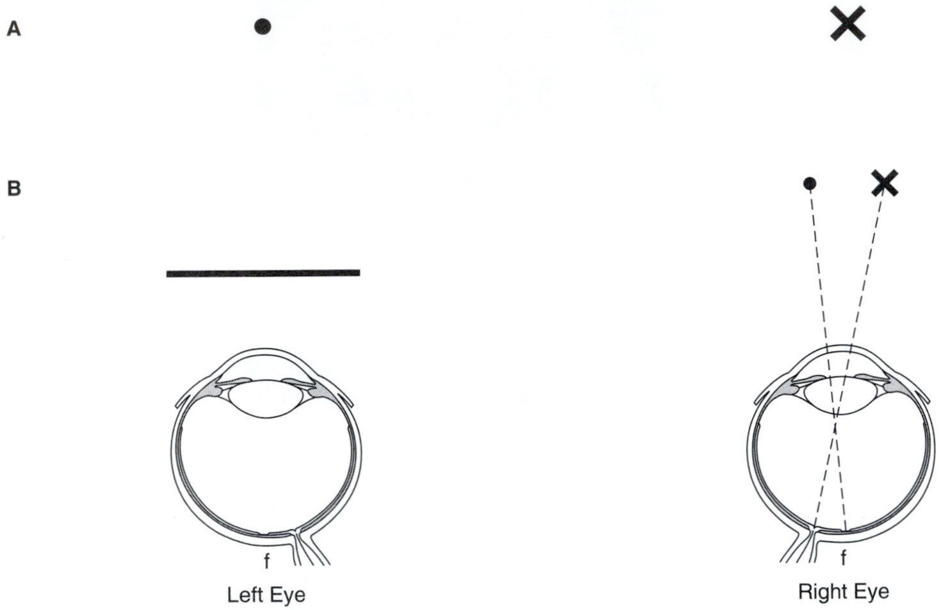


**FIGURE 2–7. A.** Demonstration of the physiologic blind spot. Close your left eye and view the dot at a distance of 8 to 10 in. Note that the X disappears. This is because the image of the X falls on the optic disk. **B.** Looking down onto the eyes, it can be seen that the optic disk is nasal to the fovea. This results in the physiologic blind spot being temporal to the fixation point.

Whereas other retinal regions are covered by the inner retinal vascular network that nourishes the inner retina, the fovea is avascular. (Observation of Figure 2–6 shows that the fovea is not covered by retinal vessels.) This adaptation prevents the scattering of light by retinal vessels and, consequently, maximizes the visual resolution provided by the fovea. Metabolic nourishment for both foveal and nonfoveal cones is provided by the choroid.

These adaptations—absence of rods, maximal density of cones, pushing aside of inner retinal elements to expose the cone outer segments to light, and absence of retinal vasculature—all contribute to the excellent resolution pro-

**TABLE 2–1. DIMENSIONS OF VARIOUS RETINAL LANDMARKS[a]**

| Anatomic Term | Clinical Term | Diameter (mm) | Diameter (degrees) |
|---|---|---|---|
| Optic nerve head | Optic disk | 1.8 | 5.0 |
| Foveola | Fovea | 0.3 | 1.2 |
| Fovea | Macula | 1.8 | 5.0 |
| Macula | Area centralis | 5.8 | 18.5 |

[a]Data from Polyak (1941).

F B

E

H M

**FIGURE 2–8.** While fixating the letter E, note that the other letters are not easily resolvable. Visual resolution is most acute in the fovea and less developed in the peripheral retina.

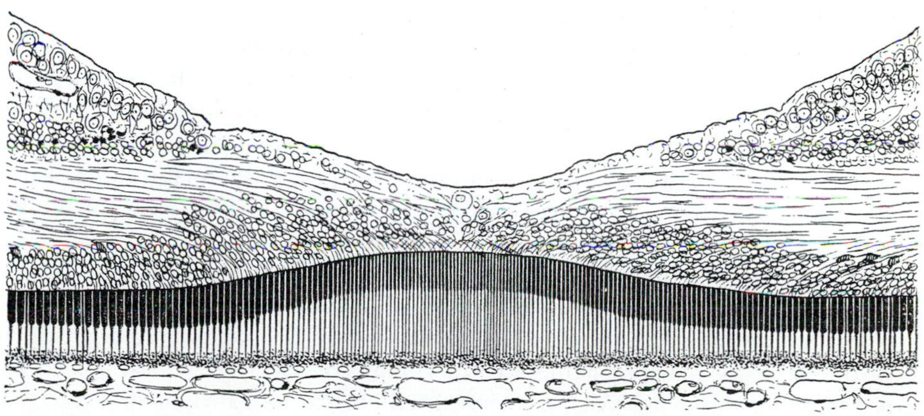

**FIGURE 2–9.** Cross-section of the human foveola. Note the pit that is formed by the pushing aside of inner retinal elements. This exposes the photoreceptors directly to light, which would be coming from the top of this diagram. (*From Polyak SL.* The Retina. *Copyright 1941. Reprinted by permission of the University of Chicago Press.*)

vided by the fovea. The fovea, although physically small, plays a very large role in the processing of visual information.

Surrounding the fovea is a region of the retina referred to as the **macula lutea.** The macula lutea contains a nonphotosensitive yellow pigment, located in the inner retina. This pigment absorbs blue light (maximal absorption is in the region of 460 nm) and may aid vision by reducing light scatter or minimizing the effects of chromatic aberration (Wald,1945).

### *Postretinal Pathways*

The axons of the retinal ganglion cells leave the eye via the second cranial nerve, the **optic nerve.** The precise course and projection of these nerve fibers are beyond the scope of this text. Rather, discussion is limited to the general course of those fibers that are central to visual perception.

At the **optic chiasm,** ganglion cell fibers from the nasal retina of each eye cross over to join the temporal fibers of the fellow eye to form the **optic tract** (Fig. 2–10). As a result, the fibers constituting the left optic tract carry information regarding the right visual field, and fibers in the right optic tract encode the left visual field.

General schemes of postretinal organization are given in Figures 2–10 and 2–11. The primary target of the optic tract is the **dorsal lateral geniculate nucleus (dLGN),** a thalamic nucleus. Most, but not all, retinal ganglion cells synapse in this six-layered structure. Layers 2, 3, and 5 receive input from the ipsilateral eye, whereas layers 1, 4, and 6 receive input from the contralateral eye (see Fig. 13–1).

The dLGN is composed of two distinct regions. The dorsal four layers, which are constituted of comparatively small neurons called parvo, or P-cells, are referred to as the **parvocellular** layers. Larger neurons, commonly called magno or M-cells comprise the ventral two **magnocellular** layers. Axons from P-cells in the retina synapse on P-cells in the dLGN forming the **parvo pathway,** while axons from retinal M-cells synapse on dLGN M-cells forming the **magno pathway.** These two pathways are referred to as parallel pathways because they each apparently process different aspects of the image that falls on the retina. As discussed in Chapter 13, the parvo pathway encodes detail and color, while the magno pathway encodes fast movement.

The cells of the dLGN send most of their axons to the cerebral cortex, the most highly evolved portion of the brain. This structure consists of two hemispheres that are connected by the corpus callosum. The cortical area in which most dLGN axons synapse is the **striate visual cortex.** This region is also referred to as visual area 1 (V1), primary visual cortex, and Brodmann's area 17. The striate cortex is dominated by foveal input, a phenomenon referred to as the cortical magnification of foveal vision.

Cells in the striate cortex send many of their axons to nearby visual cortical areas, which are collectively called the **extrastriate visual cortex.** From this

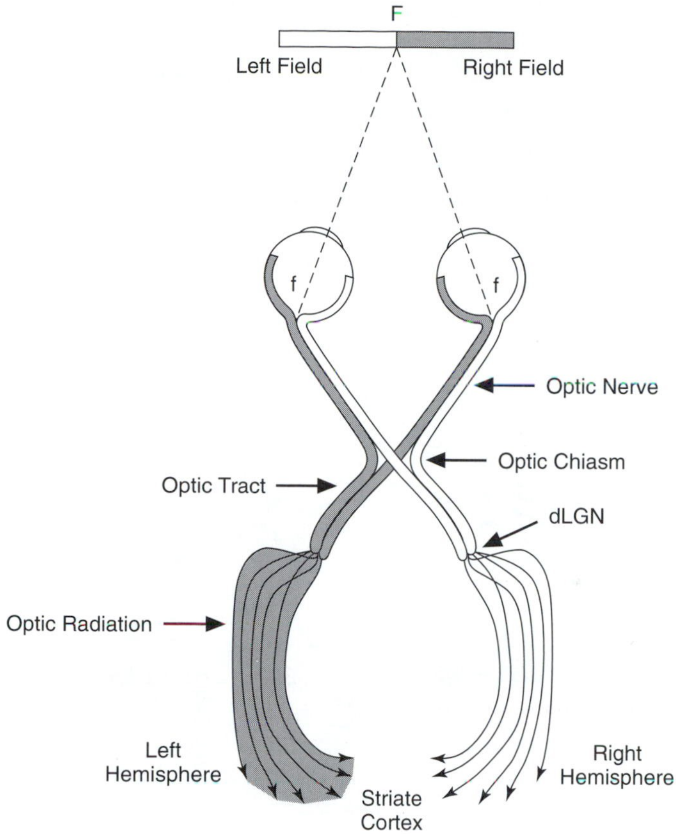


**FIGURE 2–10.** Nerve fibers that originate from the nasal half of the retina join fibers from the temporal retina of the fellow eye at the optic chiasm. Consequently, objects in the right half of the visual field are processed in the left cortical hemisphere and objects in the left half of the visual field are processed in the right cortical hemisphere. In this schematic, the foveas (f) are aligned with the fixation point (F).

point, axons are sent to a great diversity of higher cortical areas. These higher cortical areas are involved in the integration of visual information with memory and other sensory modalities. The striate cortex also sends a major projection back to the dLGN. This feedback loop can be considered analogous to the retinal centrifugal pathway.

The anatomic organization of the cortex is, in some respects, the opposite of that of the retina. Whereas the retina shows a convergence of information from the photoreceptors to the ganglion cells, once this information reaches the cortex, it is distributed to a very large number of neurons located in diverse regions of the brain and there is a divergence of information. Information is sent

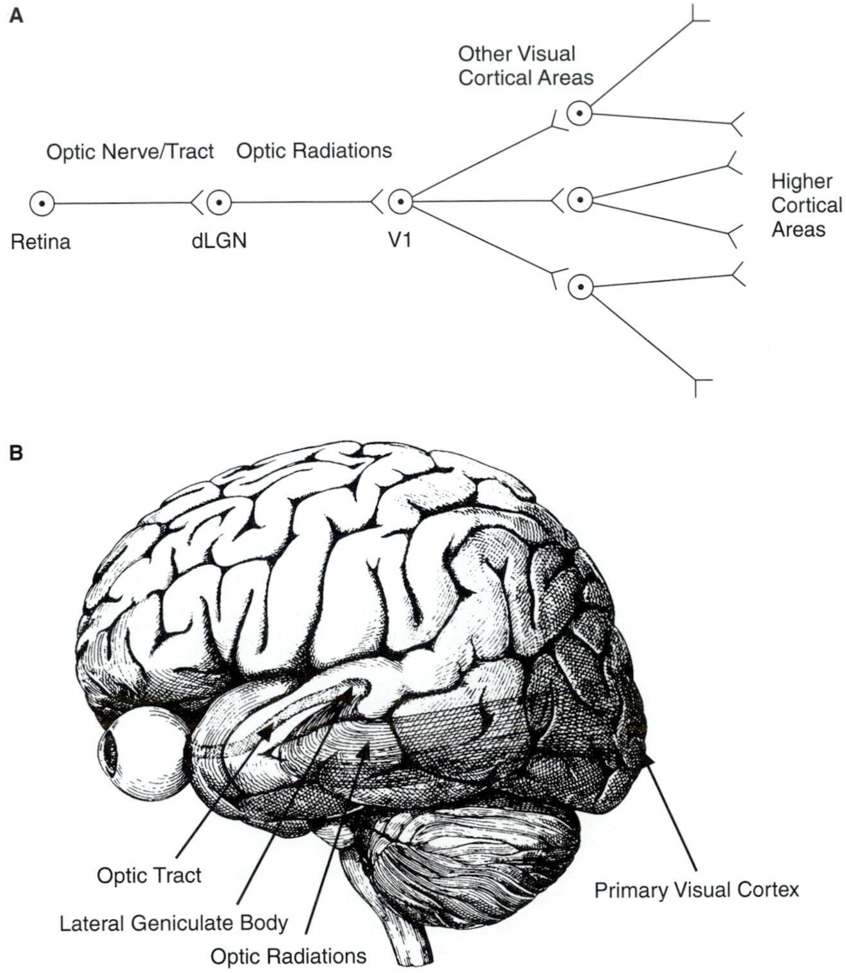


**FIGURE 2–11. A.** Schematic flow diagram of the retinocortical visual pathway. There is a divergence of information within the cortex. **B.** Sketch of the human brain showing the retinocortical visual pathway. The first postretinal synapse is at the dLGN. The dLGN projects to the striate cortex. (*Reprinted with permission from Hubel DH.* Eye, Brain, and Vision. *New York: Scientific American Library; 1988.*)

first to areas of the visual cortex that are specialized for analyzing attributes such as motion and color and then to higher centers, which combine this information with memory and other senses.

The pathway from the retina to the dLGN to striate visual cortex is referred to as the **retinocortical pathway.** While the great majority of retinal ganglion cells contribute to this pathway, a smaller percentage contribute the **retinotec-**

**tal pathway.** Ganglion cell axons in the retinotectal pathway synapse in the midbrain's superior colliculus (or tectum), bypassing the dLGN. The tectum apparently does not project to the cortex. This pathway appears to be important for encoding eye movements.

This book is concerned with the mechanisms by which visual information is analyzed by the retina and the brain proper. Before we begin our discussion of these matters, some basic characteristics of light are reviewed.

## *ELECTROMAGNETIC SPECTRUM*

Humans are capable of detecting only a small portion of the electromagnetic (EM) spectrum (Fig. 2–12). Light, or visible radiation, ranges in wavelength from about 380 to 700 nm. (One nanometer [nm] = $10^{-9}$ m.) Other wavelengths are not visible, either because they are not transmitted by the ocular media or because they are not absorbed by the retinal photopigments.

### *Wavelength and Frequency*

The electromagnetic (EM) spectrum ranges from short-wavelength radiation, such as gamma rays, to long-wavelength radiation, such as AM transmission. Wavelength and frequency of EM radiation are inversely proportional (Fig. 2–13). The relationship between wavelength and frequency is

$$\nu = c/\lambda$$

where

$\nu$ = frequency of light
$c$ = speed of light ($3 \times 10^8$ m/s)
$\lambda$ = wavelength of light

Within the visible spectrum, the wavelength of light is associated with the perception of color, and different wavelengths produce different perceptions of color. This can be demonstrated by directing a white beam of light onto a prism (Fig. 2–14). White light is a mixture of various wavelengths of light. A refracting element, such as a prism, has a different index of refraction for each wavelength. Consequently, each wavelength is deviated to a different degree, and a spectrum of wavelengths is produced. (The index of refraction and degree of deviation are inversely proportional to the wavelength.) This results in a spectrum of colors, similar to a rainbow.

Students traditionally remember the sequence of colors in the spectrum with the acronym **ROY G BIV** (red, orange, yellow, green, blue, indigo, violet). Wavelengths associated with these colors are commonly given in nanometers.

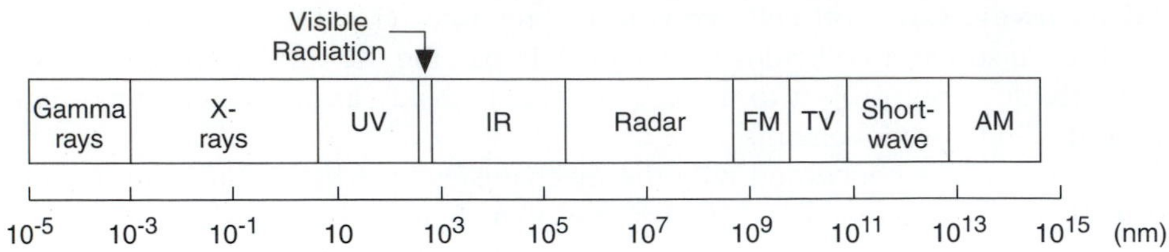


| UV | IR |
|---|---|
| A (near): 320–400 nm | Near 800–2500 nm |
| B: 280–320 nm | Mid 2500–50,000 nm |
| C: 200–280 nm | Far 50,000–$10^{6}$ nm |

**FIGURE 2–12.** The top diagram shows the electromagnetic (EM) spectrum. Note that visible radiation (light) takes up a very small portion of the EM spectrum. Below are common designations for ultraviolet (UV) and infrared (IR) radiation.

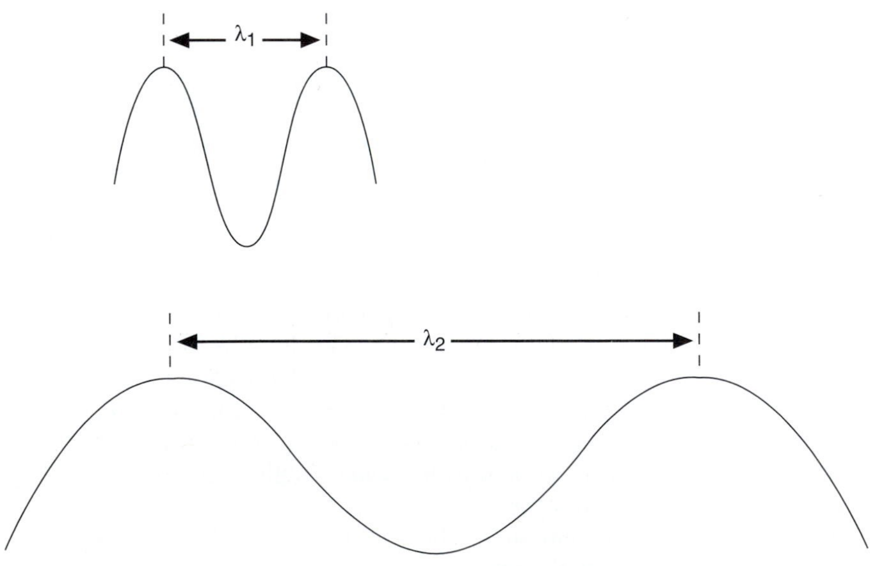


**FIGURE 2–13.** $\lambda_1$ has a shorter wavelength and a greater frequency than $\lambda_2$.

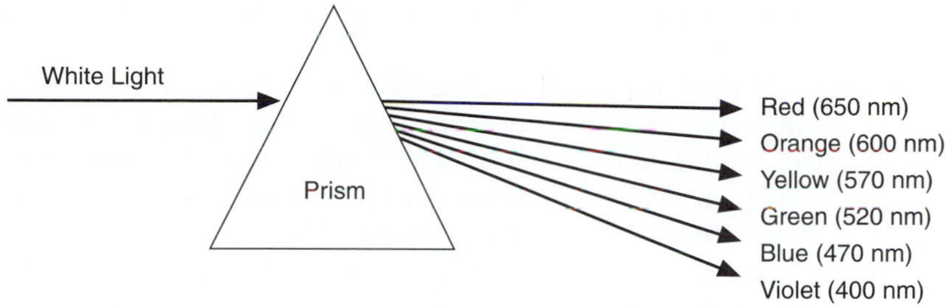


**FIGURE 2–14.** A prism breaks up white light into its various components.

### *Dual Nature of Light*

Up to now, we have discussed EM radiation only in terms of its wave nature. It is, however, often convenient to conceptualize EM radiation in terms of its quantal nature. In this conceptualization, EM radiation consists of discrete packages of energy called **quanta** or **photons** (Fig. 2–15).

The amount of energy in a quantum of light is given by the following relationship:

$$E = h\nu$$

where

$E$ = energy per quantum
$h$ = Planck's constant ($6.626 \times 10^{-37}$ J/Hz)
$\nu$ = frequency

or

$$E = hc/\lambda$$

where

$c$ = speed of light ($3 \times 10^{8}$ m/s)
$\lambda$ = wavelength

These relationships show that quanta of short wavelengths have more energy than do quanta of longer wavelengths. This is clinically important because high-

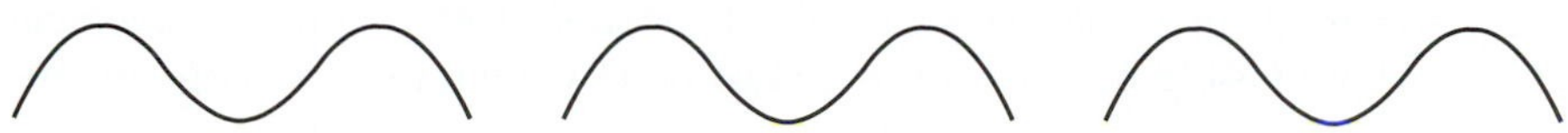

**FIGURE 2–15.** Light can be considered as consisting of packets of energy referred to as quanta or photons.

energy quanta produce more tissue damage when absorbed than do low-energy quanta.

Because of its short wavelength, ultraviolet (UV) radiation contains much energy per quantum (see Fig. 2–12). Consequently, when absorbed by the skin, this radiation can produce substantial cellular damage, including mutations that lead to malignancy. Excessive exposure to UV radiation, as occurs in sunbathing, is a preventable cause of skin carcinoma.

Ultraviolet exposure has also been associated with damage to ocular tissues. There is mounting evidence that cataract formation is promoted by exposure to UV radiation. UV radiation may also play a role in the development of age-related macular degeneration, a leading cause of irreversible blindness. For this reason, it is common for eye care practitioners to recommend spectacles that block UV radiation.

## *TRANSMISSION CHARACTERISTICS OF THE EYE*

Much of the radiation from the sun is eliminated by atmospheric scatter (short wavelengths) and absorption. To protect the sensitive retina upon which EM radiation is focused, the remaining short-wavelength radiation is largely blocked by those ocular elements that precede the retina. As long-wavelength radiation contains relatively less energy, its blockage is less critical.

The cornea absorbs much of the very short wavelength UV C radiation (< 280 nm; see Fig. 2–12) (Pitts, 1974; Lerman, 1980). Consequently, excess ocular exposure to UV C, as may occur when skiing without appropriate sunglasses, can lead to solar keratitis (i.e., corneal inflammation).

The crystalline lens provides most of the protection against the higher wavelength UV radiation—UV A and UV B. One can think of the crystalline lens as a filter that absorbs UV radiation and, thereby, protects the retina. However, this absorption of UV radiation, over many years, damages the lens and can result in cataract formation (Weale, 1983).

A clinical consideration concerns those patients who have had their crystalline lenses removed during cataract surgery. Typically, the lens is replaced with an artificial lens (lens implant). These implants contain a UV filter to protect the retina. In those instances where an artificial lens is not implanted, it is critical that UV protection be provided to the patient. This is typically done with a UV filter in the patient's spectacle lenses.

Because longer wavelengths (> 700 nm) contain little energy (compared to shorter wavelengths), their blockage by the ocular media is less critical. Nonetheless, excessive exposure to near-infrared radiation (≈ 1450 nm) can produce a so-called "glass blower's cataract" (Knowles, 1982). Longer wavelength radiation is not visible because it is not absorbed by the retinal photopigments.

## SUMMARY

Electromagnetic radiation incident on the eye is focused on the retina. Those wavelengths that may damage the retina are, for the most part, filtered out by the ocular media.

Both the cornea and the lens contribute to the focusing of light on the retina. These tissues are nourished by a complex metabolic system that is dependent on the production of aqueous by the ciliary body and its drainage by the canal of Schlemm.

From a teleological point of view, the purpose of the eye is to focus an image of the world on the retina. The retina is a multilayered neural tissue, approximately 0.2 mm thick, which is rich in both the variety of neurons it contains and the various synaptic connections between these neurons. The retina begins the process of analyzing the image that falls upon it. This analysis is an active process whereby visual information is encoded such that it is useful for the higher visual centers. In a very real sense, visual perception begins in the retina, a component of the brain.

# 3

# Duplex Nature of the Retina

The human visual system operates over an enormous range of light levels (Table 3–1). We are able to detect a star on a dark, moonless night and a jet flying in the bright midday sky. This constitutes an operational range on the order of **10 log units** (Boynton, 1979).

On first analysis, this may appear to be a trivial phenomenon. After all, it is known that the pupil changes its diameter in response to light. It could be argued that the pupil, by controlling the amount of light that reaches the retina, plays a substantial role in adaptation to different light levels.

We can determine how much of a role the pupil plays in adaptation by making some simple calculations. Suppose we go from bright conditions, with a pupil diameter of 3 mm, to dark conditions, where the pupil diameter is 9 mm. Using the formula for the area of a circle, we can calculate the degree of increase in light reaching the retina. For a 3-mm-diameter pupil, we have

$$A = \pi r^2$$
$$A_b = \pi(1.5)^2$$
$$A_b = 2.25\pi$$

When the pupil is 9 mm in diameter, the area is

$$A_d = 20.25\pi$$

The ratio of the pupil under dim illumination to that under bright illumination is

$$A_d/A_b = 20.25\pi/2.25\pi$$
$$A_d/A_b = 9.0$$

or

$$A_d/A_b \approx 1 \text{ log unit}$$

This calculation shows that changes in pupillary area account for only a small portion of adaptation; 1 log unit out of the 10-log-unit range can be explained

**TABLE 3–1. VISIBLE LIGHT INTENSITIES[a]**

| Condition | Luminance (Candelas/m$^2$) | |
|---|---|---|
| | $10^{10}$ | Tissue damage |
| Sun at noon | $10^{9}$ | ↓ |
| | $10^{8}$ | |
| | $10^{7}$ | Photopic vision |
| 100-W bulb filament | $10^{6}$ | ↓ |
| | $10^{5}$ | |
| Paper in sunlight | $10^{4}$ | |
| | $10^{3}$ | |
| | $10^{2}$ | |
| Comfortable reading | 10 | |
| | 1 | Mesopic vision |
| | $10^{-1}$ | Scotopic vision |
| Paper in moonlight | $10^{-2}$ | ↓ |
| | $10^{-3}$ | |
| Paper in starlight | $10^{-4}$ | |
| | $10^{-5}$ | |
| Threshold light | $10^{-6}$ | |

[a]Adapted from Sekuler R, Blake R. *Perception* (2nd ed.). New York: McGraw Hill; 1990.

by the pupil. The remaining adaptation is largely due to the existence and properties of two classes of retinal photoreceptors, rods and cones.

## *Basic Distinctions Between Scotopic and Photopic Vision*

**Scotopic vision** is defined as vision that occurs under dim (nighttime) lighting conditions. Under such conditions, we manifest exquisite sensitivity to very dim lights. Scotopic vision, however, is characterized by poor visual acuity (20/200 vision) and the absence of color discrimination. As we will learn in this chapter, scotopic vision is mediated by rods.

**Photopic vision,** which occurs under bright (daytime) lighting conditions, shows poor sensitivity to dim lights; however, it is characterized by both excellent visual acuity (20/20) and color discrimination. Cones mediate photopic vision.

The existence of two classes of photoreceptors, which each operate under different lighting conditions, leads to what has been referred to as a **duplex retina.** Under scotopic conditions, the retina is dominated by rods, and under photopic lighting conditions, it is dominated by cones.

Although it is often useful to consider the retina as having a duplex nature, this is a simplification. Under certain lighting conditions, such as twilight **(mesopic)** conditions, both rods and cones contribute to vision.

## *MORPHOLOGIC DISTINCTIONS BETWEEN RODS AND CONES*

Figure 3–1 displays schematic drawings of rods and cones and Figure 3–2 is a scanning electron micrograph of these two classes of photoreceptors. Note that rods and cones share several features. Both have an outer segment consisting of disk-like structures. Within these disks are photopigments that absorb light quanta and initiate those processes that ultimately lead to vision.

The outer segment is connected to the inner segment by a thin ciliary connection. Within the inner segment are cellular organelles, excluding the cell nucleus. The innermost aspect of both rods and cones consists of a synaptic ending that synapses in the outer plexiform layer.

Although there are similarities in the morphology of rods and cones, there are also important differences. Consider the outer segments. True to their respective names, rod outer segments are rod-shaped, whereas cone outer segments are cone-shaped. The outer segment disks represent infoldings of the cellular membrane. They are generated in the region of the ciliary connection and migrate outward (Young, 1970, 1971). In the rods, these disks break away and become free-floating as they migrate outward. The outer portion of the rod outer segment can be thought of as consisting of a stack of free-floating disks, somewhat like a stack of poker chips. The cone disks, as is indicated in Figure 3–1, remain attached to the cone outer segment as they migrate outward. They do not become free-floating, as is the case with the rod disks.

The outer segment disks are continuously produced, shed, and metabolized by the surrounding tissue. In essence, rod and cone disks are phagocytized by the retinal pigment epithelium (RPE), which lies outer to the rod and cone outer segments (Young, 1971). Rod disks are produced, and subsequently shed, at the rate of about 10 percent per day. Rod disks tend to be shed during the day. Cone disks tend to be shed at night (Young, 1978).

Phagocytosis of photoreceptor disks is essential to maintaining retinal health. In the absence of effective phagocytosis, metabolic waste products collect, thus damaging the rods and cones. This may be the case in **retinitis pigmentosa,** a rod-cone degenerative disease that often results in the progressive loss of vision, with scotopic vision typically affected first (Apple and Rabb, 1991).

Unfortunately, at this time there is no effective treatment for retinitis pigmentosa. One vein of laboratory work involves the transplantation of healthy retinal tissue into the abnormal retina. Early results suggest that the donor tissue maintains some degree of viability (Gouras et al, 1993), however, it seems un-

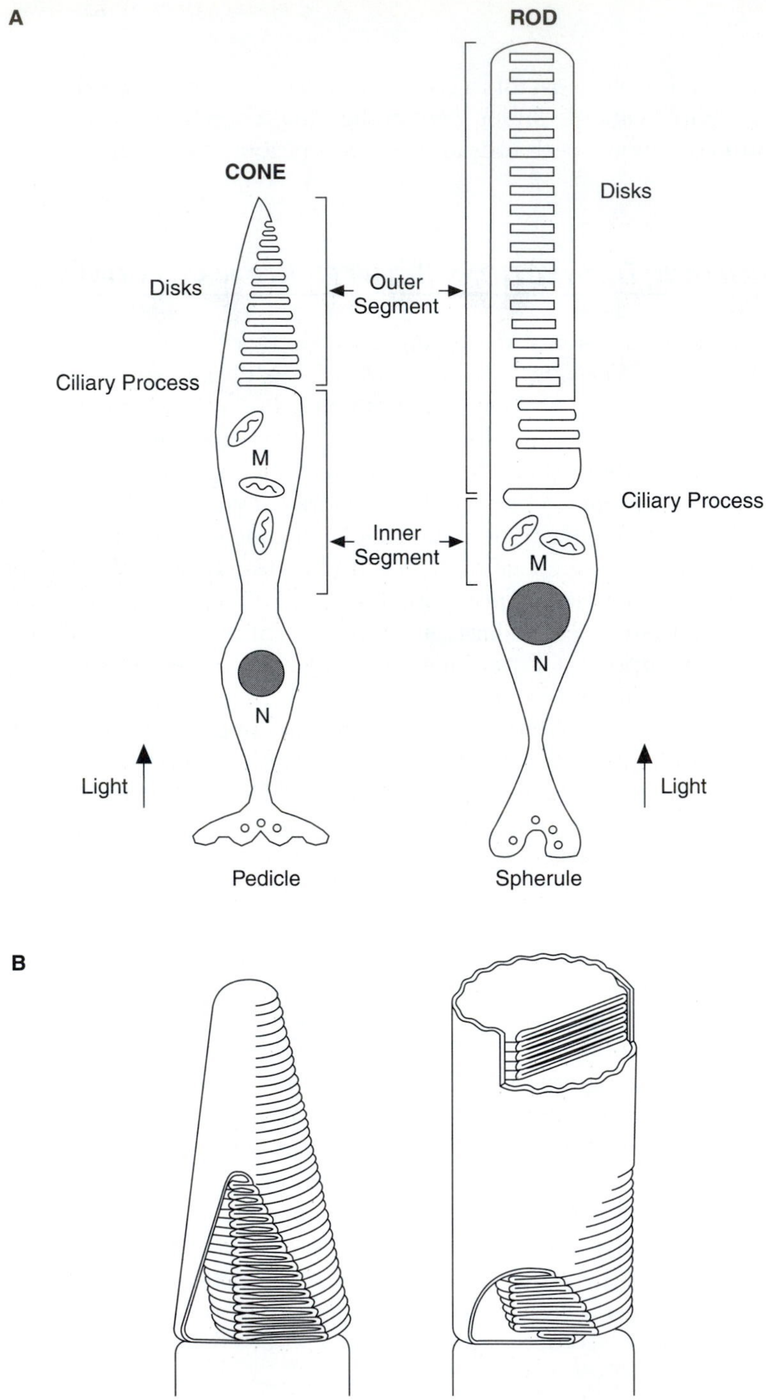


**FIGURE 3–1. A.** Schematic drawings of a cone (left) and a rod (right). The nucleus is designated by "N" and the mitochondria by "M." **B.** Schematic drawings of the outer segments of a cone and rod. (*Adapted from Young RW. Visual cells.* Sci Am. *1970;223(4):80–91.*)

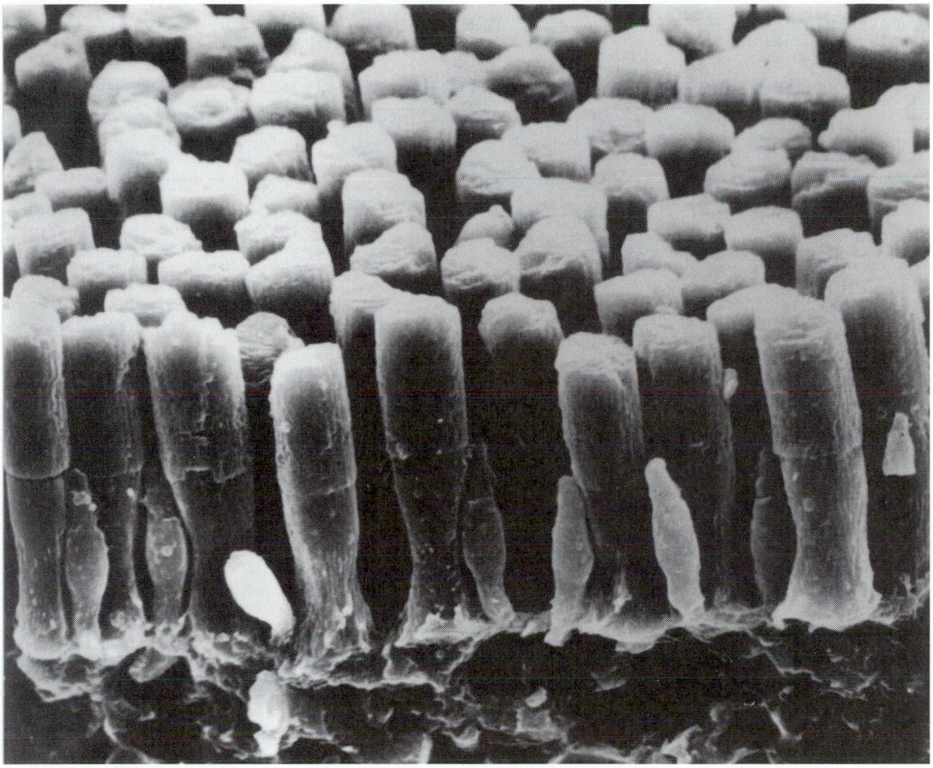

**FIGURE 3–2.** Scanning electron micrograph of the photoreceptors of the tiger salamander. The larger cells are rods and the smaller cells are cones. In humans, the rods and cones are more similar in size. (*This scanning electron micrograph was made by Scott Mittman and Maria T. Maglio, and is reprinted from Schnapf JL, Baylor DA. How photoreceptors respond to light.* Sci Am. *1987;256[4]:40–47.*)

likely that these transplants will provide anything more than the most rudimentary forms of vision. Other lines of research are directed toward determining the molecular basis for the disease.

Another distinction between rod and cone morphology concerns their synaptic endings. Rods have a roundish **spherule,** whereas cones have a flat **pedicle** (see Fig. 3–1).

## *PHOTOPIGMENTS IN RODS AND CONES*

Both rods and cones contain photosensitive pigments. These photopigments absorb light quanta and convert this light energy into electrical activity. This is the first step in a sequence of events that ultimately leads to vision.

### *Rod Photopigment*

Rods contain the photopigment **rhodopsin.** An older term for rhodopsin is **visual purple.** This photopigment is contained within the disks of the rod's outer segment. A disk contains about 10,000 molecules of rhodopsin. As each rod has about 1000 disks and an eye contains 120 million rods, there are about $10^{15}$ molecules of rhodopsin per eye (Boynton, 1979). Each molecule of rhodopsin is capable of capturing one photon of light. Consequently, the large number of rhodopsin molecules provides the eye with a tremendous ability to capture light and is the basis for our ability to detect dim objects (e.g., stars) under scotopic conditions.

Figure 3–3 shows the absorption spectrum for rhodopsin and the manner in which this curve is generated. A fixed quantity (100 quanta) of monochromatic light is incident upon a container of rhodopsin. The ratio of the transmitted light to the incident light is calculated. This procedure is repeated for many wavelengths (e.g., 400, 401, and 402 nm) across the spectrum. For each wavelength, the same number of quanta are incident upon the container. The result is a curve that shows the proportion of light transmitted as a function of wavelength.

Light quanta that are incident on the rhodopsin, but not transmitted, have been absorbed. Consequently, the absorption curve is the reciprocal of the transmission curve (see Fig. 3–3). Note that wavelengths in the region of 507 nm are most readily absorbed by this photopigment.

A molecule of rhodopsin is bleached when it absorbs light. The absorption of only one quantum of light will bleach a molecule of rhodopsin (Hecht et al, 1942). When a rhodopsin molecule is in the bleached state, it is not capable of capturing another quantum. It will transmit a quantum of light incident on it. Consequently, a bleached molecule is more transparent than an unbleached molecule. A bleached molecule will spontaneously revert back to the unbleached state. The probability that a molecule of bleached rhodopsin will revert to the unbleached state within a 5-minute period is 0.50 (Rushton, 1965a). Therefore, if a quantity of rhodopsin is bleached, 50 percent of the rhodopsin will recover in 5 minutes. In commonly used terminology, the half-life for rhodopsin regeneration is 5 minutes.

Let us consider the rhodopsin absorption spectrum in more detail. This curve shows the probability of rhodopsin absorption (indicated as log relative absorption on the ordinate) as a function of wavelength (see Fig. 3–3). Quanta of 507 nm have the highest probability of absorption. This is due to quantum mechanics: the rhodopsin molecule and a quantum of 507 nm "fit together" well, thus increasing the probability of absorption.

This does not mean that quanta of other wavelengths cannot be absorbed by the rhodopsin. Other wavelengths are absorbed, but with less probability. To illustrate this point, compare the effects of 1000 quanta of 507 nm and 1000 quanta of 580 nm that are incident on a container of rhodopsin. Assume that the rhodopsin absorption curve gives a probability of 0.20 that a quantum of

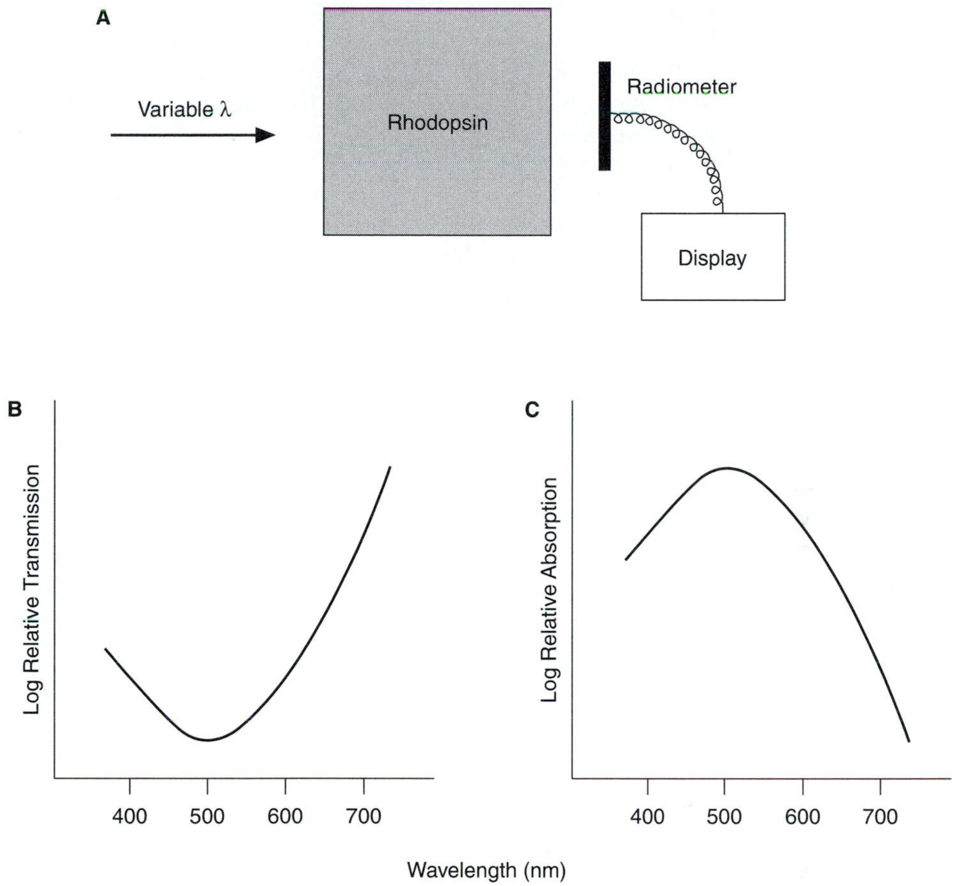


**FIGURE 3–3.** **A.** Diagram illustrating the manner in which the absorption spectrum for rhodopsin is obtained. **B.** The amount of transmitted light is determined as a function of wavelength to obtain a transmission curve. **C.** The reciprocal of this transmission curve is the absorption spectrum for rhodopsin.

507 nm will be absorbed and a probability of 0.10 that a quantum of 580 nm will be absorbed. The 507 nm will bleach 200 rhodopsin molecules, whereas the 580 nm will bleach 100 molecules. (Multiply 1000 quanta by the proportion absorbed at each wavelength.)

If the intensity of the 580-nm light was doubled to 2000 quanta, it now would produce the same number of absorptions as does the 1000 quanta of 507 nm. Consequently, 1000 quanta of 507 nm produces the same effect on the rhodopsin as does 2000 quanta of 580 nm, making it impossible to distinguish between the two stimuli based on the number of quantal absorptions. This is referred to as the **principle of univariance.** Univariance occurs because once a quantum of light is absorbed, all information regarding its wavelength is lost. Whether a molecule of rhodopsin is bleached by 580 or 507 nm, the effect is the same. An analogy is a bathroom scale that is designed to make a loud noise when it registers 100 pounds. While the sound tells us that the scale registers 100 pounds, it does not tell us what is on the scale. It could be 100 pounds of lead or 100 pounds of feathers.

### *Scotopic Spectral Sensitivity*

To determine scotopic spectral sensitivity, we dark adapt a person. This could be done by having an individual sit in a dark room for 45 minutes to allow his or her rhodopsin to maximally regenerate. Subsequently, the minimum amount of energy required for the person to detect stimuli of various wavelengths is determined. The minimum amount of energy required for detection of a stimulus is referred to as the **threshold** for that stimulus.

A curve showing threshold as a function of wavelength, under scotopic conditions, is given in Figure 3–4. Next to this threshold curve is a curve showing **sensitivity** as a function of wavelength. This sensitivity curve is simply the reciprocal of the threshold function. A low threshold indicates high sensitivity. Note that this scotopic spectral sensitivity curve has essentially the same form as the rhodopsin absorption spectrum (Wald, 1945). This similarity in form suggests that the human scotopic spectral sensitivity function is determined by the absorption characteristics of rhodopsin.

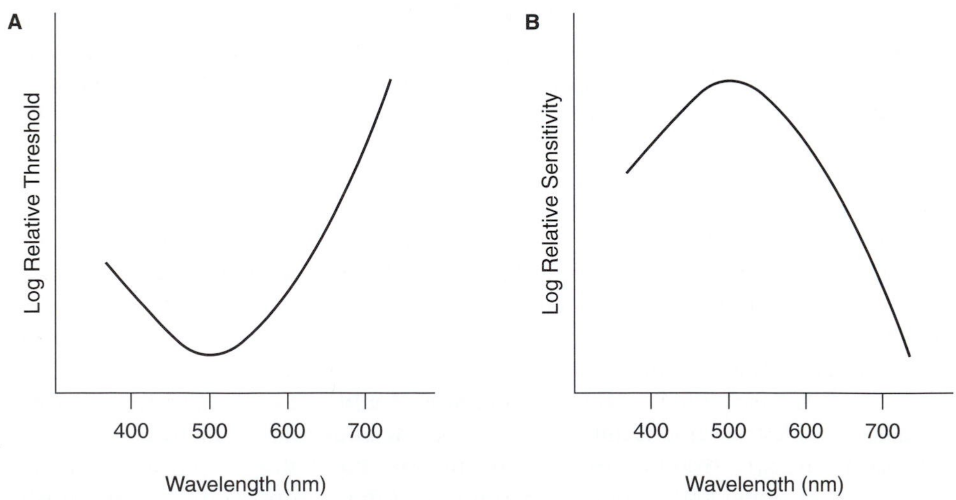


**FIGURE 3–4. A.** Scotopic threshold as a function of wavelength. **B.** Scotopic sensitivity as a function of wavelength.

### *Cone Photopigments*

Unlike rods, the human cones do not all contain the same photopigment. In a typical human eye, there are three fundamental cone photopigments, with each cone containing only one type of photopigment. The three cone photopigments are erythrolabe, chlorolabe, and cyanolabe. These photopigments typically show maximal quantal absorption in the regions 565, 535, and 430 nm, respectively (Fig. 3–5).

It is common to speak of three different classes of cones, each containing a different photopigment. The erythrolabe-containing cones are referred to as long-wavelength-sensitive cones (LWS or L-cones), the chlorolabe-containing cones as middle-wavelength-sensitive cones (MWS or M-cones), and the cones containing cyanolabe as short-wavelength-sensitive cones (SWS or S-cones). The three classes of cones are also referred to as red, green, and blue cones. The cone photopigments recover from bleaching at a faster rate than do the rods. It takes approximately 1.5 minutes for 50 percent of a cone photopigment to recover following bleaching (Rushton, 1963b).

### *Photopic Spectral Sensitivity*

The photopic spectral sensitivity curve is determined under daylight conditions. Photopic sensitivity as a function of wavelength is given in Figure 3–5. Note that the photopic spectral sensitivity curve shows a single broad peak in the region of **555 nm** (Wald, 1945).

This photopic spectral sensitivity curve apparently represents the addition of M and L-cone absorption spectra. Absorption of light quanta by either the M or L-cones contributes to photopic spectral sensitivity. Although controversial, it is thought that S-cones make little, if any, contribution to spectral sensitivity (Cavanagh et al, 1987).

### *Photochromatic Interval*

In Figure 3–6, the absolute sensitivities of the scotopic and photopic systems are plotted on the same graph. By absolute sensitivity we mean that the curves are obtained under conditions that lead to the highest possible sensitivity of each system.

Curves similar to those displayed in Figure 3–6 can be obtained under dark-adapted conditions. The individual is placed in the dark for about 45 minutes prior to the experiment. This produces maximum scotopic and photopic sensitivity because the photopigments, both rhodopsin and the cone photopigments, fully regenerate. Two thresholds are then determined at each wavelength: a threshold for colorless scotopic vision and a threshold for chromatic photopic vision. Take, for example, a stimulus of 500 nm. This stimulus is first

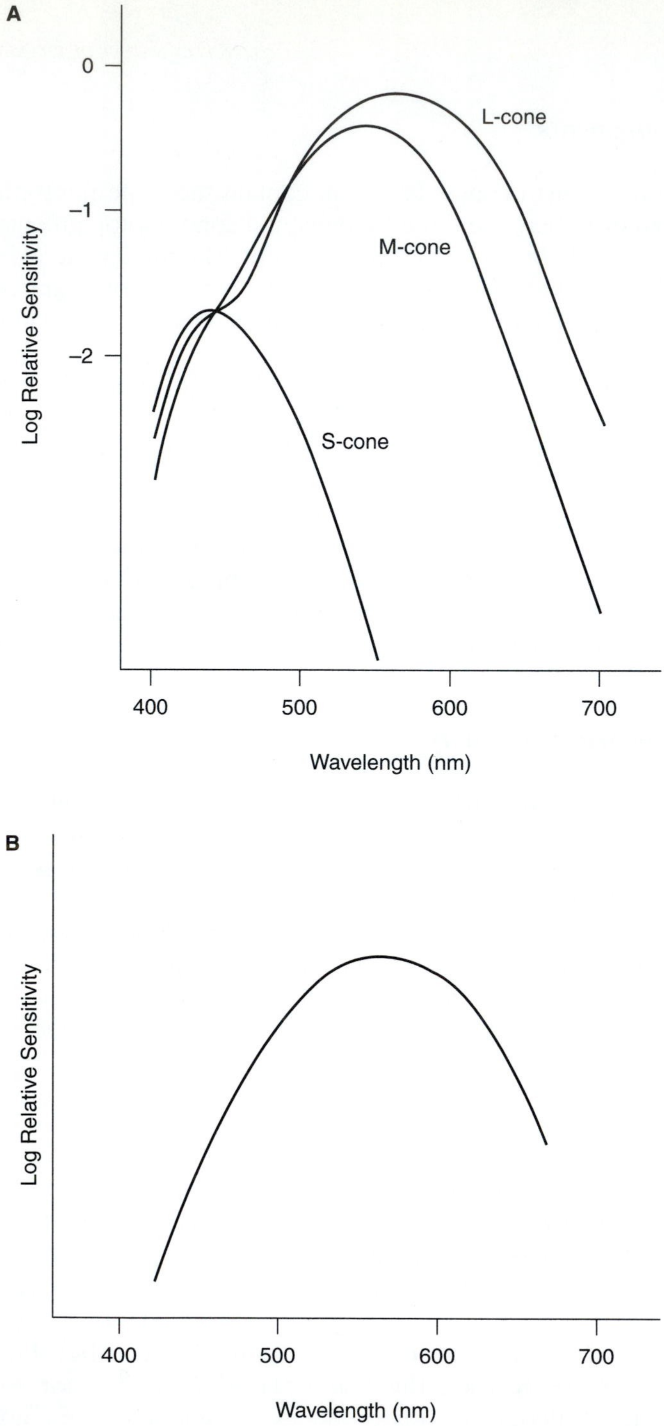


**FIGURE 3–5. A.** Approximations of the absorption spectra of cyanolabe (S-cone), chlorolabe (M-cone), and erythrolabe (L-cone) based on the data of Smith and Pokorny, 1975. (*From Boynton RM.* Human Color Vision. *New York: Holt, Rinehart, and Winston; 1979. Reprinted with permission of Dr. Boynton.*) **B.** An approximation of photopic sensitivity as a function of wavelength.

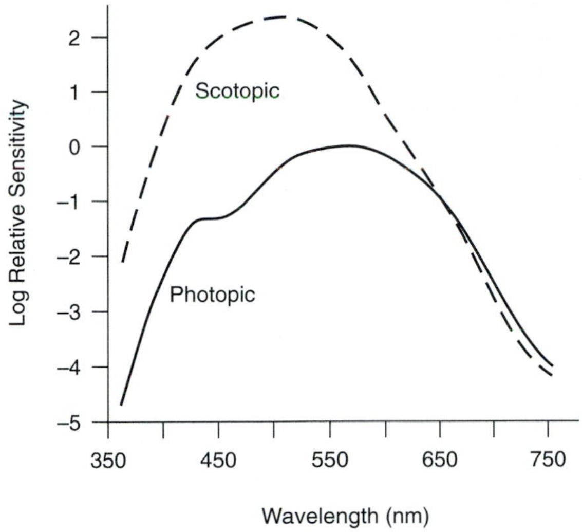


**FIGURE 3–6.** Scotopic and photopic spectral sensitivity functions. These functions represent the absolute sensitivities of the two systems. Note that for long wavelengths, the photochromatic interval is close to zero. (*Adapted from Wald G. Human vision and spectrum.* Science. *1945;101:653–658.*)

detected by the scotopic system and seen as colorless (achromatic). As the intensity of this stimulus is increased, it will eventually be seen as colored (chromatic), thus indicating detection by the photopic system. The difference in sensitivity between scotopic and photopic systems, for a given wavelength, is referred to as the **photochromatic interval (PI).**

Note that scotopic system is more sensitive than the photopic system at all wavelengths, except in the long-wavelength (red) region of the spectrum. In this area, the photochromatic interval is approximately zero and rods and cones are almost equally sensitive. (Curiously, beyond 650 nm, the photopic system is slightly more sensitive than the scotopic system.)

### *Purkinje Shift*

The scotopic and photopic spectral sensitivity curves are based on threshold data. They can, however, be used to predict the relative brightness of stimuli that are above threshold—**suprathreshold stimuli.**

Let us look at an example. A dark-adapted individual views a spectrum consisting of stimuli that all emit the same number of quanta. These stimuli are above threshold. They are, however, only slightly above threshold. This ensures that only the scotopic system detects these stimuli. The person viewing this spectrum will notice that stimuli of 507 nm appear brighter than other spectral stimuli. This is directly attributable to the absorption spectrum of rhodopsin.

This experiment can also be performed for photopic vision. The stimuli will all emit a uniformly greater number of quanta. If the stimuli are sufficiently bright, they will be detected by the photopic system. The individual will report that stimuli of 555 nm are brighter than other wavelengths. This is consistent with photopic spectral sensitivity peaking at 555 nm.

This change in peak spectral sensitivity as we go from scotopic to photopic vision is the basis for the Purkinje shift. Purkinje (1819) noted that as illumination increases, longer wavelengths appear relatively brighter. This is consistent with a shift from rod-mediated vision, with a peak sensitivity of 507 nm, to cone-mediated vision, where the peak sensitivity is 555 nm.

Let us take a specific example. A dark-adapted individual views side-by-side scotopic stimuli of 507 and 555 nm. Each stimulus emits the same number of quanta. Based on the scotopic spectral sensitivity curve, the 507-nm stimulus would appear brighter. Next, the intensity of each stimulus is increased by the same amount, such that they are now detected by the photopic system. By observation of the photopic spectral sensitivity curve, it can be seen that the 555-nm stimulus would be brighter. Therefore, by increasing the intensity of the stimuli, we increase the relative brightness of the longer-wavelength stimulus.

## RETINAL DISTRIBUTION OF PHOTORECEPTORS

Figure 3–7 shows the retinal distribution of rods and M and L-cones (Østerberg, 1935). Rods are most densely packed at about 20 degrees from the fovea, where they reach a peak density of about 150,000 rods/mm$^2$. There are no rods in the fovea. The absence of rods in the fovea results in the inability to see a small, dim object, such as a star, when it is foveally fixated under scotopic conditions. (Looking slightly to the side of a faint star increases its visibility.)

The distribution of cones is very different from that of rods. Cones are most densely packed in the fovea where their density is 150,000/mm$^2$, the same as the peak density of the rods. Note that although the density of cones is substantially reduced outside of the fovea, cones are still present all the way to the periphery of the retina. In fact, only about 4 percent of all cones are located in the fovea (Boynton, 1979).

S-cones show a different retinal distribution than do other cones (Boynton, 1979). Not only are S-cones considerably less numerous than either M and L-cones, there are no S-cones in the human fovea. Rather, their peak density lies just outside the fovea. This accounts for the inability to see very small blue objects when they are centrally fixated. The ratio of L-cones to M-cones is approximately 2 to 1 (Mollon and Bowmaker, 1992). The human retina contains approximately 120 million rods. The number of cones is about 6 million.

## DARK ADAPTATION

### The Basic Curve

Most of us have had the experience of entering a dark movie theater on a sunny afternoon. Immediately on entering the theater we are virtually blind. Yet

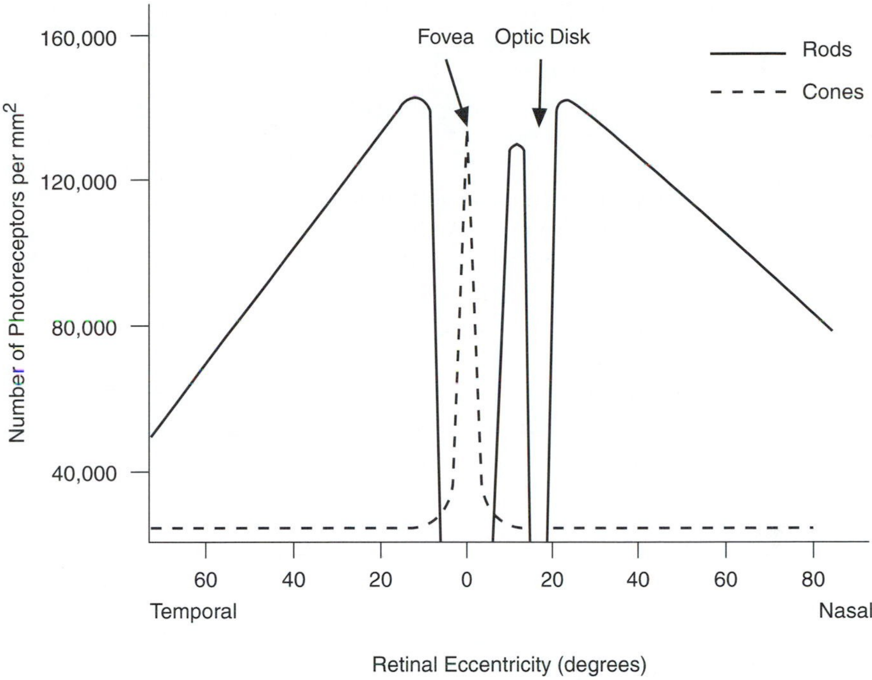


**FIGURE 3–7.** Retinal distribution of rods and M and L-cones (*Adapted from Østerberg G. Topography of the layer of rods and cones in the human retina.* Acta Ophthalmol Suppl. *1935;6:1–103.*)

after several minutes, vision recovers to the point where we can walk down the aisle and find an empty seat. This gradual improvement in vision, after exposure to a bright-adapting light (in this case the sun), is referred to as **dark adaptation.** After exposure to an adapting light, rods and cones recover sensitivity at different rates. The dynamics of this recovery are made clear in dark adaptation experiments. Dark adaptation has also proven useful in the clinical diagnosis of various retinal disorders.

Figure 3–8 is a typical dark adaptation curve. This curve was generated by the following procedure. The person is exposed to a bright-adapting light that is designed to bleach most of his or her photopigment. The adapting light is then turned off and detection threshold is determined as a function of time for stimuli flashed against a totally dark background. The stimulus is large (e.g., 10 degrees) and centrally fixated, with a wavelength of 420 nm. During these experiments, it is important that the room is perfectly black and that the individual is not exposed to ambient light.

There are several important features of the dark adaptation curve shown in Figure 3–8. Most obvious is that over a period of about 35 minutes, threshold im-

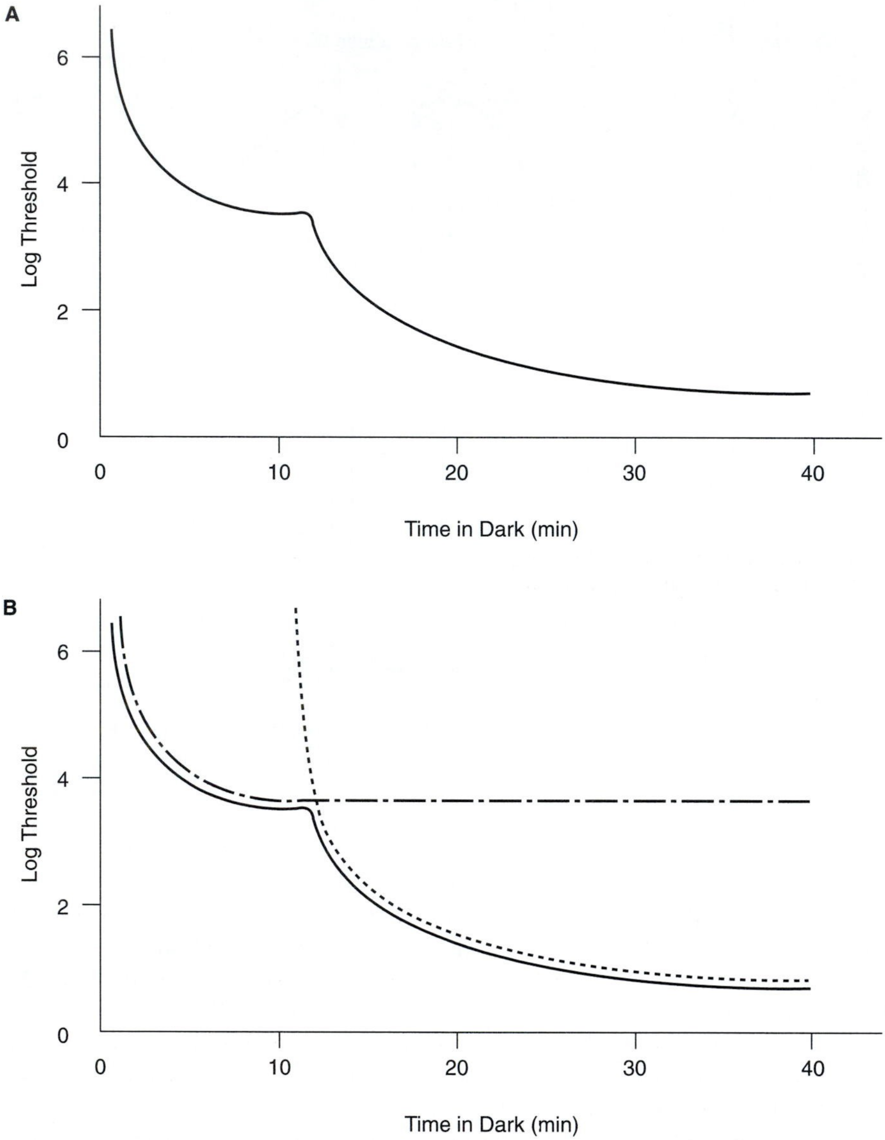


**FIGURE 3–8. A.** Typical dark adaptation curve. The stimulus is 420 nm and large. (*Adapted from Hecht S, Shlaer S, Pirenne MH. Energy, quanta, and vision.* J Gen Physiol. *1942;25:819–840.*) **B.** Dark adaptation curves for a stimulus that is detected by only rods (dots) and a stimulus detected by only cones (dot-dash). A stimulus that is detected by both rods and cones will have the form given by the solid line.

proves by about 5 log units (i.e., after about 35 minutes in the dark, the person is 100,000 times more light sensitive). Another important feature of this curve is its division into two sections. The first section shows a rapid reduction in threshold up to about 5 minutes, where the curve plateaus. This portion of the dark adaptation curve represents cone thresholds. At about 10 minutes, there is an abrupt change in the slope of the curve (Hecht et al, 1937). This break in the curve, referred to as the **rod-cone break,** is followed by a slow reduction in threshold out to about 35 minutes. This portion of the curve represents detection by the rods.

The dark adaptation curve shows the recovery of sensitivity following bleaching of the cones and rods. It shows that although cones fully recover sensitivity within about 10 minutes, it takes rods about 35 minutes to fully recover sensitivity. The rod–cone break represents that point in time when the rods become more sensitive than the cones. Prior to this point, the cones detect the stimulus. After this point, the rods detect it. Differences in cone and rod thresholds can be directly read off of a dark adaptation curve. The cone plateau (at ≈10 minutes) represents the threshold for the cone system, whereas the rod plateau (at ≈35 minutes) represents the rod threshold. Therefore, the difference between these two values (≈3 log units) represents the difference in cone and rod thresholds (the photochromatic interval).

The recovery in sensitivity that occurs during dark adaptation is related to the regeneration of photoreceptor photopigments. As we will learn, however, photopigment regeneration does not fully explain dark adaptation.

### *Effects of Stimulus Wavelength*

The dark adaptation curve given in Figure 3–8 was obtained with a stimulus of 420 nm. What form does the dark adaption curve take if the stimulus is 650 nm? Such a dark adaptation curve is given in Figure 3–9. This curve is substantially different from the curve obtained with the 420-nm stimulus. It shows only a cone portion; the rod aspect is missing. This result should not be surprising after reconsidering Figure 3–6, which shows that the photochromatic interval for 650 nm is zero. The scotopic and photopic systems are equally sensitive to this stimulus. As the scotopic system is not more sensitive to 650 nm than the photopic system, there is not an obvious rod–cone break (Hecht et al, 1937). In contrast, the 420-nm stimulus displays a large photochromatic interval. As a consequence, this stimulus produces a dark adaptation curve with a prominent rod–cone break (see Fig. 3–8).

The role of stimulus wavelength in determining the form of a dark adaptation curve is further examined in Figure 3–10. On the left of this figure are dark adaptation curves for stimuli of 465 and 610 nm. On the right are threshold scotopic and photopic functions. These threshold functions can be thought of as the reciprocal of the sensitivity curves given in Figure 3–6.

Consider the 465-nm stimulus. After about 15 minutes of dark adaptation, the cone plateau is reached. This represents the maximum sensitivity (or lowest

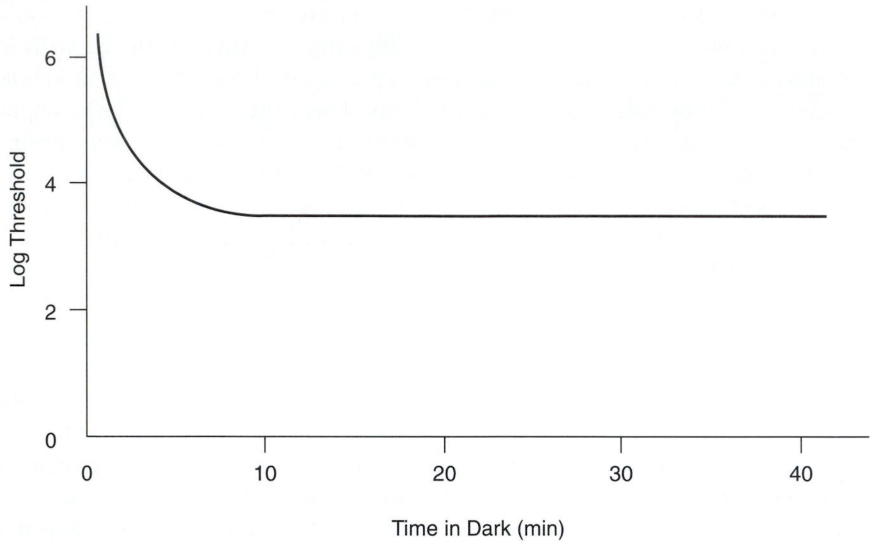


**FIGURE 3–9.** Dark adaptation curve obtained with a stimulus of 650 nm. Note the absence of a rod–cone break. (*Adapted from Hecht S, Shlaer S, Pirenne MH. Energy, quanta, and vision.* J Gen Physiol. *1942;25:819–840.*)

threshold) for cones to this stimulus. Note the dotted line, which extends from this cone plateau and intersects the photopic threshold function at 465 nm. This illustrates that the cone plateau corresponds to a specific point on the photopic threshold function. The rod portion of the dark adaptation curve for 465 nm levels off at about 40 minutes. This rod plateau has been extended to intersect the scotopic threshold function. This type of analysis is useful because it illustrates the photochromatic interval in terms of both dark adaptation curves and spectral threshold functions. For the dark adaptation curves, the photochromatic interval is the separation of the cone and rod plateaus. When viewing the spectral threshold functions, this same photochromatic interval is the difference between scotopic and photopic thresholds.

Now consider the 610-nm stimulus of Figure 3–10. Observe the spectral threshold functions and note the smaller photochromatic interval for this stimulus than for 465 nm. Note that this relatively small photochromatic interval is also given by the small separation of the plateaus of the rod and cone adaptation curves. The rod–cone break occurs later for the 610-nm stimulus than for the 465-nm stimulus. This is also explicable in terms of the photochromatic interval. Rods are substantially more sensitive to 465 nm than are cones. Consequently, they surpass the cones' sensitivity early during dark adaptation, after relatively little rhodopsin has regenerated. The situation is different for 610 nm. Although rods are more sensitive than cones, the difference in sensitivity is not

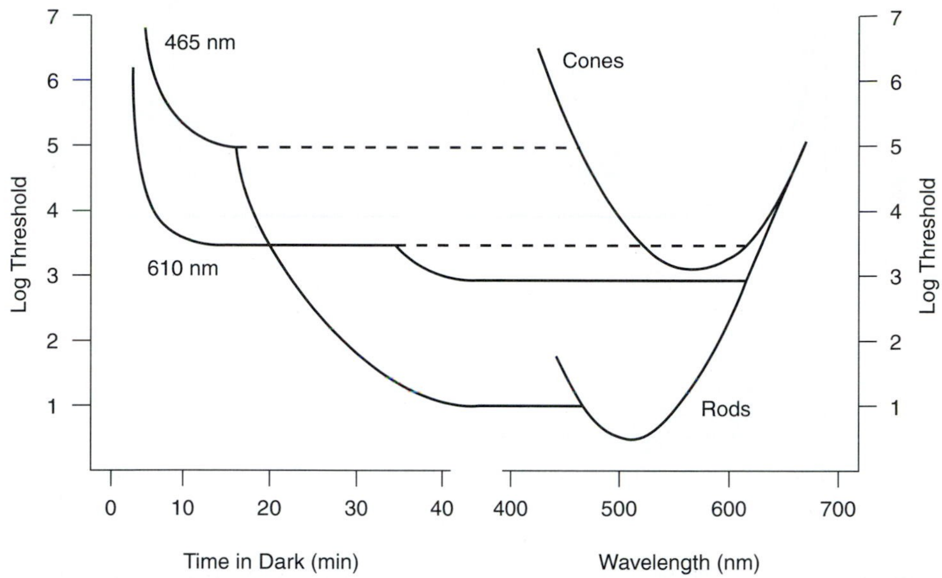


**FIGURE 3–10.** Dark adaptation curves for stimuli of 465 and 610 nm as they relate to photopic and scotopic threshold functions.

as great as for 465 nm. As a result, it takes longer for rods to recover to the point where they are more sensitive than cones. This occurs only after a relatively large amount of rhodopsin has regenerated.

### *Stimulus Size and Location*

In the preceding examples it was assumed that the stimulus was centrally fixed and that its size was such that it covered both the fovea and a portion of the surrounding retina. For example, a stimulus 10 degrees in diameter would produce the results discussed so far.

Making the stimulus very small, say 0.5 degrees, and confining it to the fovea has a predictable effect: only a cone function is obtained (Fig. 3–11). The absence of a rod function reflects the absence of rods in the fovea.

### *Physiologic Basis of Dark Adaptation*

How can we account for the slow decrease in threshold following exposure to a bright adapting light? Many of you may have assumed that this recovery in sensitivity is solely dependent on the regeneration of photopigment. This is the so-called **photochemical explanation** of dark adaptation (Hecht, 1937). Dur-

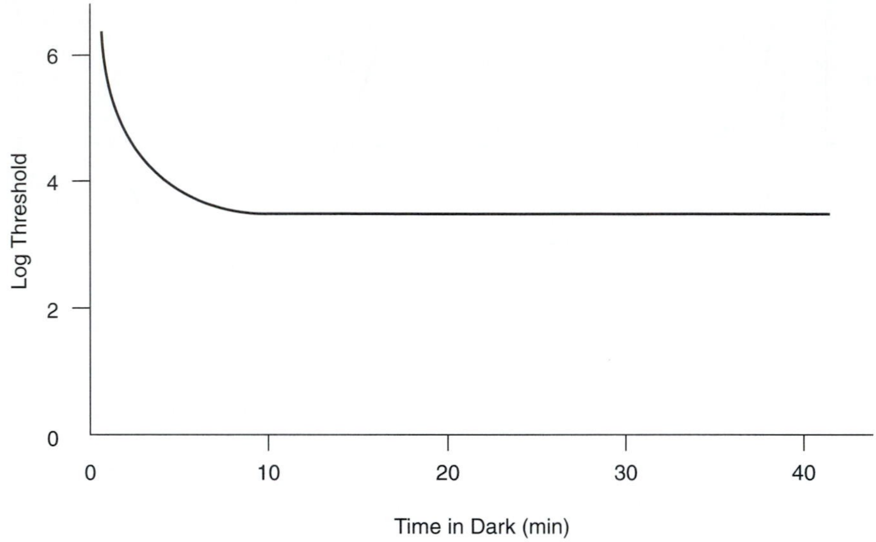


**FIGURE 3–11.** Dark adaptation curve for a small stimulus, confined to the fovea. Note the absence of a rod–cone break.

ing dark adaptation, there is a regeneration of photopigment. This regeneration of photopigment increases the probability of quantal absorptions and, therefore, threshold is reduced. The photochemical explanation of dark adaptation holds that this photopigment regeneration fully explains the recovery of sensitivity that occurs during dark adaptation.

Figure 3–12 schematically shows rods that have had one half of their rhodopsin bleached. Compared with the unbleached state, there is a 0.50 probability that a quantum of light will be captured by the rhodopsin. Therefore, based purely on photopigment considerations, a 50 percent bleaching is predicted to double the threshold. In fact, bleaching half of the rhodopsin increases the threshold by a factor of approximately $10^{10}$, or 10,000,000,000. Clearly, factors other than photopigment regeneration play a major role in dark adaptation.

Let us examine this in more detail. Figure 3–13 (circles) shows the recovery of rhodopsin in an individual who has only rods, a **rod monochromat. Retinal densitometry** was used to obtain this measurement (Rushton, 1965a). (This procedure involves shining a weak measuring light on the retina and then measuring the amount of the light reflected off of the retina. By comparing the amount of incident light with the amount of reflected light, we can determine the proportion of bleached pigment.) The solid lines show the dark adaptation curve for this individual. For comparison, the dotted line indicates the dark adaptation curve of a normal individual.

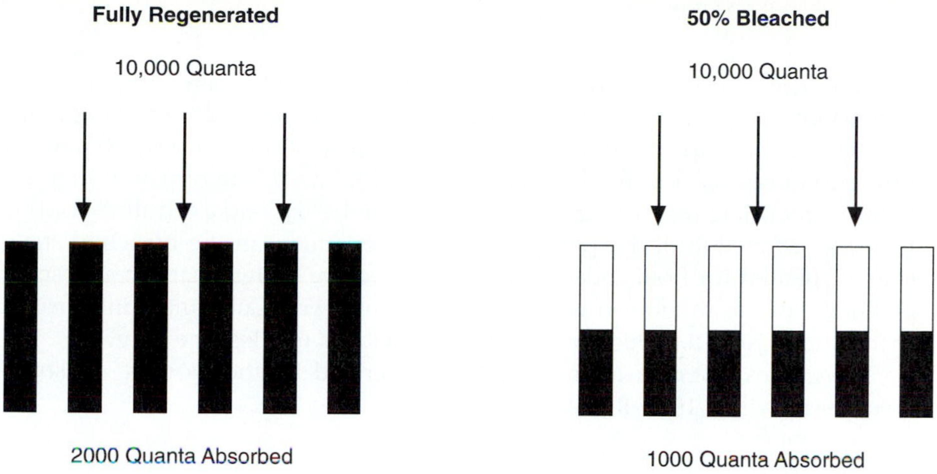


**FIGURE 3–12.** Fifty percent bleaching of rhodopsin decreases the probability of quantal absorption by a factor of one half. Yet, the threshold is increased by a factor of $10^{10}$.

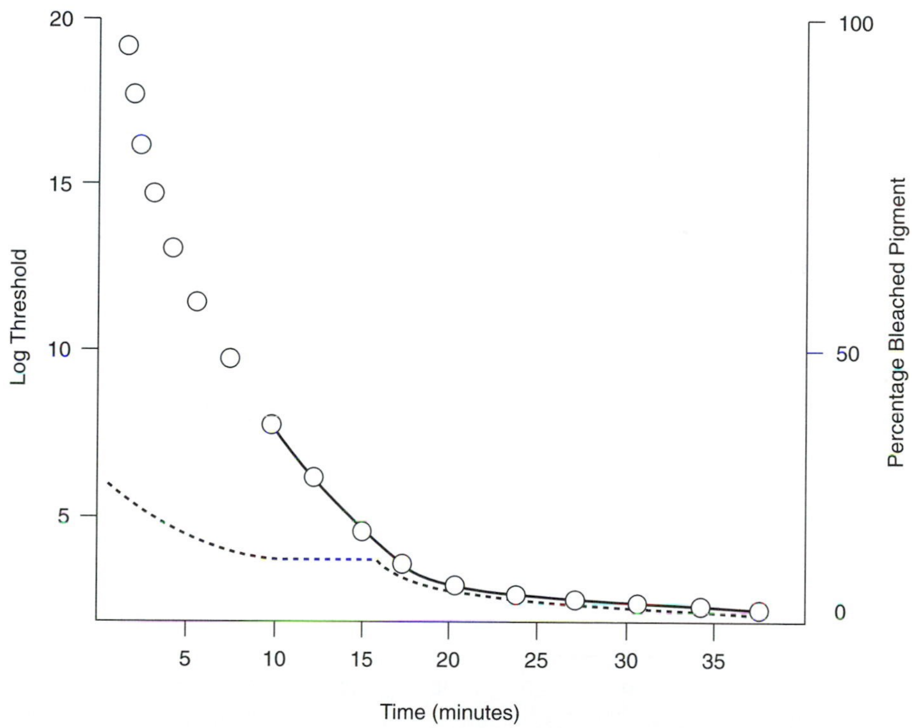


**FIGURE 3–13.** Circles show the retinal densitometry results for a rod monochromat; solid lines show the thresholds for this subject. The dots show thresholds for a normal subject. (*Adapted from Rushton WAH. The Ferrier lecture. Visual adaptation.* Proc R Soc Lond [Biol]. *1965; 162:20–46.*)

This curve illustrates a point we discussed earlier: bleaching 50 percent of the rhodopsin (right-hand ordinate scale) increases the threshold by 10 log units. It is also of interest to note that at the rod–cone break, approximately 90 percent of the rhodopsin has regenerated. Figure 3–14 displays this information in a different manner. Log relative threshold (relative to the dark-adapted threshold) is plotted as a function of the percentage of photopigment in the bleached state. Data are plotted for both rods and cones. This curve shows that when a small percentage of the rhodopsin is bleached, there is a very substantial increase in the threshold. Note that this is also true for cones, but to a lesser extent.

The curves given in Figure 3–14 are described by the Dowling–Rushton equation (Dowling, 1960; Rushton, 1961):

$$\log(I_t/I_o) = kP$$

where

$I_t$ = threshold intensity of the test flash
$I_o$ = dark-adapted threshold intensity
$P$ = proportion of pigment in the bleached state
$k$ = a constant (20 for rods, 3 for cones)

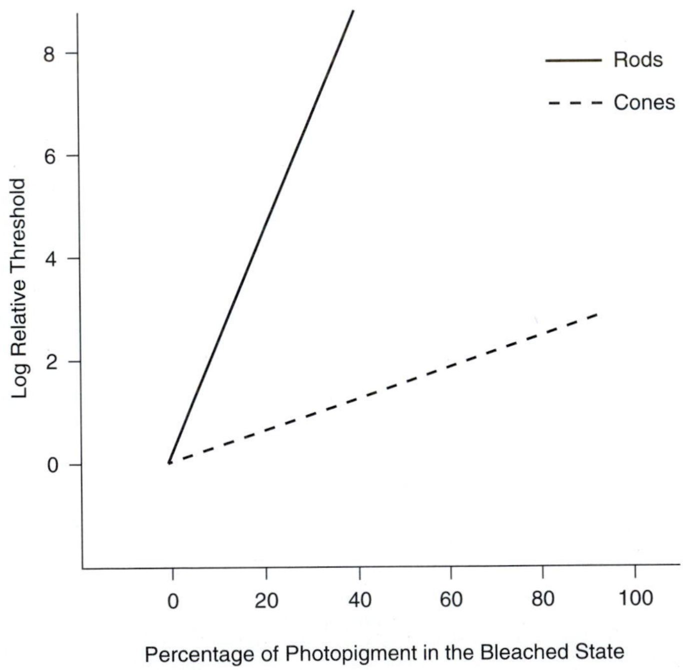


**FIGURE 3–14.** Log relative threshold (relative to dark-adapted threshold) for rods and cones as a function of the percentage of photopigment in the bleached state. (*Adapted from Cornsweet T.* Visual Perception. *New York: Academic Press; 1970.*)

This equation and the preceding graphs demonstrate that dark adaptation cannot be explained solely by photopigment regeneration. Postreceptoral and receptoral factors likely contribute to the complex dynamics of dark adaptation (Schnapf and Baylor, 1987).

## LIGHT ADAPTATION

When you step outside on a sunny day, the amount of light falling on your retinal increases by a factor of several thousand. In spite of this tremendous change in light levels, the appearance of objects remains the same (i.e., a striped shirt looks the same when viewed indoors or outdoors on a sunny day). Within a very brief period—so fleeting that you are unaware of it—your visual system fully adapts to the change in illumination levels, a process referred to as **light adaptation.**

In the laboratory, light adaptation is studied with an **increment threshold procedure.** The stimulus for such an experiment and the results are given in Figure 3–15. Basically, a threshold is determined for an increment that is presented on a background of a given intensity. After a threshold has been determined, the background intensity is increased and the threshold measurement is

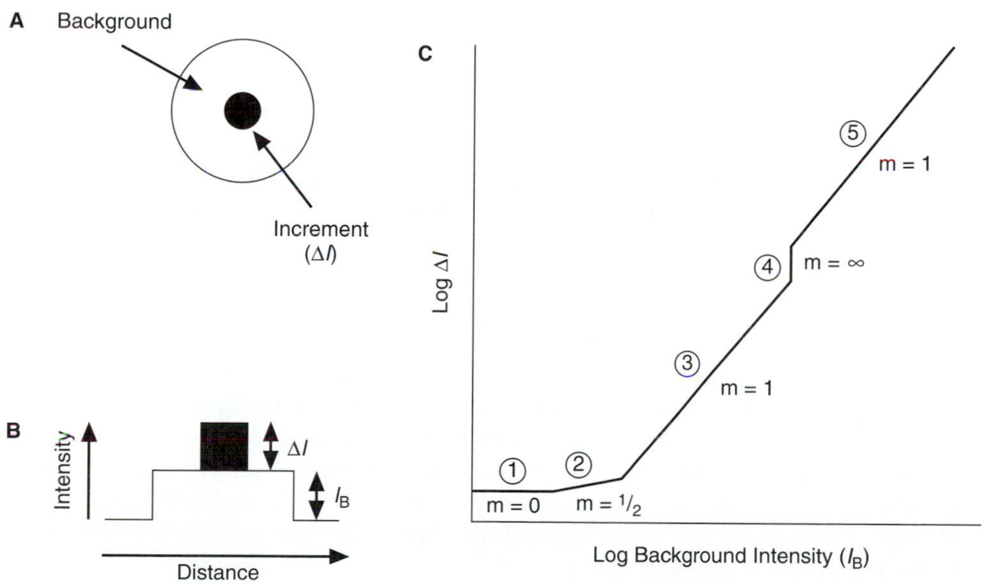


**FIGURE 3–15.** For a light adaptation experiment an increment, $\Delta I$, is presented on a background with an intensity of $I_B$. **A.** Stimulus for such an experiment. **B.** Intensity profile of this stimulus. **C.** Simplified light adaptation curve.

repeated. This procedure is performed for background light levels ranging from darkness to extreme brightness. The result is a curve showing increment threshold ($\Delta I$) as a function of the background adapting ($I_B$) intensity.

### *Scotopic Portion*

Sections 1, 2, 3, and 4 represent the scotopic portion of this function. The explanations for the first two sections are rather technical and they are only briefly touched on in this chapter. Section 1, for which the slope (m) is zero, is that range of light levels where detection is limited by the neural noise inherent within the visual system. The background is practically black, and neural noise produces as much so-called "dark light" as does the background itself (Fechner, 1860; Barlow, 1956). (To experience this "dark light," simply close your eyes and note that you do not see pure darkness, but see various visual phenomena.)

The second section, having a slope of 1/2, reflects quantal fluctuations in the background (DeVries, 1943; Rose, 1948). The background is so dim that fluctuations inherent in the light source that produces the background play a primary role in determining threshold. This is frequently expressed as the **DeVries–Rose law,** which predicts that $\Delta I$ is equal to $(I_B)^{1/2}$.

The third section, which covers a 4-log-unit range, has a slope of approximately 1 (Aguilar and Stiles, 1954; Barlow, 1965; Walraven and Valeton, 1984). A slope of 1 indicates that **Weber's law** is followed.

Although Weber's law is discussed in detail in Chapter 11, let us apply it to the situation at hand. Weber's law implies that as the background brightness is increased, the increment intensity must be increased such that the ratio of the increment intensity ($\Delta I$) to the background intensity ($I_B$) remains constant. This constant ratio, $\Delta I/I_B$, is referred to as Weber's fraction or Weber's constant.

The Weber fraction for scotopic vision is approximately 0.14 (Cornsweet, 1970). If we start with a background of 100 units of intensity, the increment must have an intensity of 14 units ($\Delta I = 14$) to be detected. If the background is increased to 1000 units of intensity, the increment must increase to a value of 140 units ($\Delta I = 140$) to maintain a Weber fraction of 0.14 and be detected.

The visual system has evolved to distinguish objects from the background in which these objects reside. When an object is sufficiently more intense than its background, it can be detected. This so-called just noticeable difference (JND) increases as illumination increases (Weber's law is followed). As is discussed in detail in Chapter 7, the ratio of the increment intensity to the background intensity is referred to as contrast. Saying that the visual system follows Weber's law is the same as saying that the threshold contrast remains constant as the illumination changes.

Weber's law reveals that as background illumination increases, there is a corresponding increase in the increment threshold (i.e., JND). There is a reduction in the absolute sensitivity (and no change in the contrast sensitivity) of the visual system with increasing levels of illumination. This is referred to as **sensitivity regulation.** The physiologic basis of sensitivity regulation, at the level of the photoreceptor, is beginning to be elucidated. Although not fully understood, it appears that calcium plays an important role in this process (Fain and Matthews, 1990).

The final section of the scotopic portion of the light adaptation curve, section 4, has a slope of infinity. This indicates that the rods are saturated (Aguilar and Stiles, 1954). At these high background illuminations, it is not possible for the rods to signal the stimulus, no matter how bright it is. The rods are overwhelmed by the brightness of the background. On first analysis, you might suppose that **rod saturation** occurs when all the rod photopigment has been bleached. In actuality, only 10 percent of the rhodopsin is bleached at the point of rod saturation (Rushton, 1965a).

As we will learn in Chapter 12, the bleaching of a rhodopsin molecule results in the closure of sodium channels located in the rod outer segment. This reduces the flow of sodium into the outer segment and leads to rod hyperpolarization. The degree of this hyperpolarization is dependent, up to a point, on the intensity of the stimulus. The number of sodium channels in a rod outer segment is limited. This limits the possible magnitude of the rod hyperpolarization (Baylor et al, 1984). When approximately 10 percent of the rhodopsin molecules are bleached, a critical number of the sodium channels are closed. Consequently, further bleaching of rhodopsin produces no further hyperpolarization as the rods are saturated.

### *Photopic Portion*

Section 5 shows the photopic section of the light adaptation curve. The slope of 1 indicates that the photopic system follows Weber's law. The photopic Weber fraction is about 0.015 (Stiles, 1953). This tells us that photopic system is more sensitive to contrast than is the scotopic system.

Note (see Fig. 3–15) that the cones do not show a saturation effect (Walraven et al, 1990). Although cone saturation can be demonstrated to occur, very specific stimulus conditions are required to elicit this saturation (Shevell, 1977).

## SPATIAL RESOLUTION AND SPATIAL SUMMATION

### *Basic Concepts*

Do we see better under photopic or scotopic conditions? One's first response may be that our vision is better under photopic conditions. The ability to resolve detail—visual resolution—is substantially superior under daylight conditions (photopic visual acuity is on the order of 20/20, whereas scotopic acuity is about 20/200, a 1-log-unit difference).

But visual resolution is not the whole story. Recall from the discussion of dark adaptation, that the ability to detect a stimulus is much superior under scotopic conditions than under photopic conditions. For a 420-nm stimulus to be detected under photopic conditions, it must be 3 log units (1000 times) more intense than is required for detection under scotopic conditions (see Fig. 3–8). Therefore, while visual resolution is superior under photopic conditions, we are more sensitive under scotopic conditions. This trade-off between visual resolution and visual sensitivity, to a large extent, is due to the manner in which the rods and cones are connected to the postreceptoral elements of the retina. Rods are connected in such a manner as to sum up information over space. This produces great sensitivity, but poor resolution. Cones, on the other hand, manifest connections that maximize visual resolution at the expense of sensitivity.

Figure 3–16 schematically illustrates rod and cone connections to a ganglion cell. Rods and cones do not actually synapse on a ganglion cell, but this simple model is useful for illustrative purposes. A major distinction between the scotopic and photopic systems, as illustrated by this diagram, is the number of photoreceptors that communicate with a single ganglion cell. Many more rods communicate with a ganglion cell than is the case for cones. This illustrates that the scotopic system, to a greater extent than the photopic system, sums up information over space. In other words, the scotopic system manifests greater **spatial summation.**

The large amount of scotopic spatial summation produces high scotopic sensitivity, as illustrated by the following example. Suppose that for a ganglion cell to signal an event, a total of 10 quanta must be absorbed, with each photoreceptor absorbing only 1 quantum. Furthermore, assume that these quanta are delivered in two flashes of light, separated by the distance $x$, and each spot contains 5 quanta (see Fig. 3–16). Finally, assume that all the incident quanta are absorbed.

By observation of Figure 3–16, it is seen that this stimulus arrangement causes the scotopic system to reach threshold. The two spots of light produce a total of 10 quantal absorptions, and this information is summed up by the ganglion cell to produce a signal. This ganglion cell signals the presence of a single light. It does not signal the presence of two lights; this information is lost due to spatial summation. In other words, the spatial summation of the scotopic system produces excellent sensitivity (a stimulus is seen), yet produces poor spatial resolution (only one stimulus is seen).

Now consider the situation for the photopic system with the same stimuli (see Fig. 3–16). In these circumstances, no stimulus is seen. This is because the limited spatial summation of the photopic system prevents it from adding up the information contained in both spots of light. A ganglion cell requires 10 quantal absorptions to signal an event, but each of the ganglion cells in this example only has input reflecting 5 absorptions. Therefore, the ganglion cell threshold is not met.

What happens if we double the number of quanta contained in each spot of light. The two ganglion cells, in the photopic case, each reach threshold and

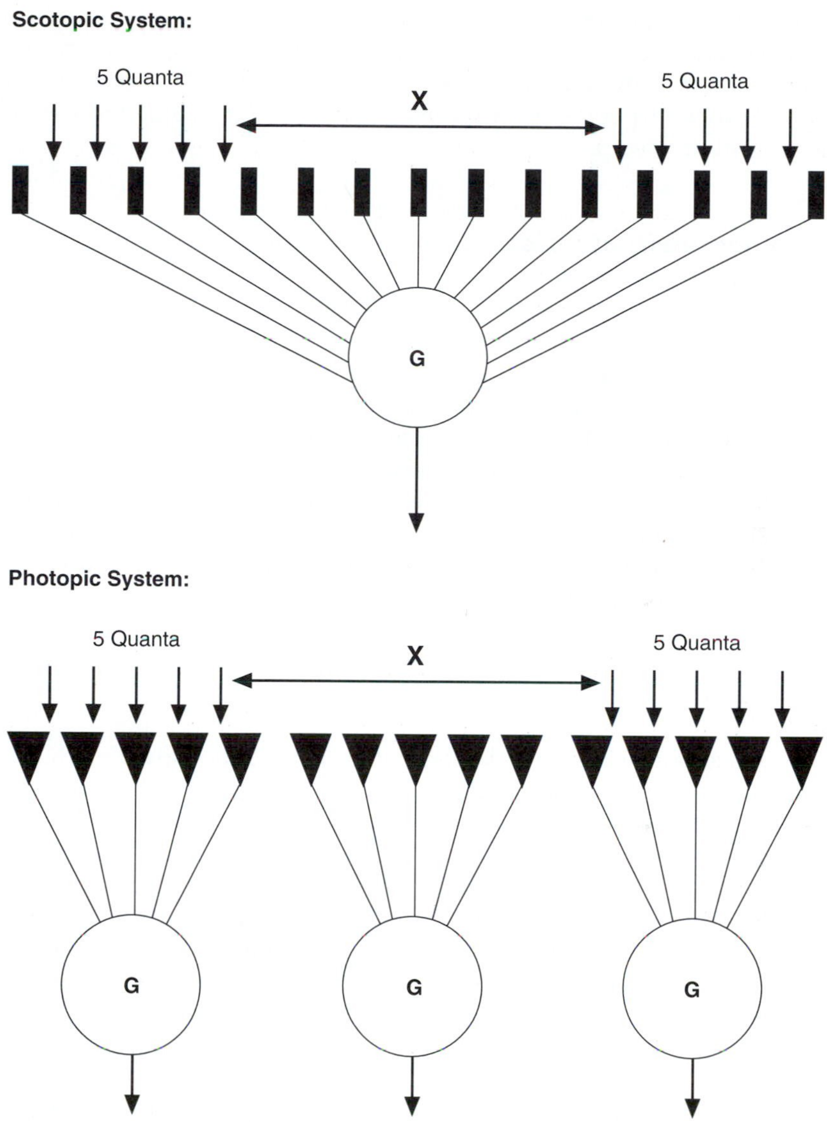


**FIGURE 3–16.** Schematic illustrations of scotopic and photopic retinal organization. The scotopic system manifests greater spatial summation than the photopic system. The simplified explanation in the text, which is associated with these diagrams, is best applied to the peripheral retina.

signal the presence of a stimulus. Consequently, two stimuli are seen. For the scotopic condition, the ganglion cell also reaches threshold; however, because all the rods converge on only one ganglion cell, the two spots of light are not resolved, and only one stimulus is seen.

In summary, the scotopic system shows excellent spatial summation. This contributes to its high sensitivity, but results in poor spatial resolution. Consequently, we can see a dim star at night, yet have a scotopic acuity of only 20/200. In contrast, the photopic system shows relatively less spatial summation. This results in poor sensitivity, yet allows a system capable of excellent spatial resolution (20/20).

### *Absolute Sensitivity of Vision*

Although it may be difficult to believe, the details given in the preceding example are largely correct. One quantal absorption is sufficient to cause activation of one rod. Ten such activated rods are sufficient to activate a ganglion cell, with the result that the stimulus is detected. However, a stimulus that emits only 10 quanta is not visible. This is because many quanta are either reflected or absorbed by pre-retinal elements or not absorbed by the rhodopsin. Less than 20 percent of the quanta incident on the retina are absorbed by rhodopsin (Hecht et al, 1942). For 10 quantal absorptions to result in detection, they must occur within certain space and time constraints. These constraints reflect the limits of spatial and temporal summation of the visual system.

### *Ricco's Law*

Spatial summation is classically demonstrated by the following experiment. An observer is presented with a small spot of light. The threshold number of quanta necessary to perceive this light is determined. The experiment is then repeated with spots of increasing size. The results of such an experiment are given in Figure 3–17, which shows the threshold number of quanta required for detection as a function of test spot diameter. These data are for the scotopic system. Note that for stimuli up to 10′ of arc in diameter, the total number of quanta necessary for detection is constant (Barlow, 1958). This means that the threshold number of quanta could be delivered in a 1′ arc test spot or spread out over a larger area, up to 10′ arc. Up to 10′ arc, the **critical diameter,** the scotopic system manifests total spatial summation.

Total spatial summation is represented mathematically by Ricco's law:

$$IA = K$$

where

$I$ = stimulus intensity (quanta/area)
$A$ = stimulus area
$K$ = constant

The difference in spatial summation between the scotopic and photopic systems is reflected by the difference in the critical diameters for these two systems. It

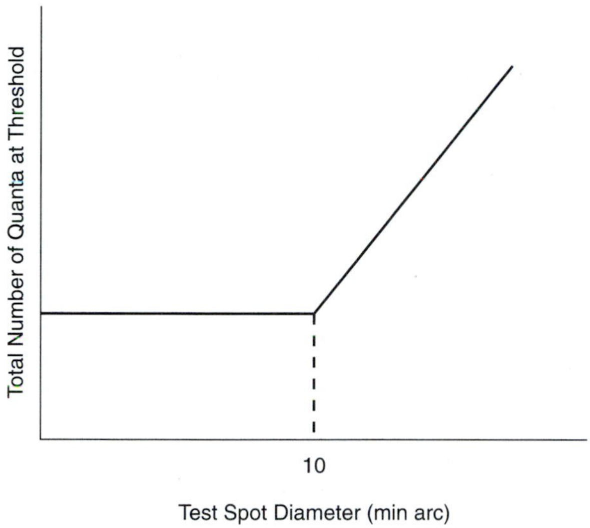


**FIGURE 3–17.** Classic expression of Ricco's law regarding spatial summation (scotopic conditions).

should not be surprising that the critical diameter of the photopic system is smaller than that for the scotopic system. This reflects the reduced spatial summation capability of the photopic system.

## TEMPORAL RESOLUTION AND TEMPORAL SUMMATION

In addition to manifesting differences in spatial resolution and summation, scotopic vision and photopic vision also demonstrate significant differences in temporal (time-related) resolution and summation. The scotopic system sums up information, over time, to a greater extent than the photopic system; it shows greater temporal summation. However, the photopic system is better able to distinguish two flashes of light separated by a brief interval in time. This shows that the photopic system has superior temporal resolution.

Let us examine this in more detail. Figure 3–18B shows two subthreshold pulses of light presented under scotopic conditions. Each pulse of light, by itself, will not be seen. Assume that these pulses are separated by an interpulse interval (IPI) of 90 milliseconds and that the temporal summation period of the scotopic system is 100 milliseconds. On the basis of this information, it is expected that the two subthreshold flashes will be summed up to reach threshold; the subject will report seeing a stimulus. As both pulses occur during the temporal summation period, however, the subject reports only one flash of light, not two.

Increasing the intensity of the pulses such that they are above threshold (suprathreshold), as indicated in Figure 3–18C, still does not allow the subject to perceive two flashes of light. The scotopic system's high degree of temporal summation limits its ability to resolve distinct temporal events. Only when these

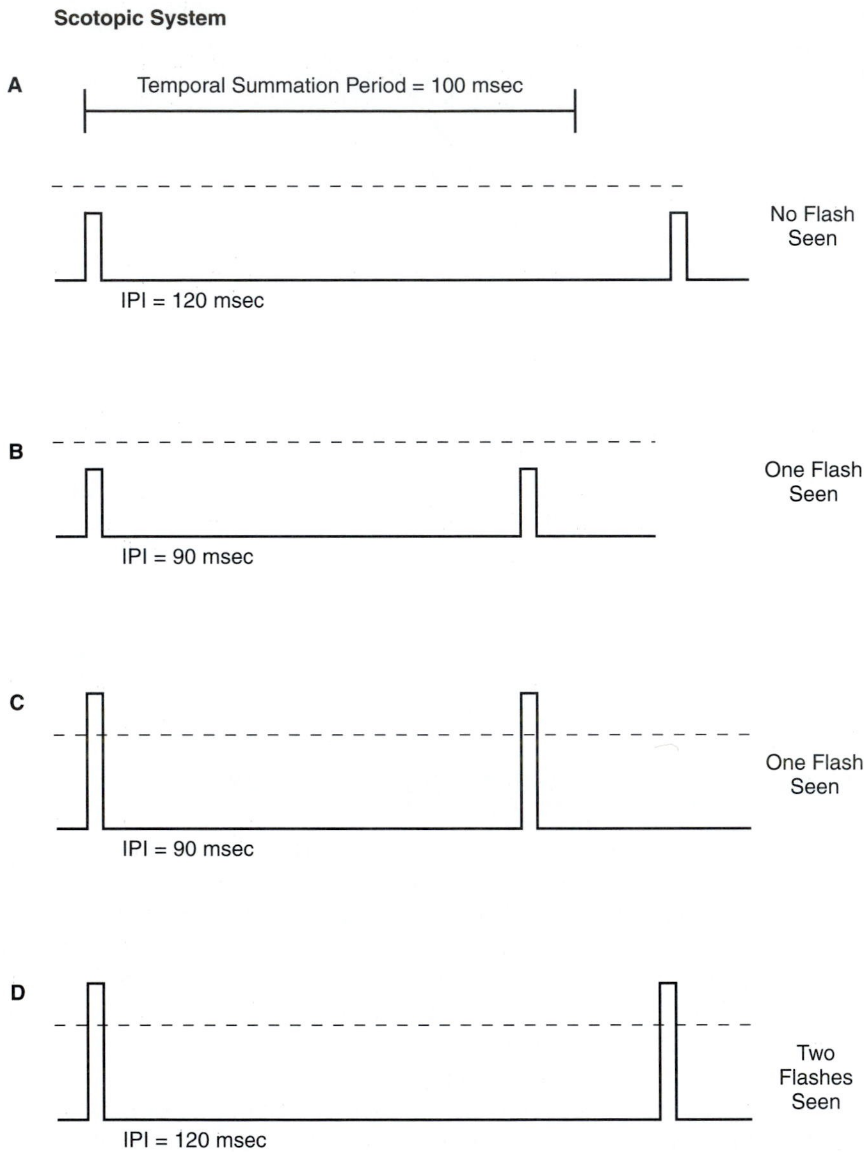


**FIGURE 3–18.** Temporal properties of the scotopic system assuming a temporal summation period of 100 milliseconds. The dashed line represents threshold for a single pulse. **A.** Two subthreshold pulses, separated by an interpulse interval (IPI) of 120 milliseconds, do not sum to reach threshold. A stimulus is not perceived. **B.** Two subthreshold pulses, presented within the temporal summation period, result in the perception of a single flash. **C.** Two suprathreshold pulses, presented within the temporal summation period, result in the perception of only a single flash. **D.** Two suprathreshold pulses, presented with an IPI of 120 milliseconds, are perceived as two flashes.

two suprathreshold pulses are separated by greater than 100 milliseconds, as indicated in Figure 3–18D, are two flashes seen.

The photopic system, as indicated in Figure 3–19A, shows a shorter period of temporal summation. As a consequence, the two subthreshold stimuli are not summed up to reach threshold. They need to be presented closer in time, as indicated in Figure 3–19B, to produce a percept of a single flash of light.

Although the photopic system demonstrates poor temporal summation, it does manifest superior temporal resolution. As indicated in Figure 3–19C, two suprathreshold pulses, separated by only 50 milliseconds, are distinguishable as two flashes. The scotopic system, with its high degree of temporal summation, would not be able to resolve these stimuli.

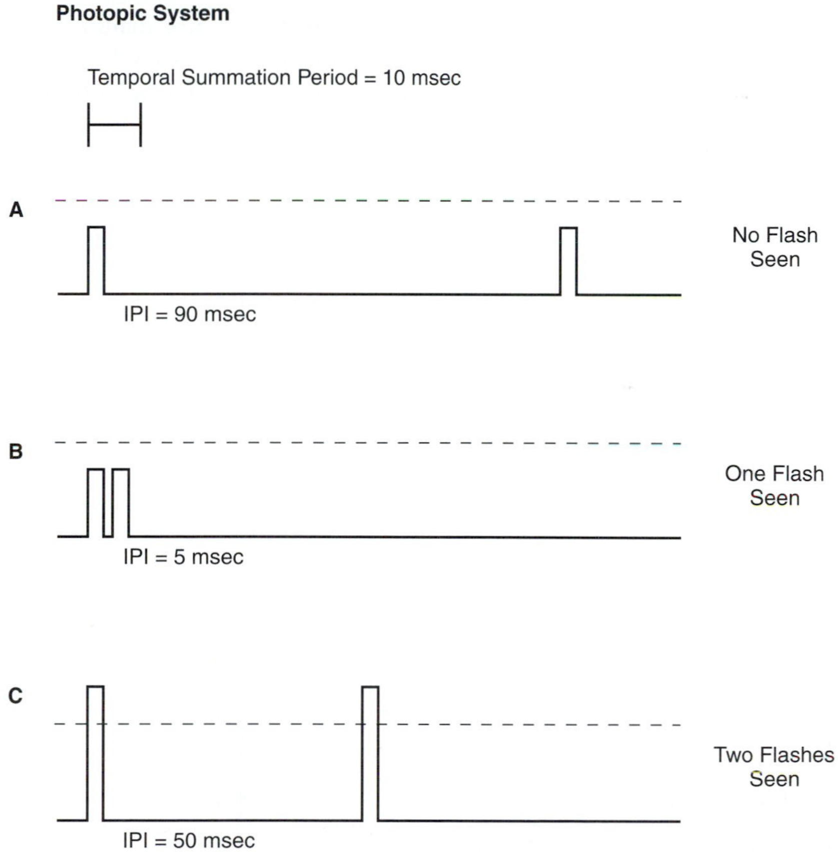


**FIGURE 3–19.** Temporal properties of the photopic system assuming a temporal summation period of 10 milliseconds. **A.** Two subthreshold pulses, presented with an interpulse interval of 90 milliseconds, do not sum to reach threshold. **B.** Two subthreshold pulses, presented within the summation period, are summed to reach threshold. **C.** Two suprathreshold pulses, separated by 50 milliseconds, are perceived as two flashes.

The high degree of temporal summation of the scotopic system is consistent with its greater sensitivity. The scotopic system sums information over both space (spatial summation) and time (temporal summation) to obtain excellent sensitivity. In contrast, the photopic system shows limited spatial and temporal summation. This, however, provides the photopic system with excellent spatial and temporal resolution. It is evident that there is a trade-off between summation and resolution.

### Bloch's Law

Bloch's law is the temporal equivalent to Ricco's law and is illustrated in Figure 3–20. This graph shows that within the so-called **critical duration,** or **critical period,** there is total temporal summation. As long as the threshold number of quanta are delivered within this critical duration, it does not matter how they are delivered. They could be presented in one or more flashes. Of course, multiple flashes presented within this critical duration are not resolved and only one flash is seen.

This graph can be mathematically expressed by Bloch's law as follows:

$$It = K$$

where

$I$ = stimulus intensity (quanta/time)
$t$ = stimulus duration
$K$ = constant

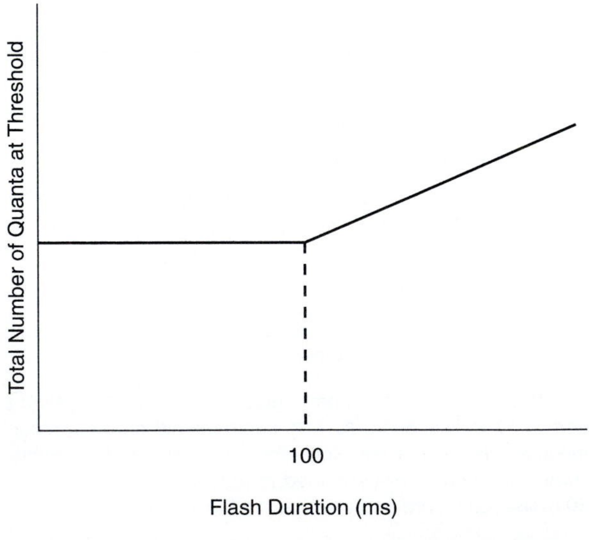


**FIGURE 3–20.** Classic expression of Bloch's law regarding temporal summation (scotopic conditions).

As we expect, the scotopic and photopic systems manifest different critical durations. Scotopic vision, with its greater degree of temporal summation, shows a critical duration of 100 milliseconds, whereas photopic vision manifests a critical duration on the order of 10 to 50 milliseconds (Sperling and Jolliffe, 1965; Krauskopf and Mollon, 1971; Swanson et al, 1987).

## STILES–CRAWFORD EFFECT OF THE FIRST KIND

Rods and cones respond in a different manner to light rays that do not strike them perpendicular (orthogonal) to their surface. This can be demonstrated by using a pinhole, as indicated in Figure 3–21. If the pinhole is centered in front of the pupil, the light rays strike the photoreceptors perpendicular to their surface. If, however, the pinhole is decentered, as in the bottom diagram, the light rays strike the same photoreceptors at an angle.

If the preceding experiment is performed under scotopic conditions, the subject notes relatively little change in brightness (Van Loo and Enoch, 1975). This tells us that the angle at which light rays are incident on rods is relatively insignificant.

The same experiment repeated under photopic conditions produces a very different result. Light rays that strike cones perpendicular to their surface are perceived as brighter than those that do not strike perpendicular to the surface. This effect, which is strongly manifested by cones, is referred to as the Stiles–Crawford effect of the first kind (Stiles, 1939). (The Stiles–Crawford effect of the second kind refers to a change in hue and saturation of monochromatic light as the point of entry into the pupil is changed.)

The Stiles–Crawford effect of the first kind is probably due to waveguide properties of the cones (Enoch and Fry, 1958). The physical dimension of a quantum of light is such that it approaches the size of a cone. This closeness in physical size between a quantum of light and a cone makes the angle of entry of the ray of light into the funnel-shaped cone critical. Any deviation from an orthogonal entry reduces the effectiveness of light rays in bleaching photopigment and, consequently, reduces the perceived brightness of these rays.

In normal circumstances, cones point toward the center of the pupil. This maximizes their effectiveness. An interesting question concerns an eye with a decentered pupil, illustrated in Figure 3–22. (A decentered pupil can be congenital or secondary to trauma.) Do the cones point toward the normal pupil position, or do they point toward the location of the displaced pupil? The Stiles–Crawford effect manifested by these eyes suggests that the cones point toward the location of the displaced pupil (Applegate and Bonds, 1981; Enoch and Birch, 1981). In fact, one can take an adult individual with a normally centered Stiles–Crawford effect and decenter the effect by fitting him or her with a contact lens that has a displaced pupil. The cones return to their original state once the contact lens is removed. These results tell us that the cones are mobile and that they orient themselves to light. If the pupil becomes decentered, the cones reorient them-

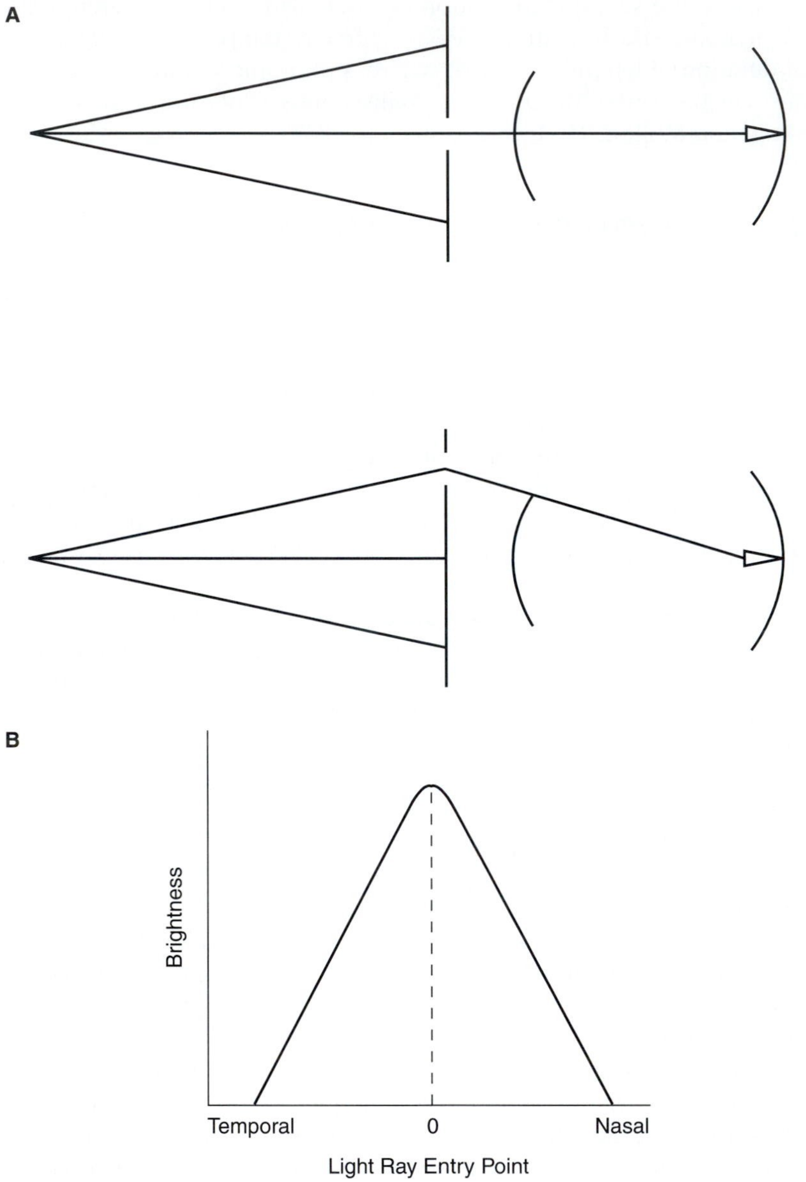


**FIGURE 3–21.** Stiles–Crawford effect of the first kind. **A.** A centered pinhole (top) causes light rays to strike cones perpendicular to their surface, whereas a decentered pinhole (bottom) causes light rays to strike cones at an angle. **B.** Under photopic conditions, the centered pinhole produces a brighter image than the decentered pinhole.

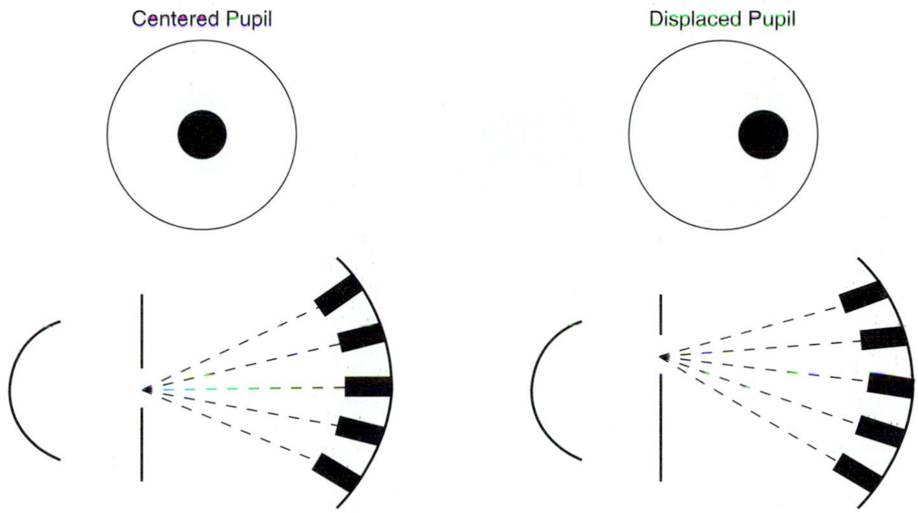


**FIGURE 3–22.** The cones migrate to point toward the center of the pupil when the pupil is displaced.

selves such that they now point toward the center of the pupil. This maximizes their effectiveness in capturing photons of light.

## *Clinical Considerations*

### *Visual Field Testing*

Visual field testing is a common and important clinical procedure. It plays a critical role in the diagnosis of many disorders of the visual system, including glaucoma and other neurologic diseases. In visual field testing, visual sensitivity is determined as a function of retinal location. The patient views a fixation point, and sensitivity is determined at a large number of retinal locations. Lighting conditions are typically photopic, but not overwhelmingly so. The stimulus is essentially an increment on a steady background, similar to that used in a light adaptation experiment.

In normal circumstances, a sensitivity profile similar to that given in Figure 3–23 is obtained. As expected, under photopic conditions sensitivity is greatest centrally, in the fovea. Sensitivity falls off in the periphery of the retina, making the sensitivity profile appear like a hill. Consequently, this sensitivity profile is often referred to as the **hill of vision.**

Modern visual field devices determine thresholds for a large number of retinal points and compare these values with those for age-matched normals. Com-

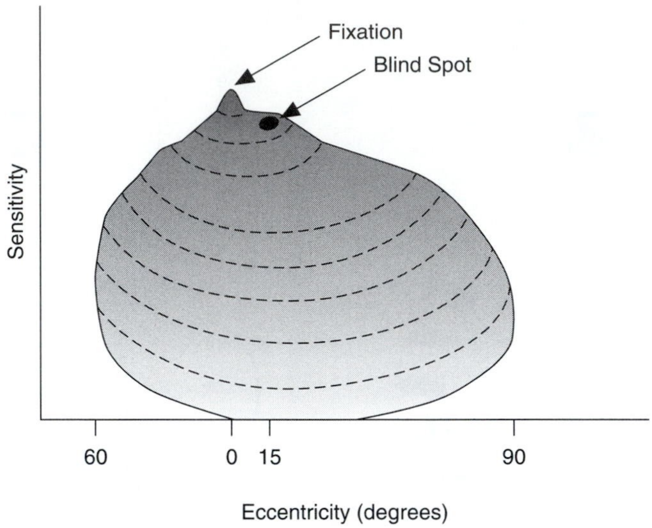


**FIGURE 3–23.** Hill of vision obtained under photopic conditions for a right eye. Note the fixation peak for the fovea and the blind spot produced by the optic disk. As we approach old age, increment sensitivity decreases; this is manifested as a "sinking" of the hill of vision.

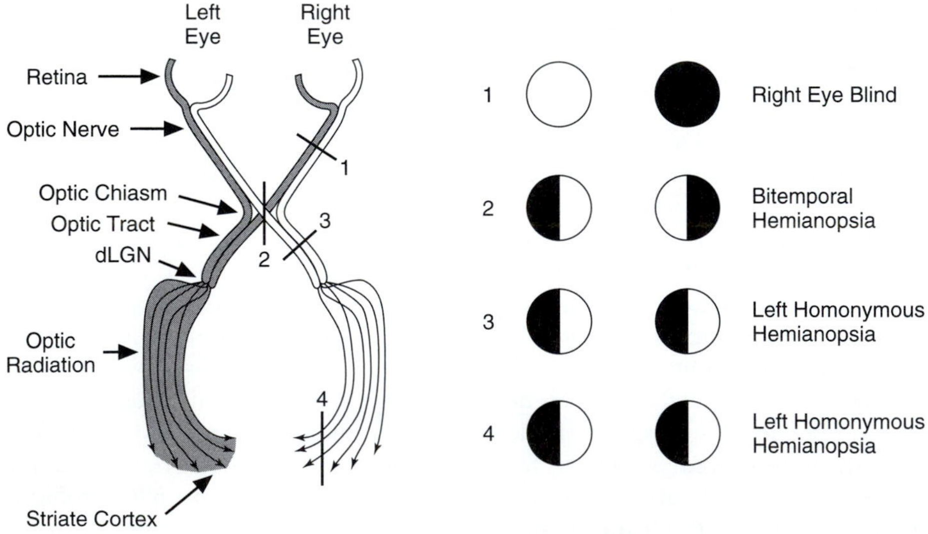


**FIGURE 3–24.** The location of a lesion within the visual pathway determines the nature of the field defect.

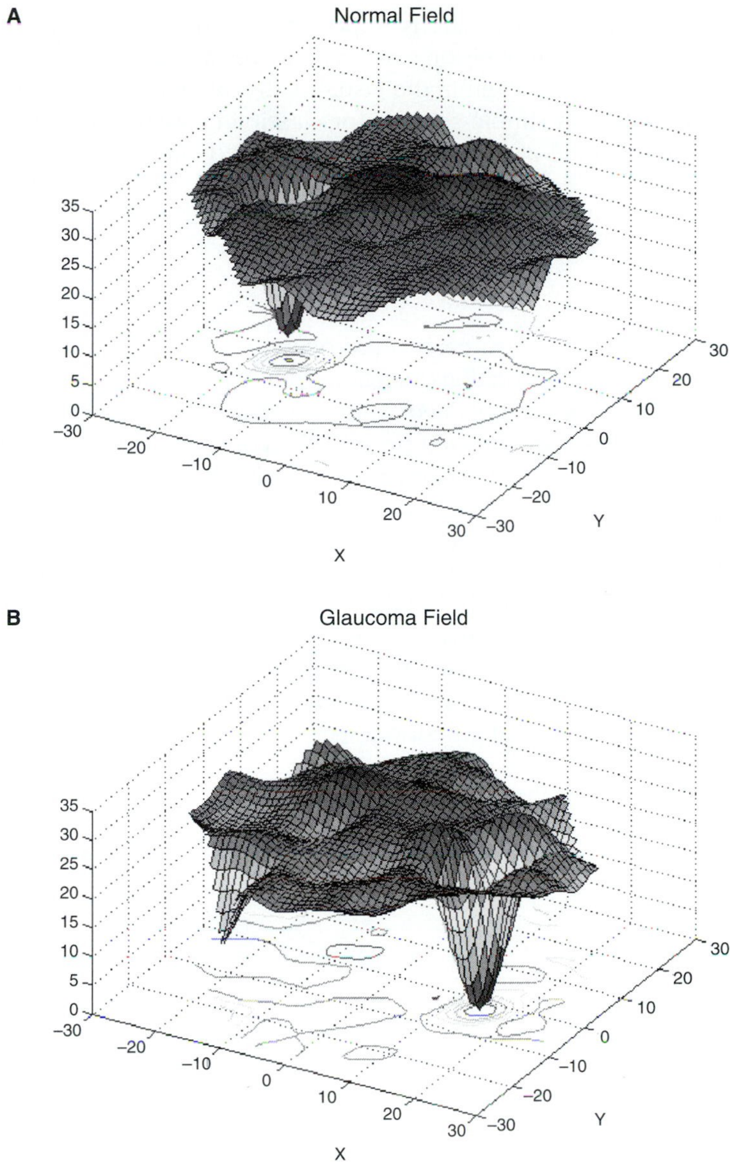


**FIGURE 3–25.** Visual field profiles as measured clinically with the Humphrey Visual Field Analyzer. **A.** A normal visual field for a left eye. Note the central foveal peak and the temporal pit, which represents the blind spot. **B.** A visual field for a right eye showing moderate glaucomatous damage. The blind spot is enlarged and there is a reduction in sensitivity in the inferonasal region of the field. (*These visual fields were kindly provided by Humphrey Systems in San Leandro, California.*)

parison with age-matched normals is important because increment sensitivity decreases with age; the hill of vision sinks with increasing age (Weale, 1992).

The location of a lesion within the visual pathway determines the nature of the visual field defect. A simple scheme for classifying such lesions is given in Figure 3–24. An example of a visual field as measured clinically is given in Figure 3–25.

### *Dark Adaptation*

Clinical dark adaptation measurements are occasionally useful in the diagnosis of certain rod–cone degenerations, such as retinitis pigmentosa (RP). These measurements are typically obtained using a Goldmann–Weekers dark adaptometer. In RP, the rods are affected prior to the cones, sometimes leading to a dark adaptation curve with an abnormal rod portion relatively early in the disease (Fig. 3–26). This rod portion may take an unusually long time to level off and plateau at a higher than normal threshold.

This abnormal rod section of the dark adaptation curve is consistent with these patients' symptoms of night blindness and slow visual recovery following exposure to a bright light. This is particularly evident following ophthalmoscopy. The intense ophthalmoscope light bleaches the rods and they recover unusually slowly. The result is that the patient is visually incapacitated for several minutes following ophthalmoscopy.

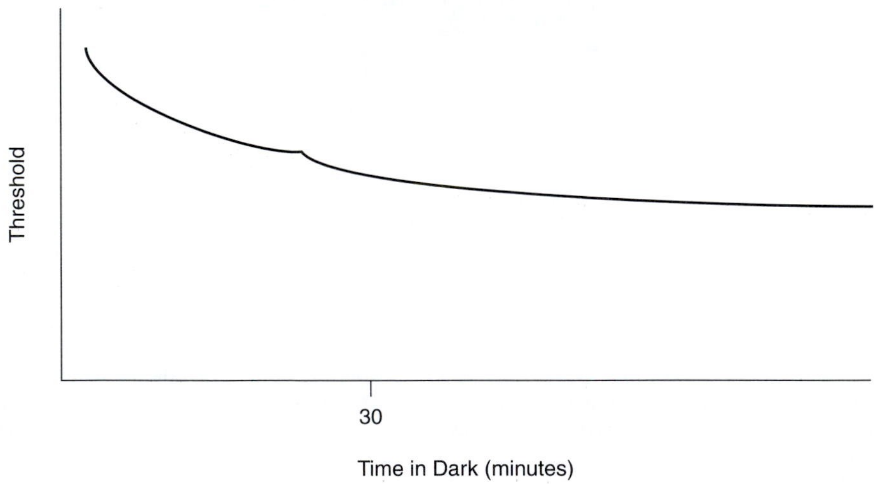


**FIGURE 3–26.** Dark adaptation curve for a hypothetical patient in the early stages of retinitis pigmentosa. Note the slow rate of recovery and elevated rod threshold.

## SUMMARY

Rods and cones show differences in morphology, photopigments, and retinal distribution (Table 3–2). Moreover, these photoreceptors differ in their connections to postreceptoral elements. The consequence of all these differences is a duplex retina: a rod-dominated system operates under dim (scotopic) lighting conditions and a cone-dominated system functions under daylight (photopic) conditions. This duplex retina allows us to have usable vision on both a dark evening and a sunny day, even though there may be up to a 10-log-unit difference in the light levels provided by these two conditions.

Scotopic vision shows great sensitivity largely because of its high degree of spatial and temporal summation; however, this high degree of spatial and temporal summation limits scotopic spatial and temporal resolution. Photopic vision, on the other hand, displays substantially greater spatial and temporal resolution, but poorer spatial and temporal summation.

**TABLE 3–2. SUMMARY OF FEATURES OF THE SCOTOPIC AND PHOTOPIC SYSTEMS**

| Property | Scotopic System | Photopic System |
|---|---|---|
| Receptor | Rods | Cones |
| Outer segment morphology | Separate disks | Disks formed by infoldings of membrane |
| Weber's fraction | 0.140 | 0.015 |
| Photopigment(s) and peak absorption | Rhodopsin (507 nm) | Erythrolabe (565 nm)<br>Chlorolabe (535 nm)<br>Cyanolabe (430 nm) |
| Maximal sensitivity of the system | 507 nm | 555 nm |
| Chromatic discrimination | Colorblind | Color discrimination |
| Sensitivity | Very sensitive to dim lights, not to bright lights | Not sensitive to dim lights, but sensitive to brighter lights |
| Spatial resolution (resolution acuity) | Poor (20/200) | Excellent (20/20) |
| Spatial summation | Excellent | Poor |
| Temporal resolution (CFF[a]) | Poor (20 Hz) | Excellent (70 Hz) |
| Temporal summation | Excellent | Poor |
| Contrast sensitivity | Low | High |
| Stiles–Crawford effect | Minimal | Yes |

[a]Critical flicker fusion frequency.

# Q Self-Assessment Questions

1. Rod monochromat eyes are missing most of their cones; vision is dominated by rods. **A.** Describe the symptoms you expect a patient who is a rod monochromat to manifest. **B.** What color sunglasses would you recommend for a patient who is a rod monochromat?

2. Stimuli of 507 and 555 nm are placed side-by-side. These stimuli are bright and are detected by the photopic system. An observer is asked to adjust the intensities of the stimuli so that they are equally bright. The intensities of these two stimuli are then reduced by the same amount such that they are detected by the scotopic system. Under these scotopic conditions, which stimulus appears brightest?

3. Name the wavelength that is most effective at bleaching rhodopsin. Explain.

4. Refer to Figure 3–10. **A.** After 20 minutes of dark adaptation, what is the color of the 610-nm stimulus at threshold. **B.** Answer the same question for the 465-nm stimulus. Explain.

5. Refer to Figure 3–10. **A.** After 1 hour of dark adaptation, what is the difference in sensitivity between the rods and cones for a stimulus of 465 nm? **B.** Answer the same question for the 610-nm stimulus.

6. **A.** The cones are exposed to a bright light source that bleaches much of their photopigment. After 3 minutes in the dark, what percentage of the bleached cone photopigment has recovered? **B.** What percentage of the rod photopigment has recovered at the rod–cone break for 610 nm (see Fig. 3–10).

7. Refer to Figure 3–8. **A.** What is the rod threshold after about 11 minutes of dark adaptation for a large 420-nm stimulus? **B.** For the same 420-nm stimulus, what is the cone threshold after 20 minutes of dark adaptation? **C.** What is the photochromatic interval for 420 nm?

# Q

**8. A.** Two patches of light are adjacent to each other. The conditions are scotopic. One patch emits light of 507 nm and the other emits light of 620 nm. Both patches produce 40 quanta of light. Which patch is brighter? **B.** A patch of 507 nm and a patch of 620 nm each bleach 30 rhodopsin molecules. Which patch is brighter?

# 4

# Photometry

The provision of routine eye and vision care requires the practitioner to understand how light is measured and specified—the topics of this chapter. The clinical relevance of this material becomes particularly obvious after considering that most clinical procedures are performed under specified lighting conditions and that ophthalmic lenses are frequently specified in terms of their spectral transmission characteristics.

This material also has application to **visual ergonomics,** the design of a safe and comfortable work environment. Issues addressed in this field include the proper illumination for work spaces and the design of highway signs such that their visibility is maximized.

## *PHOTOMETRY AND RADIOMETRY: BASIC CONCEPTS AND UNITS*

**Radiometry** refers to the measurement of the power produced by a source of electromagnetic radiation. **Photometry,** in comparison, refers to the effect this radiation has on the visual system. This distinction can be understood by observing Figure 4–1, which displays the photopic luminosity curve, $V(\lambda)$. This curve shows luminous efficiency as a function of wavelength. Luminous efficiency is closely related to brightness. Note that this function has a form that is very similar to the photopic spectral sensitivity function (see Chap. 3).

Let us discuss this in more detail. Figure 4–2 shows two stimuli, one of 400 nm and the other of 600 nm. Both produce 10 W of radiant power. (One watt [W] is equal to one joule [J] per second.) Although these two stimuli have the same radiant power, they have very different effects on the visual system. The 400-nm stimulus has a luminous efficiency approaching zero; the 600-nm stimulus has an efficiency of 0.62. Therefore, although these two stimuli are radiometrically equal, they are photometrically different. The 400-nm stimulus is

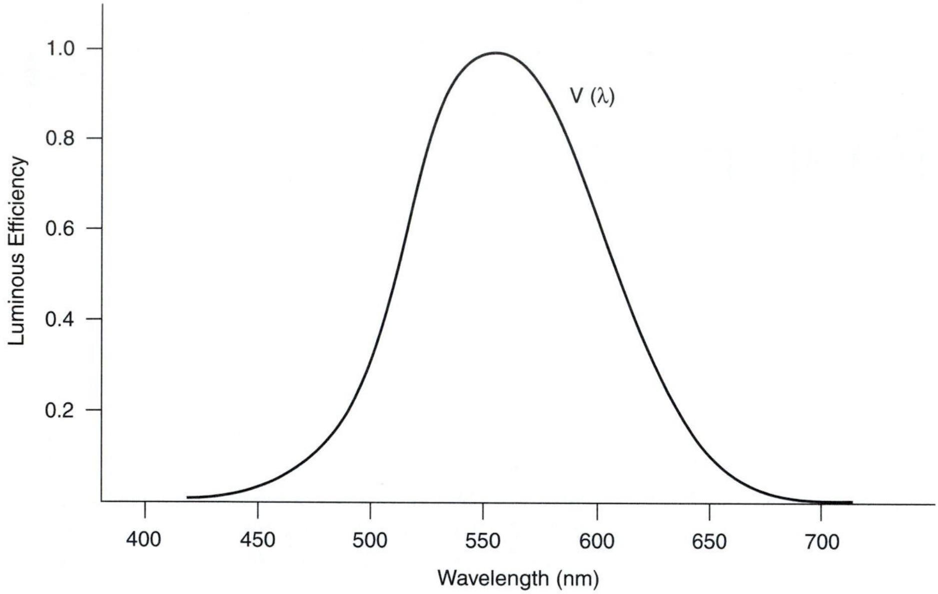


**FIGURE 4–1.** Photopic luminosity function, *V*(λ). Luminous efficiency, which is related to brightness, is plotted as a function of wavelength.

practically invisible (it produces almost no light), whereas the 600-nm stimulus is visible.

### *Lumens*

A basic unit of photometry is the lumen. A lumen is a measure of **luminous power,** as compared with a watt, which is a unit of **radiant power.** By convention, there are 680 lumens per watt at 555 nm. (There are actually 683 lumens per watt at 555 nm; however, to simplify calculations, in this text we use the approximation of 680 lumens per watt at 555 nm.) Wavelengths other than 555 nm are less efficient and yield fewer lumens per watt proportionate to their position on the *V*(λ) curve. For example, at 650 nm there are (0.1)(680 lumens/W), or 68 lumens/W. (The value of 0.1 is the luminous efficiency of 650 nm, and is read off the *V*(λ) curve.)

Let us return to our earlier example, given in Figure 4–2, in which patches of 400 and 600 nm each emit 10 W of radiant power. As the luminous efficiency of 400 nm is essentially zero, this patch emits almost zero lumens. This stimulus has radiant power, but almost no luminous power. The 600-nm patch produces (0.62)(680 lumens/W)(10 W), or 4216 lumens. This patch, although of the same radiant power as the 400-nm patch, has substantial luminous power. In fact,

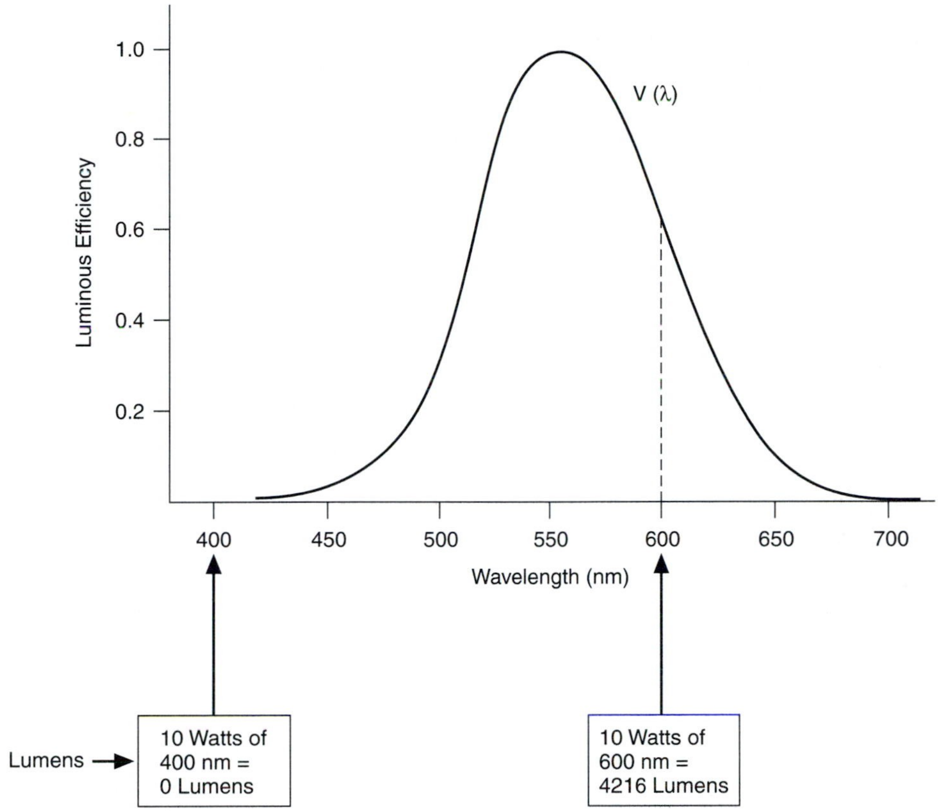


**FIGURE 4–2.** Ten watts (power) of 400 nm produces close to zero lumens of light, whereas 10 W of 600 nm produces 4216 lumens. Although both stimuli have the same power, they have different effects on the visual system because of their differing luminous efficiencies.

whereas the 400-nm patch produces virtually no light, the 600-nm patch produces significant light.

### *Abney's Law of Additivity*

Monochromatic stimuli are rarely encountered. Rather, most objects emit (or reflect) a mixture of many different wavelengths. A simplified example of the spectral distribution of such a stimulus is given in Figure 4–3. The total number of lumens produced by this stimulus is determined by calculating the number of lumens produced by each wavelength in the mixture and then adding these values together. This is done as follows:

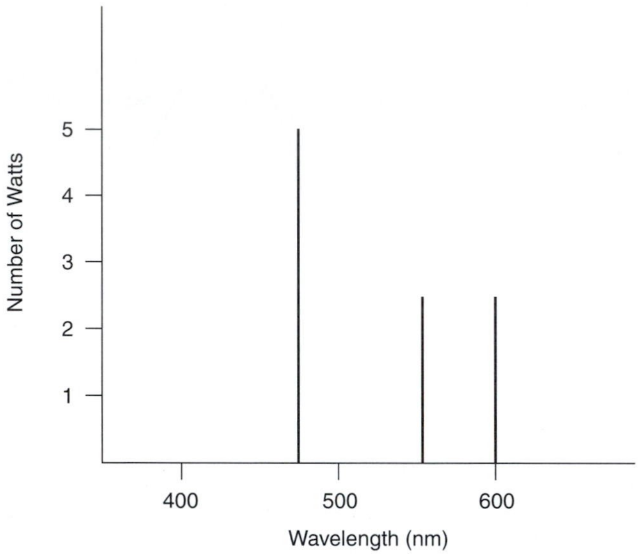


**FIGURE 4–3.** Spectral distribution of a stimulus composed of 5 W of 475 nm, 2.5 W of 555 nm, and 2.5 W of 600 nm.

| | |
|---|---|
| 5 W of 475 nm: | (0.1) (680 lumens/W) (5 W) = 340 lumens |
| 2.5 W of 555 nm: | (1.0) (680 lumens/W) (2.5 W) = 1700 lumens |
| 2.5 W of 600 nm: | (0.62) (680 lumens/W) (2.5 W) = 1054 lumens |
| Total = | 340 lumens + 1700 lumens + 1054 lumens |
| Total = | 3094 lumens |

We can add these different values together because the photometric system we use is **additive.** This property is referred to as **Abney's law of additivity** (Abney, 1913).

### *Luminous Intensity*

Luminous power is a nondirectional measure. It is useful for expressing the total light power produced by a light source in all directions. Household light bulbs are typically specified in terms of the number of lumens they produce.

Luminous intensity, in contrast, refers to the number of lumens produced in a given direction by a point light source. A light bulb may produce a total of 1000 lumens in all directions, however, its luminous intensity is specified in one particular direction (Fig. 4–4).

The units for luminous intensity are **lumens per steradian.** One lumen per steradian is equal to one **candela (cd).** A steradian (ω or Sr) is a solid an-

| | Definition | Common Units | Radiometric Equivalent and Units |
|---|---|---|---|
| **Luminous Power** 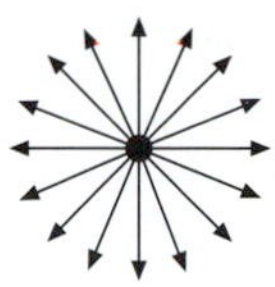 | Total light power produced by a source | Lumens | Radiant power (joules/second or watts) |
| **Luminous Intensity** 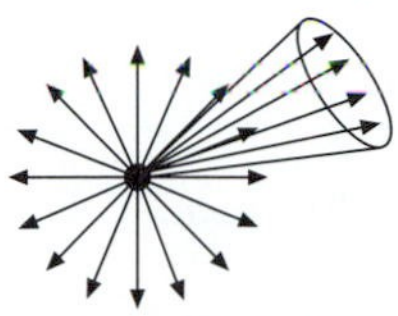 | Light power produced in a solid angle by a point source | Lumens/steradian<br>Candelas<br>(1 lumen/steradian = 1 candela) | Radiant intensity (watts/steradian) |
| **Luminance** 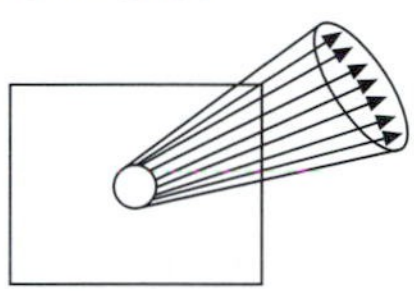 | Luminous intensity per unit projected area of an extended source | Candelas/square meter<br>Foot-lamberts | Radiance (watts/steradian/square meter) |
| **Illuminance** 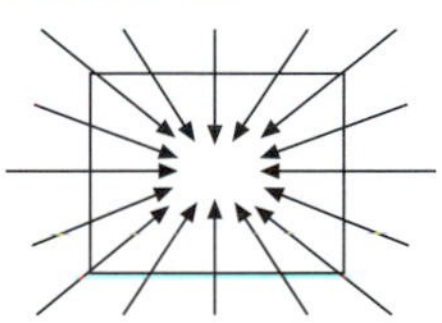 | Luminous power falling on a surface | Lumens/square meter<br>Lumens/square foot | Irradiance (watts/square meter) |

**FIGURE 4–4.** Various terms, definitions, and units common in photometry and radiometry.

gle. It is a conic section of a sphere (Fig. 4–5). Mathematically, a steradian is defined as

$$\omega = A/r^2$$

where

$r$ = radius of the sphere
$A$ = surface area of sphere subtended

Given the intensity of a point source, the total number of lumens produced by this source may be calculated *if* the source is uniform in its output. This calculation is based on the fact that a light source with an intensity of 1 cd, which has equal output in all directions, produces a total power of $4\pi$ lumens. Conse-

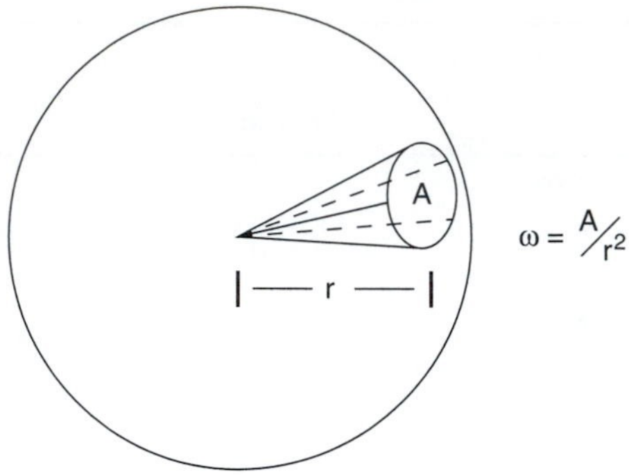


**FIGURE 4–5.** A steradian, or solid angle, is defined as $A/r^2$. The symbol ω or the abbreviation Sr is typically used to denote a steradian.

quently, if a uniform point source has an intensity of 10 cd, its total luminous output is expected to be (10 cd)(4π lumens/cd), or 127 lumens.

### *Luminance*

Luminance is similar to luminous intensity, except that it refers to an extended source (see Fig. 4–4). An extended source is a large source, such as a wall, which may be thought of as consisting of an infinite number of point sources. One can think of luminance as being similar to the brightness of a surface. The units for luminance are candelas per projected area of the light source. Common units are **candelas per square meter** ($cd/m^2$) and **foot-lamberts.**

Just as the brightness of a surface does not change with viewing distance, luminance does not change with viewing distance. As the viewing distance increases, the projected surface area (i.e., the area of the surface as imaged on, for example, the retina) decreases at the same rate as does the number of candelas contained within the projected surface. This results in a constant ratio of candelas to projected surface area and therefore, the luminance remains constant.

### *Illuminance*

Illuminance refers to the luminous power that falls on a surface (see Fig. 4–4). Typical units are **lumens per square meter (lux)** and **lumens per square foot (foot-candles).** Think of illuminance as being analogous to rain. The greater the density of rain drops (lumens) the harder it is raining (the greater the illuminance). Note that illuminance is unrelated to the surface on which the light is falling. Referring back to the rain analogy, the intensity of rain is unrelated to the surface on which the rain falls.

Lighting standards have been established for certain facilities and activities

(Table 4–1). These standards specify the amount of light that should fall upon a surface (the illuminance) to provide satisfactory vision. A standard illuminance meter can be used to determine if lighting conditions meet industrial standards.

It is easy to confuse the definitions of luminance and illuminance. Luminance is a property of a surface under a given set of lighting conditions and refers to the light coming off a surface, whereas illuminance refers to the amount of light falling (raining) on a surface. A desk may have the same illumination across its entire surface, but the luminance of the objects on which the light falls may vary. The luminance of a white piece of paper on the desk will be greater than that of a black book on the desk. This is because the white paper reflects more light than the black book.

### *Photometric Units*

A plethora of units are used for luminance and illuminance. Conversions between various units are simple and require only a conversion factor. Common conversion factors are given in Table 4–2. It should be pointed out that the Système International d'Unités recognizes the metric units of $cd/m^2$ and lux for luminance and illuminance, respectively. This standardization body does not rec-

**TABLE 4–1. RECOMMENDED ILLUMINANCE VALUES**

| | Illumination | |
|---|---|---|
| **Area or Activity** | ***Lux*** | ***Footcandles*** |
| General residential lighting | 50–100 | 5–10 |
| Exhibition hall | 100–200 | 10–20 |
| Elevator | 100–200 | 10–20 |
| Hotel corridor | 100–200 | 10–20 |
| Residential dining room | 100–200 | 10–20 |
| Restroom | 100–200 | 10–20 |
| Library stack | 200–500 | 20–50 |
| Residential reading | 200–500 | 20–50 |
| Industrial wrapping, packing, labeling (general) | 200–500 | 20–50 |
| Classroom | 500–1000 | 50–100 |
| School science laboratory | 500–1000 | 50–100 |
| Eye surgery | 1000–2000 | 100–200 |
| Clothes fitting area | 1000–2000 | 100–200 |
| Dental procedures | 5000–10000 | 500–1000 |

Adapted from Rea, MS (ed). *Lighting Handbook: Reference and Application.* New York: IESNA; 1993.

**TABLE 4–2. CONVERSION FACTORS FOR COMMON UNITS OF ILLUMINANCE AND LUMINANCE**[a]

**Illuminance Conversion Factors**

| | | *Lux ($lm/m^2$)* | *Phot* | *Milliphot* | *Footcandle* | | *Lumen (per square unit of area)* | *Abbreviation* |
|---|---|---|---|---|---|---|---|---|
| 1 Lux | = | 1 | $10^{-4}$ | $10^{-1}$ | $9.290 \times 10^{-2}$ | = | 1 $lm/m^2$ | [lx] |
| 1 Phot | = | $10^4$ | 1 | $10^3$ | $9.290 \times 10^2$ | = | 1 $lm/cm^2$ | [ph] |
| 1 Milliphot | = | 10 | $10^{-3}$ | 1 | $9.290 \times 10^{-1}$ | = | $10^{-3}$ $lm/cm^2$ | [mph] |
| 1 Footcandle | = | $1.076 \times 10$ | $1.076 \times 10^{-3}$ | 1.076 | 1 | = | 1 $lm/ft^2$ | [fcd] |

**Luminance Conversion Factors**

| | | *Nit ($cd/m^2$)* | *Stilb* | *Apostilb* | *Lambert* | *Millilambert* | *Footlambert* | *Candela $ft^{-2}$* | *Candela $in^{-2}$* | | *Candela (per square unit of area)* | *Abbreviation* |
|---|---|---|---|---|---|---|---|---|---|---|---|---|
| 1 Nit | = | 1 | $10^{-4}$ | 3.142 | $3.142 \times 10^{-4}$ | $3.142 \times 10^{-1}$ | $2.919 \times 10^{-1}$ | $9.290 \times 10^{-2}$ | $6.452 \times 10^{-4}$ | = | 1 $cd/m^2$ | [nt] |
| 1 Stilb | = | $10^4$ | 1 | $3.142 \times 10^4$ | $3.142 \times 10^3$ | $3.142 \times 10^3$ | $9.919 \times 10^3$ | $9.290 \times 10^2$ | 6.452 | = | 1 $cd/m^2$ | [sb] |
| 1 Apostilb | = | $10^{-1}$ | $10^{-5}$ | 1 | $10^{-4}$ | $10^{-1}$ | $9.290 \times 10^{-2}$ | $2.957 \times 10^{-2}$ | $2.054 \times 10^{-4}$ | = | $(1/\pi)$ $cd/m^2$ | [asb] |
| 1 Lambert | = | $3.183 \times 10^3$ | $3.183 \times 10^{-1}$ | $10^4$ | 1 | $10^3$ | $9.290 \times 10^2$ | $2.957 \times 10^2$ | 2.054 | = | $(1/\pi)$ $cd/cm^2$ | [L] |
| 1 Millilambert | = | 3.183 | $3.183 \times 10^{-4}$ | 10 | $10^{-3}$ | 1 | $9.290 \times 10^{-1}$ | $2.957 \times 10^{-1}$ | $2.054 \times 10^{-3}$ | = | $10^{-3}$ $(1/\pi)$ $cd/cm^2$ | [mL] |
| 1 Footlambert | = | 3.426 | $3.426 \times 10^{-4}$ | $1.076 \times 10$ | $1.076 \times 10^{-3}$ | 1.076 | 1 | $3.183 \times 10^{-1}$ | $2.210 \times 10^{-3}$ | = | $(1/\pi)$ $cd/ft^2$ | [fL] |
| 1 Candela/$ft^2$ | = | $1.076 \times 10$ | $1.076 \times 10^{-3}$ | $3.382 \times 10$ | $3.382 \times 10^{-3}$ | 3.382 | 3.142 | 1 | $6.944 \times 10^{-3}$ | = | 1 $cd/ft^2$ | [$cdft^{-2}$] |
| 1 Candela/$in^2$ | = | $1.550 \times 10^3$ | $1.550 \times 10^{-1}$ | $4.869 \times 10^3$ | $4.869 \times 10^{-1}$ | $4.869 \times 10^2$ | $4.524 \times 10^2$ | $1.44 \times 10^2$ | 1 | = | 1 $cd/in^2$ | [$cdin^{-2}$] |

**Other Equivalent Units**

| | | |
|---|---|---|
| 1 equivalent phot | = | 1 lambert |
| 1 equivalent lux | = | 1 blondel = 1 apostilb |
| 1 equivalent footcandle | = | 1 footlambert |

[a]For example, $X$ footlamberts = $X \times 3.426 \times 10^{-4}$ stilbs.

From Wysecki G, Stiles WS. *Color Science: Concepts and Methods, Quantitative Data and Formulae.* Copyright 1982. Reprinted by permission of John Wiley & Sons, Inc.

ognize units such as foot-lamberts and lumens/ft$^2$, which are based on English measurement units.

### Radiometric Units

The radiometric equivalents of luminous power, luminous intensity, luminance, and illuminance are, respectively, radiant power, radiant intensity, radiance, and irradiance (see Fig. 4–4). These radiometric terms do not take into account the luminous efficiency of the visual system.

## COSINE DIFFUSERS

A cosine surface shows the same luminance regardless of the angle at which its luminance is measured. Cosine surfaces are also referred to as **Lambert surfaces, perfectly diffusing surfaces,** or **matte surfaces.** A good example of a cosine surface is a piece of nonglossy paper. From whatever angle you view this paper, its brightness is the same, as is its luminance. A mirror is an example of a surface that is not perfectly diffusing. The luminance of a mirror varies depending on the direction at which it is measured. This type of surface is referred to as a **specular surface.**

Cosine diffusers have the advantage that their luminance can be easily calculated if the reflectance factor of the surface (a nondimensional unit that ranges from 0 to 1), along with the illumination falling on the surface, is known (Fig. 4–6). The equation for this calculation is

$$L = rE$$

where

$L$ = luminance in foot-lamberts
$r$ = reflectance factor (nondimensional, no units)
$E$ = illumination in foot-candles (lumens/ft$^2$)

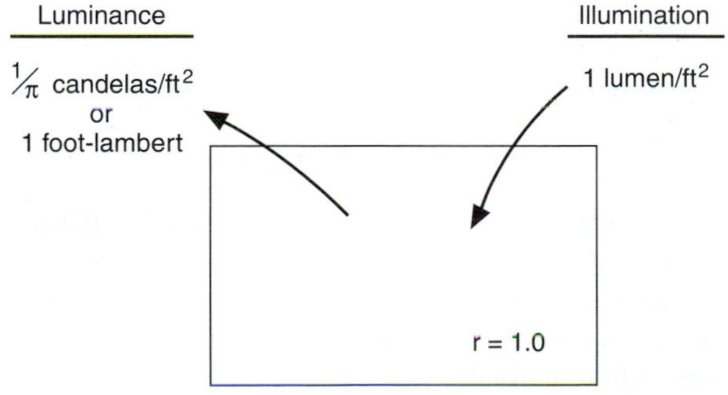


**FIGURE 4–6.** A cosine surface with a reflectance factor of 1 will have a luminance of 1 foot-lambert when the illumination falling on it is 1 lumen/ft$^2$.

The basis for this relationship is that an illumination of 1 lumen/ft$^2$, falling on a matte surface with a reflectance factor of 1, produces a luminance of 1/π cd/ft$^2$. To avoid the 1/π factor, 1 foot-lambert is defined as 1/π cd/ft$^2$. Consequently, an illumination of 1 lumen/ft$^2$ falling on a surface with $r = 1$ produces a luminance of 1 foot-lambert.

## INVERSE SQUARE LAW

As a surface is moved away from a point source, the number of lumens falling on the surface decreases with the square of the distance, resulting in a decrease in illumination (of the surface). This is illustrated by Figure 4–7A. Mathematically, this inverse square law is expressed as

$$E = I/d^2$$

where

$E$ = illumination falling on the surface
$I$ = intensity of the point source
$d$ = distance from the point source to the surface

This formula assumes that the surface is normal to the light source. If the surface is tilted, as indicated in Figure 4–7B, fewer lumens fall on it, with a resultant decrease in illumination. The reduction in illumination falling on the surface is proportional to the cosine of angle of tilt of the surface. This cosine law of illumination is

$$E = (I/d^2) \cos \theta$$

or

$$E_2 = E_1 \cos \theta$$

where

$E_1$ = illumination falling on the surface when it is normal to the light source
$E_2$ = illumination falling on the tilted surface

## RETINAL ILLUMINATION

Vision scientists often specify stimuli in terms of retinal illumination. This term takes into account the area of the eye's pupil. This is important because when viewing the same surface, the retinal illumination of an eye with a larger pupil is greater than that of an eye with a smaller pupil. This difference in retinal illumination could affect the state of retinal adaptation.

The basic unit for retinal illumination is a troland, defined as

$$T = LA$$

where

$T$ = retinal illumination in trolands (td)
$L$ = luminance of the surface that is viewed
$A$ = pupil area

Consequently, if the retinal illumination for an experiment is specified as a given number of trolands, all subjects should have the same amount of light falling on their retinas regardless of pupil diameter.

## SCOTOPIC UNITS

Our discussion of photometry, up to this point, has concerned photopic vision. On occasion, however, it is necessary to specify visual stimuli in terms of sco-

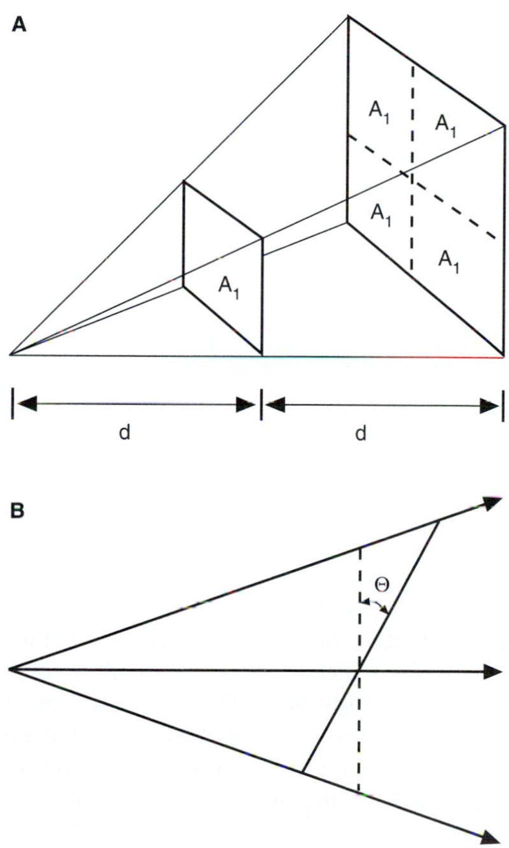


**FIGURE 4–7. A.** The illumination falling on an area $A_1$ decreases by the square of the distance. **B.** The illumination falling on a surface decreases with the cosine of the angle.

topic units. For instance, if a stimulus is to be viewed under very low light level conditions, where only rods are operative, scotopic units are most appropriate.

The basic unit of scotopic photometry is the **scotopic lumen.** A scotopic lumen is a unit of **scotopic photometric power.** By convention, there are 680 scotopic lumens per watt at 555 nm. The number of scotopic lumens per watt for other wavelengths is determined by the scotopic luminosity function, $V'(\lambda)$, which is given in Figure 4–8. For example, at 507 nm, the peak of the scotopic luminosity function, the number of scotopic lumens per watt is determined by a proportionality:

$$\frac{\text{luminous efficiency of 555 nm}}{\text{680 scotopic lumens/W}} = \frac{\text{luminous efficiency of 507 nm}}{X \text{ scotopic lumens/W}}$$

$$\frac{0.4}{680} = \frac{1.0}{X}$$

$$X = 1700 \text{ scotopic lumens/W at 507 nm}$$

For 575 nm, the calculation is

$$\frac{0.4}{680} = \frac{0.2}{X}$$

$$X = 340 \text{ scotopic lumens/W at 575 nm}$$

Scotopic lumens can be confusing. It is important to keep in mind that by definition, there are 680 scotopic lumens per watt at 555 nm, the peak of $V(\lambda)$, rather than at 507 nm, the peak of $V'(\lambda)$.

## DERIVATION OF THE PHOTOPIC LUMINOSITY FUNCTION

In our discussion of the photopic luminosity function, $V(\lambda)$, the assumption has been made that this function is related to brightness. This is true, but it does not convey the complete story.

If the $V'(\lambda)$ function truly represents brightness, it could be determined by a direct brightness matching procedure as illustrated in Figure 4–9. One wavelength, say 555 nm, is chosen as a standard, and all other wavelengths (sample wavelengths) are matched to this standard for brightness. The observer adjusts the radiance of a sample wavelength such that its brightness matches the standard. This is done across the spectrum. Such an experiment is difficult to perform. The reason is obvious when you think of the task. The individual must match for brightness two stimuli of different colors. As it is difficult to ignore color differences, this is not an easy task. Consequently, there is much variability in the matches a person will make and this method has poor reliability (Boynton, 1979; Pokorny et al, 1979).

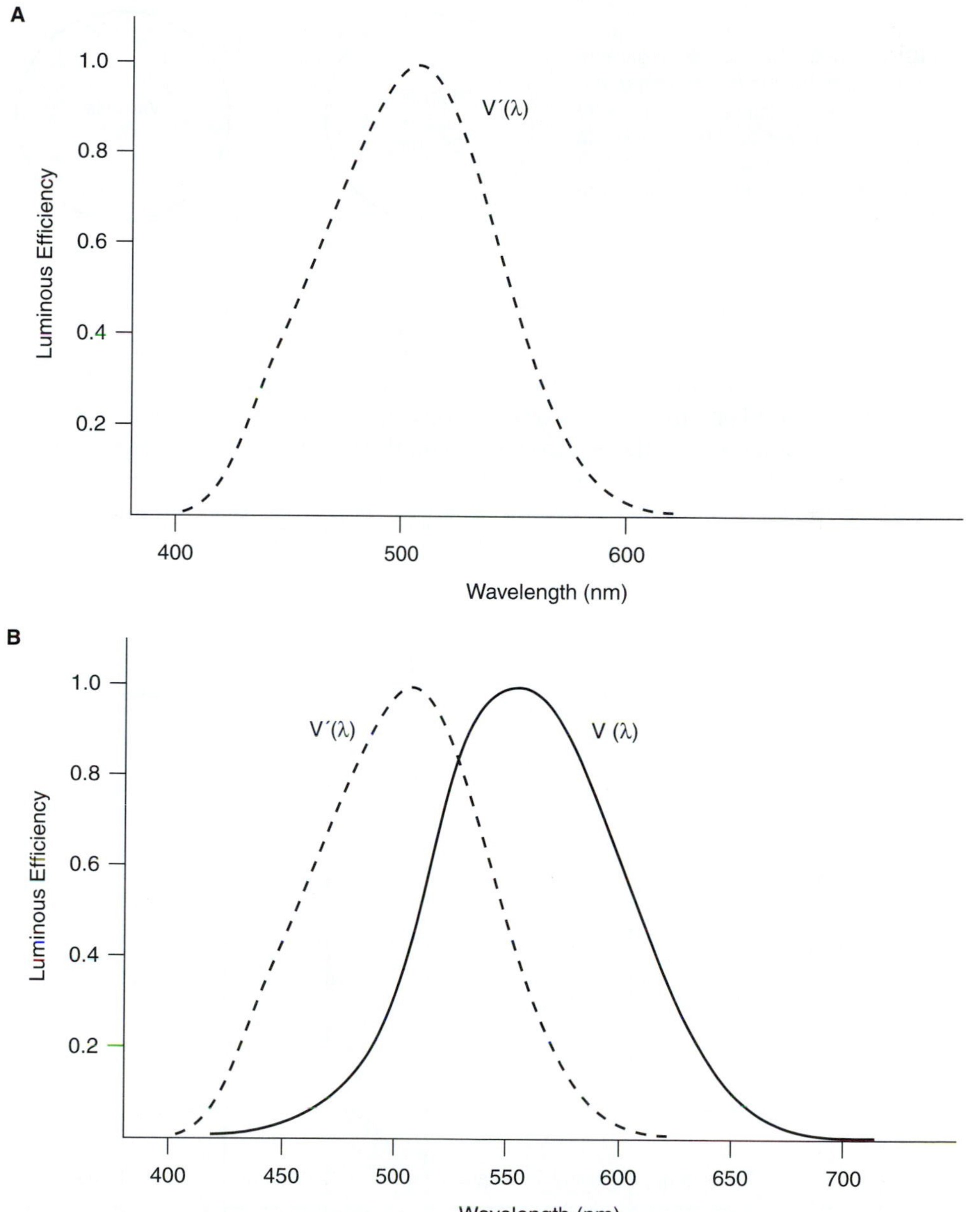


**FIGURE 4–8. A.** Scotopic luminosity function, $V'(\lambda)$. **B.** Both the scotopic $V'(\lambda)$ and photopic $V(\lambda)$ luminosity functions plotted on the same coordinates.

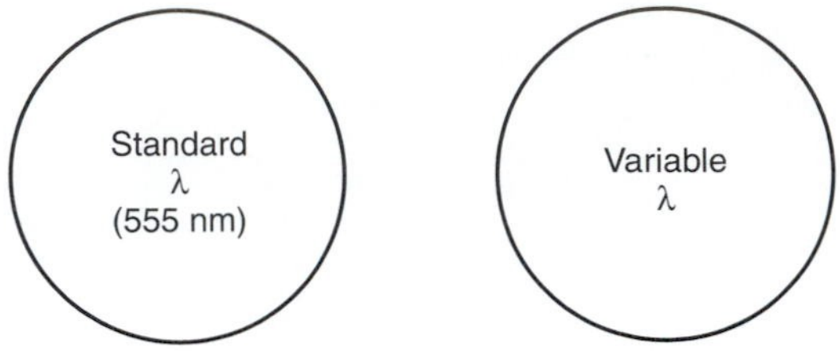


**FIGURE 4–9.** Stimulus arrangement for a direct brightness matching experiment. The observer's task is to adjust the radiance of the sample (variable) wavelength such that it matches the brightness of the standard wavelength.

Other methods of determining the photopic luminosity function that overcome this problem have been developed. Perhaps the most widely known method is that of heterochromatic flicker photometry (HFP) (Wagner and Boynton, 1972). In this method, a standard wavelength stimulus, say 555 nm, is temporally exchanged with the sample wavelength stimulus, for example, 650 nm (Fig. 4–10). The rate of flicker is moderate, about 15 cycles per second. This produces color fusion and only one color is seen. In this case, the 555 nm (green) and 650 nm (red) fuse such that an orange color is perceived.

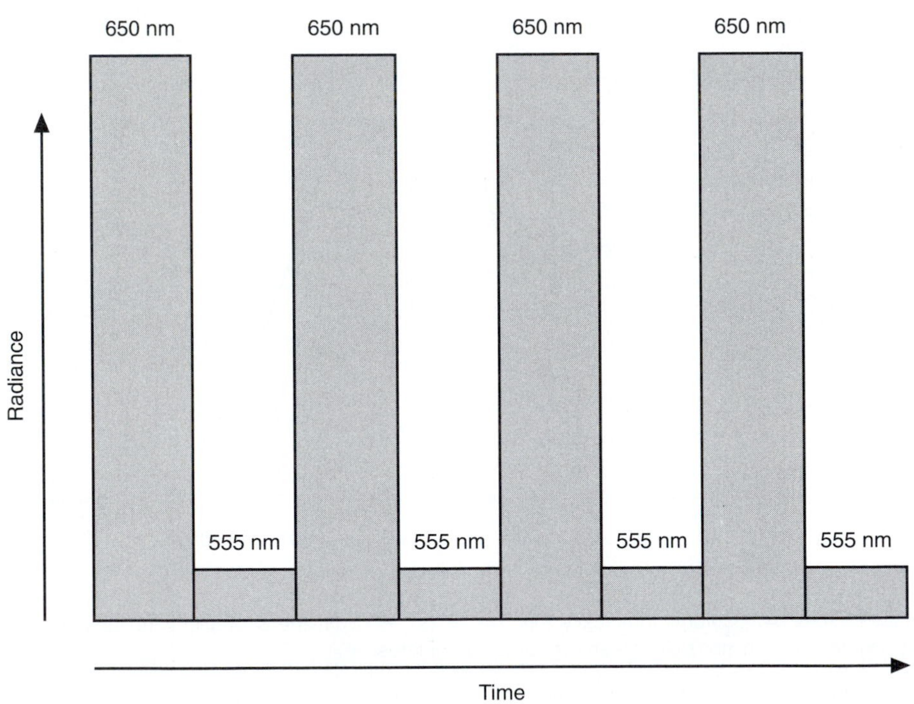


**FIGURE 4–10.** In heterochromatic flicker photometry, two monochromatic stimuli are temporally alternated. The observer's task is to adjust the radiance of one of these stimuli such that the perception of flicker is minimized.

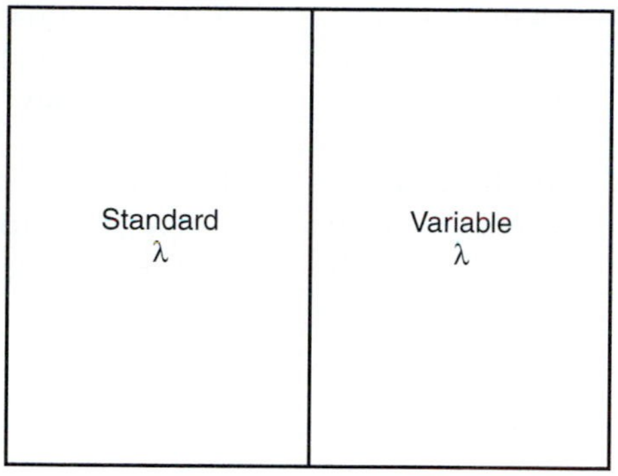


**FIGURE 4–11.** In the minimally distinct border method of determining $V(\lambda)$, the observer adjusts the radiance of the sample (variable) wavelength such that the border made with the standard is minimized.

This orange color, however, is not seen as steady; it is perceived as flickering. The flicker is due to a mismatch in the luminance of the two stimuli. The task in HFP is to adjust the radiance of the sample stimulus such that the flicker is minimized. When this is done, the standard and sample wavelength are at equal luminance. This procedure, when repeated across the spectrum, yields a photopic luminosity function. HFP produces very reliable results.

Another approach to determining $V(\lambda)$ is the minimally distinct border (MDB) method devised by Boynton (1973) and illustrated in Figure 4–11. In this method, the standard wavelength and sample wavelength are placed side by side such that a border is formed where they meet. The observer's task is to adjust the radiance of the sample so that the visibility of the border is minimized. When repeated across the spectrum, a photopic luminosity function is obtained. As with HFP, MDB produces highly reliable results.

The HFP and MDB methods produce very similar results, and these results differ from those obtained using direct brightness matching (Wagner and Boynton, 1972). Importantly, the results of HFP and MDB follow Abney's law of additivity, whereas the results of direct brightness matching do not.

The $V(\lambda)$ curve represents data obtained largely with HFP. This photopic luminosity function was derived from the data of several laboratories and was standardized by the Commission Internationale de L'Eclairage (CIE). As such, the CIE $V(\lambda)$ curve does not represent luminosity for any one individual, but for an ideal standard observer. Without such a standard luminosity function, it would not be possible to have a workable photometric system. It is important to keep in mind that $V(\lambda)$ is closely related to brightness. For the reasons outlined earlier, it is not precisely the same as brightness.

## SPECIFICATION OF LIGHT SOURCES

Modern light sources are divided into two categories: incandescent sources and luminescent sources. Household light bulbs that contain a filament are examples of **incandescent light sources.** By definition, an incandescent source generates light by being heated. In the case of a common light bulb, a voltage differential across a filament causes the filament to become hot and generates light.

A frequently encountered **luminescent light source** is the fluorescent light tube. These tubes are filled with gases whose molecules are energized into an excited state by a voltage differential applied across the tube. The unstable gas molecules release energy when they spontaneously return to their unexcited state. This energy is in the form of low-wavelength ultraviolet radiation. The ultraviolet radiation is absorbed by a phosphor, which coats the inside of the bulb, and emitted as longer-wavelength visible light. This phosphor can be varied to produce the desired spectral emission characteristics.

Figure 4–12 shows the spectral distributions of typical incandescent and fluorescent light sources. Note that the incandescent source shows a relative concentration of energy at long wavelengths. The fluorescent source, in contrast, does not show such a skewing of power toward the long-wavelength region of the spectrum. It does, however, show energy spikes across the spectrum. The spikes produced by *certain* fluorescent light bulbs may render them unsuitable for administering color vision tests.

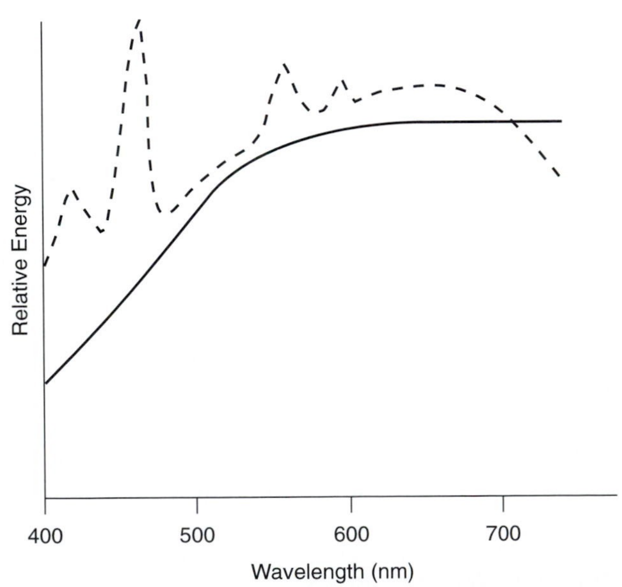


**FIGURE 4–12.** The solid curve represents the spectral distribution of a tungsten (incandescent) light bulb, and the dashed curve, the spectral distribution of a fluorescent light tube. Note the energy spikes in the fluorescent tube's spectral distribution.

### *Blackbody Radiators and Color Temperature*

A blackbody radiator is a theoretical source. It is a perfect radiator of electromagnetic energy. As such, blackbody radiators are ideal sources that do not actually exist. This concept, however, does have practical applications for specifying the spectral distribution of light sources.

Figure 4–13A shows the spectral distribution of a blackbody radiator at three different temperatures. A convenient feature of a blackbody radiator is that its spectral output is totally defined by its temperature. This relationship between spectral output and temperature ($T$) is quantified by Wein's displacement law:

$$\text{Peak Wavelength} \propto 1/T$$

and the Stefan–Boltzman law:

$$\text{Total Power} \propto T^4$$

The application of these laws is seen by observing the effects of temperature on the curves in Figure 4–13A. Wein's displacement law states that as the temperature increases, the peak wavelength decreases. The Stefan–Boltzman law states that the area under the spectral distribution curve, which represents power, increases with the fourth power of the temperature.

When it comes to specifying light sources, that portion of the blackbody radiator's spectral output that is of most interest is in the visible spectrum. This region is indicated by the dashed lines in Figure 4–13A. The three spectral distributions are replotted in Figure 4–13B so that differences in output in the visible region of the spectrum are highlighted. Note that a blackbody radiator with a temperature of 2000 kelvin (K) has most of its power concentrated at longer wavelengths. In comparison, a blackbody radiator with a temperature of 10,000 K has its power concentrated at shorter wavelengths.

Let us see how the concept of blackbody radiators is used to specify the spectral distribution of commonly encountered light sources. Suppose we have a tungsten–halogen light bulb, as is found in an ophthalmoscope, and we wish to specify its spectral output. One approach is to provide a graph of its spectral output. Another approach is to provide the temperature of the blackbody radiator with a spectral output that matches that of the ophthalmoscope bulb. In other words, the spectral output of the bulb is determined and then matched to the spectral output of a blackbody radiator. The temperature in degrees kelvin (K) of the blackbody radiator with an output that most closely matches the bulb is referred to as the **color temperature (CT)** of the bulb.

Commercially available light sources are frequently specified by their color temperature. Even without examining the spectral distribution of a source, much information is obtained from knowledge of its color temperature. For example, although sources of 2000 K and 10,000 K both appear white, they do not match each other in appearance. From reviewing Figure 4–13, it is seen that the 2000 K source will appear yellow-white, whereas the 10,000 K source will

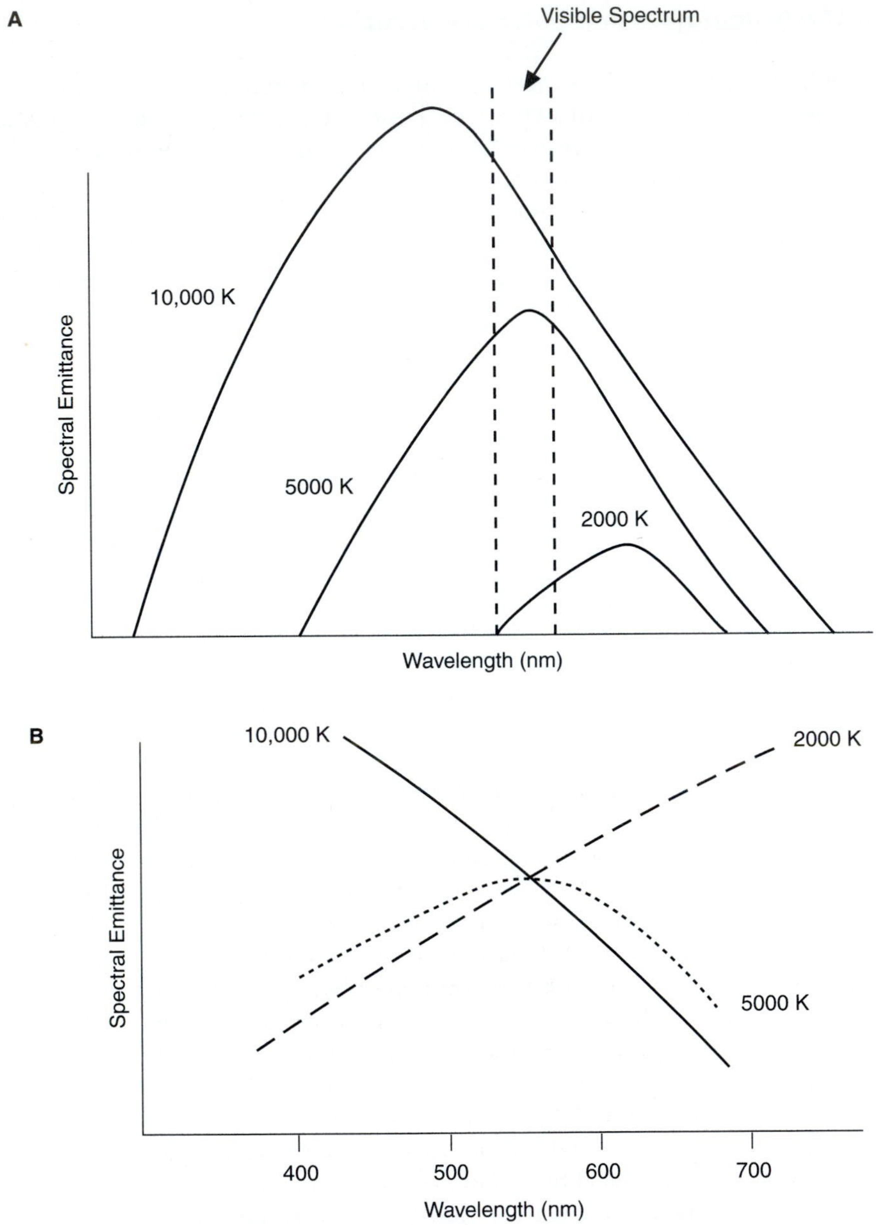


**FIGURE 4–13. A.** Approximate spectral distributions for blackbody radiators with temperatures of 2000 K, 5000 K, and 10,000 K. The dashed lines show the range of the visible spectrum. **B.** Approximate relative spectral distributions, for visible wavelengths, of the sources given in A. These distributions have been normalized to 555 nm.

appear blue-white. This is because the 2000 K source has relatively more energy in the long-wavelength region of the spectrum, whereas the 10,000 K source has relatively more energy in the low-wavelength region.

The term color temperature is only appropriate when specifying incandescent light sources. For the specification of nonincandescent sources, such as fluorescent bulbs, the proper term is **correlated color temperature.** The correlated color temperature of a fluorescent light tube depends on the nature of the phosphor that coats the bulb.

Merchandisers frequently illuminate products with bulbs with color temperatures that show their products to maximum advantage. For instance, a butcher may illuminate beef using a relatively low color temperature to accentuate the fresh, red color of the meat, while a jeweler may choose to illuminate his or her diamond display with a high color temperature to highlight the bluish nature of the diamonds.

### *Standard Illuminants*

Several standard illuminants have been defined by international convention. The spectral distributions of certain standard illuminants are given in Figure 4–14. Standard illuminant A, with a CT of 2854 K, represents an incandescent light bulb. Illuminants B and C represent sources with higher blue contents. Illuminant C is recommended for administering most color vision tests (see Chap. 6).

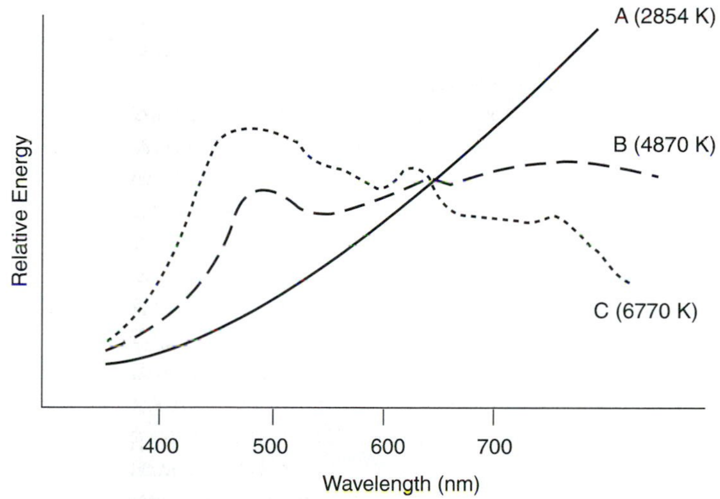


**FIGURE 4–14.** Approximate spectral distributions of standard illuminants A, B, and C, along with their color temperatures.

## *FILTERS*

### *Colored Filters*

A colored filter absorbs some wavelengths that are incident upon it and transmits other wavelengths. The result is that the spectral distribution of the light emerging from the filter is not the same as that incident on the filter.

Figure 4–15A shows a filter that is illuminated by a tungsten bulb. The light incident on the filter will appear white, but the light emerging from the filter will be green. This is because the filter strongly absorbs most wavelengths, except those in the region of 540 nm. These wavelengths are transmitted and give the filter its green appearance.

The filter in Figure 4–15A is an example of a **narrow-band filter;** this filter passes only a narrow spectral band of light. Filters of this type are typically

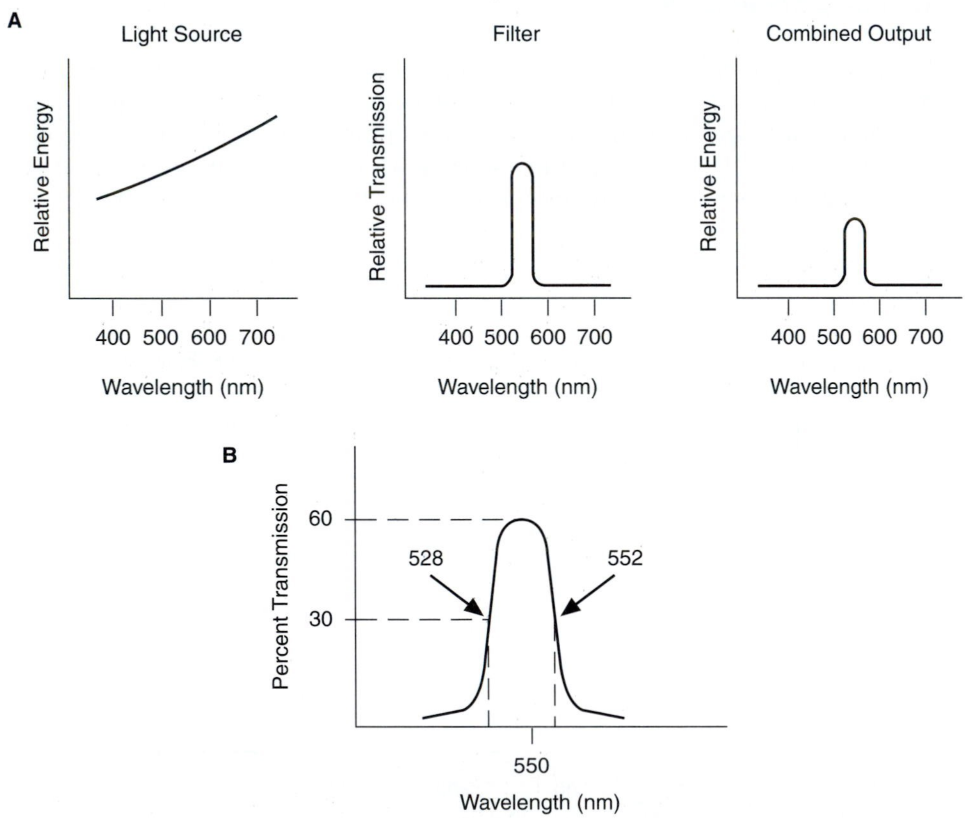


**FIGURE 4–15. A.** A band-pass filter, when illuminated with a tungsten source, transmits a band of light. The filter will appear green because the wavelengths it transmits are centered at 540 nm. **B.** The half-height bandwidth for this filter is 552 nm – 528 nm = 24 nm.

specified by the location of their peak and their half-height bandwidth. As indicated in Figure 4–15B, the half-height bandwidth of a filter represents the spectral range over which the filter transmits 50 percent or more of its peak transmission percentage. The smaller the half-height bandwidth, the more selective is the filter.

**Interference filters** often have very small half-height bandwidths. They are so narrow in their transmission characteristics that, for practical purposes, they can be thought of as transmitting only a single wavelength of light. They are essentially monochromatic. Such filters have important applications in vision research.

**Broad-band filters,** as illustrated in Figure 4–16A, transmit a broad range of wavelengths. Like narrow-band filters, broad-band filters have a band-pass nature. Both transmit a band of wavelengths; however, the width of the band is greater for a broad-band filter.

**Long-pass filters** do not transmit short wavelengths, yet do transmit long wavelengths. An example is provided in Figure 4–16B.

### *Subtractive and Additive Color Mixtures*

Two colored filters, when placed in sequence, produce a subtractive color mixture. An example is given in Figure 4–17. The first filter transmits a broad band of light centered at about 570 nm, whereas the second filter is centered at 470 nm. When placed in sequence, the only light transmitted by the filter combination is that light represented by the overlap of the two transmission curves. In this case, the resultant spectral distribution peaks at about 520 nm.

Note that the filter combination transmits less light than either filter by itself. This is a natural result of the manner in which these filters work; they absorb light. Consequently, this is referred to as a subtractive color mixture. Subtractive color mixtures are commonly encountered. The pigments present in common paints, when mixed together, produce a subtractive mixture.

Subtractive mixtures should be distinguished from additive color mixtures. In an additive color mixture, light from two different sources is added together. For example, if we shine a light through each of the two filters in Figure 4–17 and then combine the output on a screen, we have an additive mixture (Fig. 4–18). The additive mixture contains more light than that emitted by either of the filters. Most projection systems, such as televisions and motion picture projectors, use additive light mixtures.

### *Neutral Density Filters*

A neutral density filter has a flat transmission curve, as illustrated in Figure 4–19A. These filters have the same transmission characteristics for all wavelengths; therefore, they are neutral with respect to wavelength. An advantage of

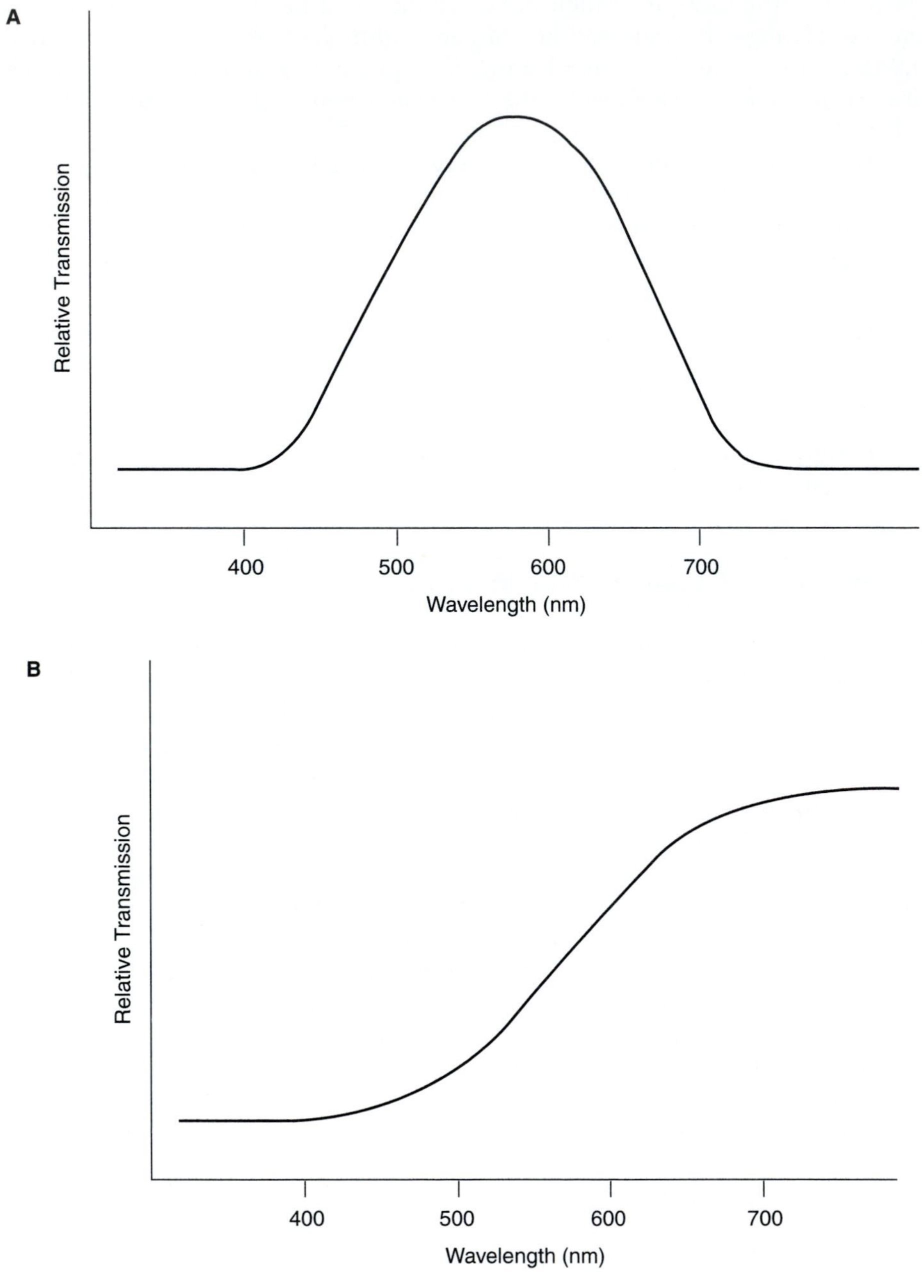


**FIGURE 4–16.** **A.** Broad-band filter. **B.** Long-pass filter.

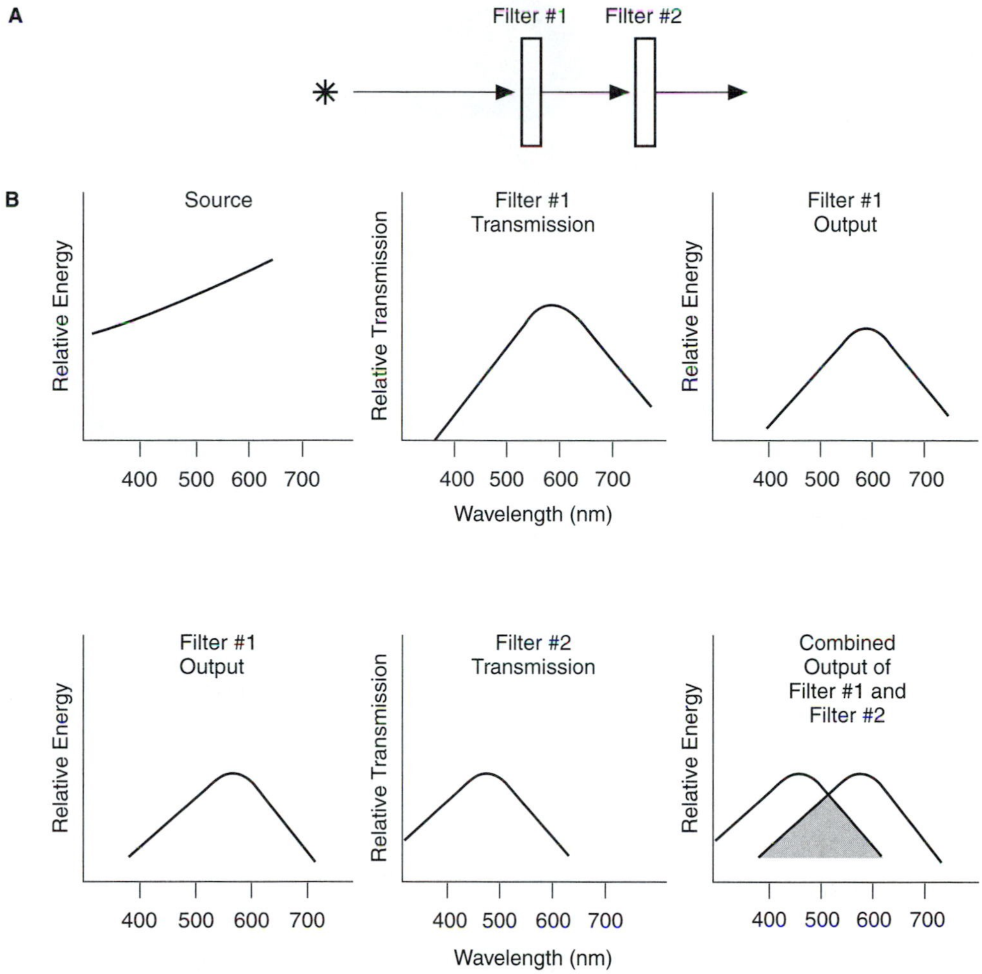


**Figure 4–17. A.** A tungsten source illuminates two band-pass filters in sequence. The first filter shows maximal transmission at 570 nm and the second at 470 nm. **B.** The top row shows the output of the first filter when illuminated with the tungsten source. Because the filter has a peak transmission of 570 nm, the peak output of this filter is at 570 nm. The bottom row shows the output of this same filter incident on the second filter. The second filter has its peak transmission at 470 nm. Only that light common to the two filters is transmitted. This is given by the shaded area of overlap of the two spectral distributions. This is an example of a subtractive color mixture.

neutral density filters is that they minimize color distortion. Filters that are selective in their transmission properties alter the color of a viewed scene. For example, objects viewed through a long-pass filter tend to appear yellowish or red. Neutral density filters, because they transmit all wavelengths equally, do not typically alter the color of objects viewed through them.

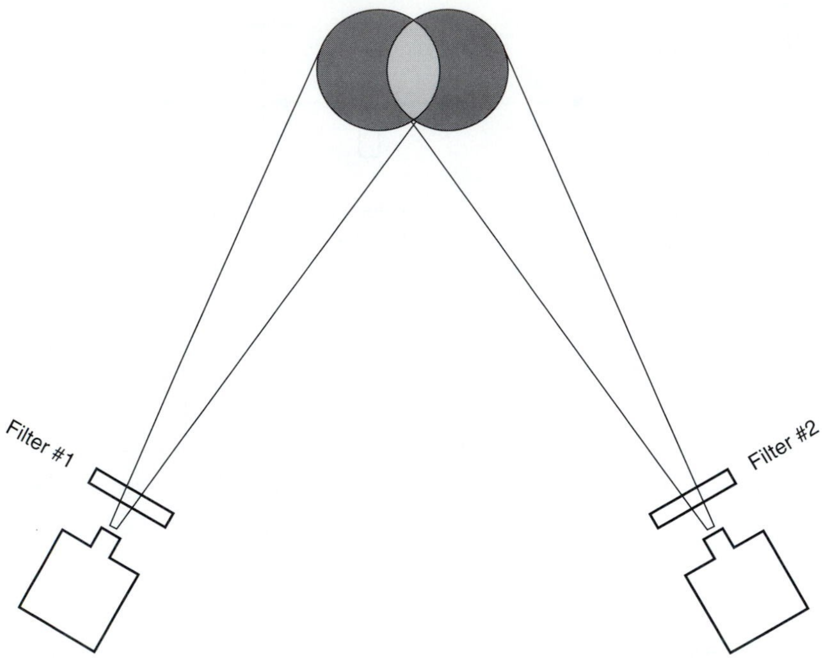


**FIGURE 4–18.** The output of two separate light sources is combined on a screen to produce an additive light mixture.

The density of a neutral density filter is referred to as optical density. Optical density (OD) is expressed in log units as defined by

$$OD = \log(1/T)$$

where $T$ is the fraction transmittance of the filter.

Take an example. A neutral density filter transmits 10 percent of the light incident on it. What is its OD?

$$OD = \log(1/0.10)$$
$$OD = 1$$

The advantage of specifying optical density in log units is that these values are additive. If we place a 1 log filter and a 2 log filter back to back, the combination is a 3 log filter (Fig. 4–19B). Using the formula for OD, we calculate the percentage transmitted by this filter to be 0.1 percent.

## CLINICAL CONSIDERATIONS

The crystalline lens absorbs high-energy ultraviolet (UV) radiation and, thereby, helps protect the retina; however, the absorption of UV radiation by the lens is

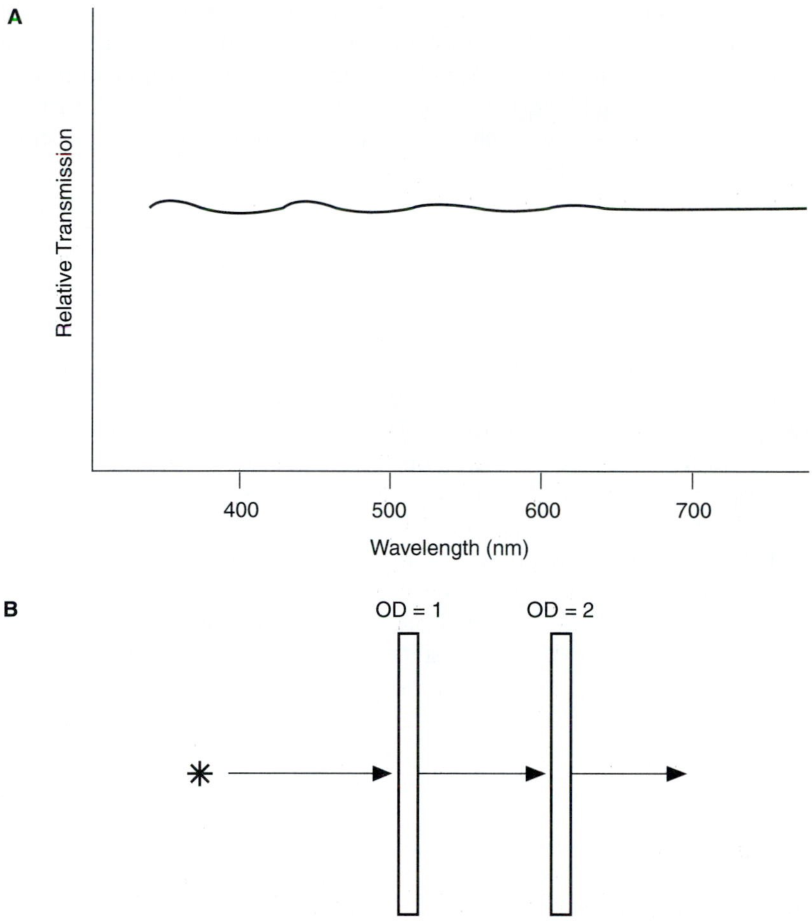


**Figure 4–19. A.** Relatively flat transmission curve of a neutral-density filter. **B.** A combination of neutral density filters with optical densities of 1 and 2 produces an optical density of 3. This combination transmits 0.1 percent of the incident light.

thought to promote cataract formation (Weale, 1983). For this reason, it is common to prescribe spectacles that block UV radiation.

To produce a UV block, an ophthalmic lens is either coated or saturated with a substance that acts as a long-pass filter. This substance should block both UV A and UV B. The result is a clear or slightly yellow lens. The lens appears slightly yellowish if the filter blocks some low-wavelength visible radiation (e.g., blue light). Because they tend to block some blue light, in addition to UV radiation, these spectacles are occasionally referred to as blue-blockers. These spectacles do not substantially block visible radiation; therefore, they are not sunglasses. To provide patient comfort in the form of sunglasses, visible radiation must also be blocked. This is done by the addition of various colored filters. Neutral density filters are especially suitable for this application because they block all wavelengths equally. Consequently, there is little color distortion. Certain color sunglasses (e.g., yellow sunglasses) can interfere with distinguishing red from green traffic signals.

## SUMMARY

Radiometry refers to the power produced by electromagnetic sources. It does not take into account the visibility of these sources. Photometry, in comparison, takes into account the visibility of light sources. This is done through the use of the $V(\lambda)$ photopic luminosity function. This standardized function provides the basis for an additive photometric system.

The spectral distribution of a light source can be given by specifying the source's color temperature or correlated color temperature. The spectral distribution of this source can be altered by projecting it through filters that, in combination with the light source, produce a subtractive light mixture.

The discussion in this chapter represents a basic summary of photometry and radiometry. A more detailed discussion may be found in Wyszecki and Stiles (1982).

# Self-Assessment Questions

1. A light source and filter combination produces 1000 lumens. The filter is monochromatic with peak transmission at 600 nm. How many watts are transmitted by the filter?

2. A source produces 10 W at 500 nm, 5 W at 550 nm, and 20 W at 650 nm. How many lumens are produced?

3. For the data in question 2, give the number of scotopic lumens produced.

4. An illuminance probe is used to measure the illuminance in a classroom. The reading obtained is 70 foot-candles. The probe measures $3 \times 3$ cm. How many lumens are incident on the surface of the probe?

5. A device measures irradiance. You would like to convert this device into an illuminance probe. How do you do this?

6. A point source has an intensity of 100 cd. What illumination does it produce at a distance of 2 ft? Give your answer in both foot-candles and lux (lumens/$m^2$). (Assume there are 10 lux per foot-candle.)

7. A point source of 50 cd is 1 ft from a sheet of paper. Another point source at 3 ft from this same piece of paper illuminates the paper equal to the first source. What is the intensity of this unknown point source?

8. An illuminance meter is tilted 60 degrees from the perpendicular position with respect to a point source of light. The meter reads 100 lux and is 2 ft from the source. What is the intensity of the point source?

9. A neutral density filter absorbs 75 percent of the light incident on it. What is the optical density of the filter?

10. A 0.5 neutral density filter is combined with a 1.0 neutral density filter. **A.** How much light (as a percentage) does the combination transmit? **B.** How much is absorbed?

# Q

**11.** A matte surface with a reflectance factor of 0.7 has a luminance of 50 foot-lamberts. What is the illuminance falling on the surface?

**12.** By use of the inverse square law and an illuminance device, the intensity of a point source is determined to be 25 cd. Assume this uniform point source produces the same amount of light in all directions. How many total lumens does it produce?

**13.** A light source is located 3 ft from a matte surface. The illumination falling onto the surface is 100 lux. The luminance of this surface, at an angle of 30 degrees, is 5 foot-lamberts. What is the reflectance factor of this surface?

# 5

# Color Vision

One of the most striking features of our visual world is the presence of color. As you look out the window or glance around the room, notice the great variety of colors you perceive. This ability to perceive fine gradations in color enormously enhances our visual capabilities.

To gain some appreciation of the significance of color vision for survival purposes, imagine being totally colorblind. Moreover, imagine that you lived many thousands of years ago, perhaps in the jungle or on a prairie. Under these conditions, the lack of sophisticated color discrimination would threaten your survival. It would be difficult to see the tiger stalking you in the tall grass, or the crocodile patiently waiting for you down the trail, or the coral snake sunning itself next to your favorite resting spot. You would find it difficult to distinguish poisonous berries from safe berries. You would find it difficult to see camouflaged parasites hiding on you or your mate.

Color vision has evolved to a very high level in primates because of its survival value. Although it may not be as critical in modern-day civilization as it was in prehistoric times, the ability to distinguish colors immeasurably enriches our visual world.

Color vision has been extensively studied for two centuries. It is an area of vision science where we have made great progress. Importantly, this knowledge can be applied to the diagnosis and treatment of eye disease.

## TRICHROMATIC THEORY

### Historical Considerations

From Chapter 2, we know that color is a wavelength-dependent perception. As we change the wavelength of a stimulus, its color also changes. The question we wish to answer is: what are the physiologic mechanisms that produce this relationship between wavelength and color?

Early investigators postulated that each color was coded by a different type of cone, each with a different spectral sensitivity. The problem with this model is that humans are capable of perceiving thousands of colors. For this model to be true, we would need thousands of different cone types, each coding a different color, at all retinal locations. Given all the other stimulus characteristics that must be encoded and the finite processing capabilities of the retina, this model is not plausible.

Thomas Young, in 1802, proposed an alternative model of color vision. In Young's own words:

> As it is almost impossible to conceive each sensitive point of the retina to contain an infinite number of particles, each capable of vibrating in perfect unison with every possible undulation, it becomes necessary to suppose the number limited; for instance to the three principal colours . . . and that each of the particles is capable of being put in motion more or less forcibly by undulations differing less or more from perfect unison. Each sensitive filament of the nerve may consist of three portions, one for each principal colour (MacAdam, 1970, p. 51).

Although the terminology is dated, Young formulated a theory on which modern color vision science is based. Young postulated that color information is coded by a limited number of cone types, perhaps three. It was thought that the relative activities of these different cone types encoded color. The theory that embodies this and related concepts is referred to as the **trichromatic theory.** Much of the support for the trichromatic theory comes from psychophysical color matching experiments, our next topic.

## *Monochromacy*

The first step in grasping the trichromatic theory is to understand why a person with only one photopigment has no color discrimination. Such a person is referred to as a **monochromat.** Figure 5–1 shows the absorption spectrum for the hypothetical photopigment of such an individual. This absorption spectrum displays the probability of a quantum being absorbed as a function of wavelength. For example, a quantum of $\lambda_b$ has a 50 percent chance of being absorbed, whereas a quantum of $\lambda_a$ has only a 25 percent chance of being absorbed.

Although $\lambda_b$ is more likely to bleach a molecule of this photopigment than $\lambda_a$, the photopigment does not encode which wavelength it absorbed. Once a quantum of light has been absorbed, all information regarding its wavelength is lost. This is referred to as the principle of **univariance.**

Is this individual, who has only one photopigment, able to make wavelength-based discriminations? In other words, if we show this person two patches of light, one patch consisting of $\lambda_a$ and the other of $\lambda_b$, can he or she distinguish between these two patches? This question can be answered by observing Figure 5–2. This figure illustrates two patches of light, $\lambda_a$ and $\lambda_b$, each of which emits 100 quanta of light. Because the probabilities of absorption of

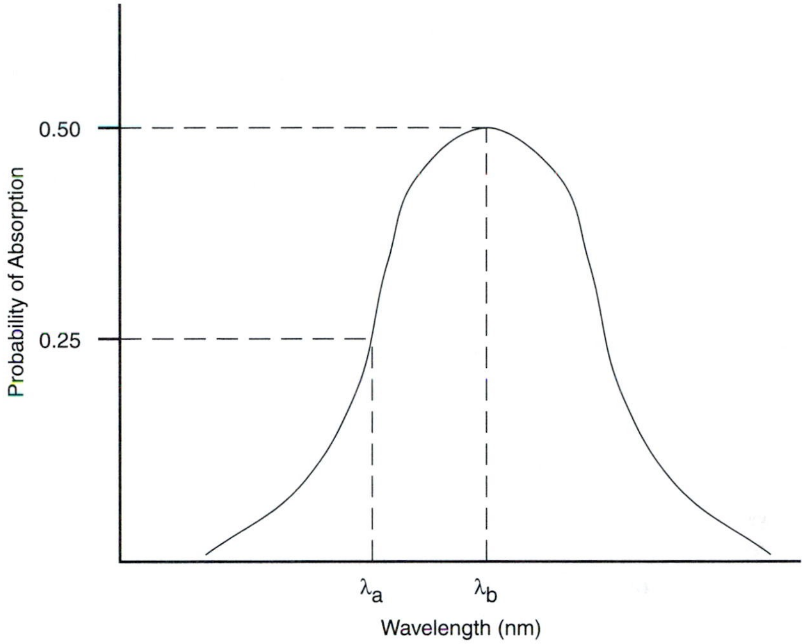


**FIGURE 5–1.** Absorption spectrum for the photopigment of a hypothetical monochromat.

these two wavelengths are different, each patch results in a different number of quantal absorptions. For $\lambda_a$ the probability of absorption is 0.25. Therefore, the patch containing $\lambda_a$ produces 25 absorptions. Likewise, for the patch containing $\lambda_b$, a probability of 0.50 results in 50 quantal absorptions.

Because these two patches of light result in different numbers of quantal absorptions, they look different. They are distinguishable on the basis of a brightness difference. As the patch with $\lambda_b$ produces twice as many quantal absorptions, it appears brighter than the patch containing $\lambda_a$. This may be interpreted by the subject as a color difference, but can be thought of as a brightness difference.

Let us take this a step further. What happens if we were to double the intensity of the patch with $\lambda_a$ such that it now emits 200 quanta. We keep $\lambda_b$ at the same intensity. As shown in Figure 5–2, this results in 50 quantal absorptions for both wavelengths. Because both patches produce the same effect on the visual system, they are indistinguishable. This example shows that a person with one photopigment cannot make wavelength-based discriminations because different wavelengths *can always be made to appear identical by adjusting their intensity*. This is the condition of monochromacy. The individual is totally colorblind; he or she is unable to distinguish objects on the basis of wavelength alone.

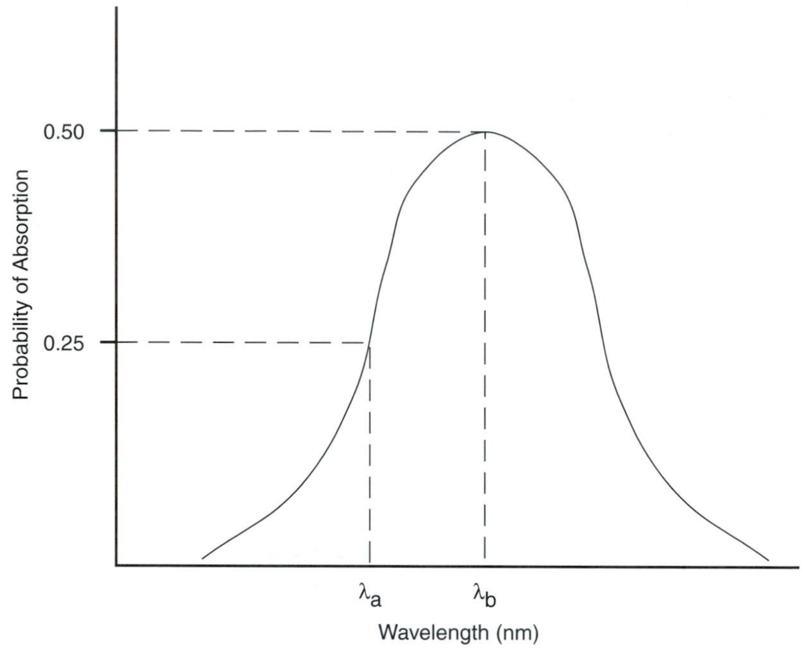


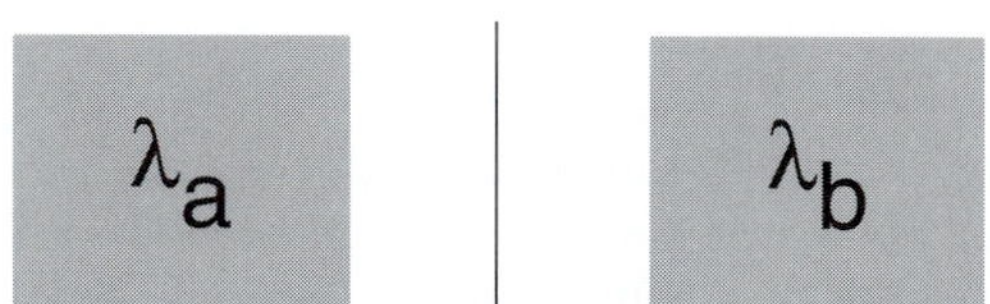


| Number of Quanta Emitted | Number of Quanta Absorbed | Number of Quanta Emitted | Number of Quanta Absorbed |
|---|---|---|---|
| 100 | 25 | 100 | 50 |
| 200 | 50 | 100 | 50 |

**FIGURE 5–2.** These two patches of light will be indistinguishable to this monochromat when each patch produces the same number of quantal absorptions.

Although we know that people with monochromatic vision are unable to make distinctions based on wavelength, they may very well be able to correctly label colors. Although, this may seem to contradict the preceding discussion, it is perfectly consistent with that analysis. Consider the case of a **rod monochromat.** This individual has only rods. As we learned in Chapter 3, the rhodopsin contained in rods peaks at 507 nm. Say that we show this person three patches of light as indicated in Figure 5–3. Each patch emits 5000 quanta of light. The 600-nm patch will appear very dim, the 570-nm patch substantially brighter, and the 505-nm patch the brightest. We tell the subject that one patch is red, one is yellow, and the other is blue-green. If we ask the subject to assign these color labels to the patches of light, he or she is likely to do so correctly.

How does the subject apply these color labels? The subject uses brightness to label colors. All of his or her life, this rod monochromat has noticed that other people label dim objects as red and bright objects as green. Therefore, he

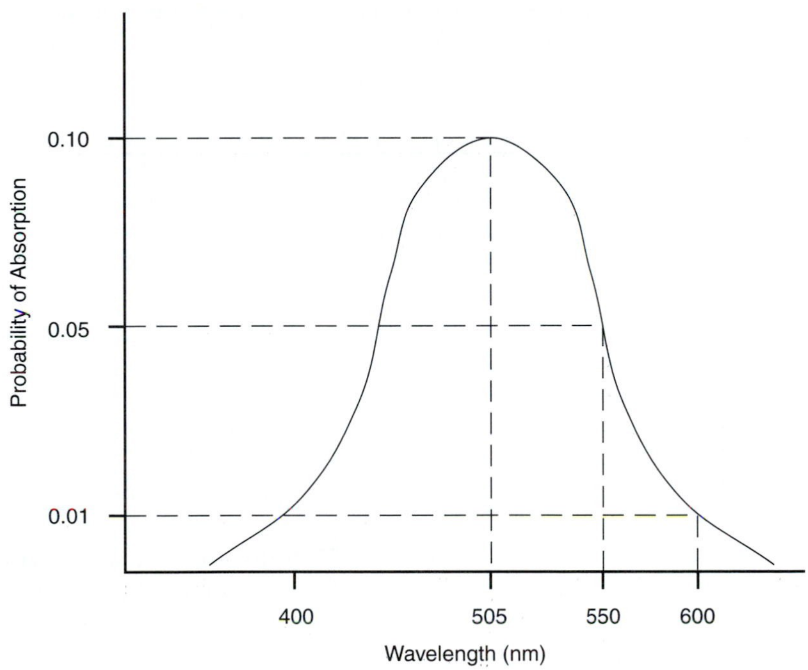


| | 505 nm | 550 nm | 600 nm |
|---|---|---|---|
| Number of Quanta Emitted | 5000 | 5000 | 5000 |
| Number of Quanta Absorbed | 500 | 250 | 50 |

**FIGURE 5–3.** A rod monochromat assigns color labels to these patches of light based on brightness differences.

or she has learned to label colors on the basis of brightness. When confronted with natural objects, such as apples and bananas, the task of color labeling may be made easier by the presence of other cues, such as the shape of the fruit.

Does this subject see or perceive colors? We have no way of answering this question. After all, I cannot even be sure that you and I are perceiving the same color when we observe a red tomato. We do, however, know that monochromats can be fooled if we adjust the intensities of stimuli: they do not have the ability to distinguish stimuli on the basis of the wavelength alone.

### Dichromacy

Consider the photopigment arrangement in Figure 5–4. The individual has two photopigments, M and L, which peak at different wavelengths and which overlap through much of the spectrum. In the following analysis, we will determine if this person is able to make wavelength-based discriminations.

Suppose the person is given two patches of light, one patch consisting of $\lambda_a$ and the other patch of $\lambda_b$. The person is then asked to adjust the intensity of $\lambda_b$ such that the two patches appear identical. If the individual is capable of matching these two wavelengths, he or she does not have the ability to make wavelength-based discriminations. If, however, the person is unable to match these two patches of light, he or she possesses the ability to make discriminations based purely on wavelength.

From a study of Figure 5–4, it is clear that it is not possible to adjust the intensity of $\lambda_b$ such that it will match $\lambda_a$. This is because the number of quanta absorbed by M and L for $\lambda_b$ never equals the number absorbed by these same photopigments for $\lambda_a$. No matter how we adjust the intensity of these two patches of light, they never have identical effects on the visual system. They are distinguishable and, moreover, they are distinguishable solely because they are different wavelengths.

Now consider the situation in Figure 5–5. In this case we again have two patches of light; however, one patch consists of $\lambda_b$ and the other consists of an additive mixture of $\lambda_a$ and $\lambda_c$. The individual is able to control the intensity of each wavelength, independent of the other wavelengths. For example, he or she can adjust the intensity of $\lambda_c$ without affecting the intensity of $\lambda_a$ or $\lambda_b$. Given this situation, will the person be able to adjust the intensities of the various wavelengths such that the patch on the left is identical to that on the right? That is, can the intensity of the various wavelengths be adjusted such that each patch of light results in the same number of quantal absorptions by pigments M and L?

Careful examination of Figure 5–5 shows that it is indeed possible to adjust the intensities such that *each patch has the same effect on the visual system.* (Each patch produces 200 quantal absorptions by photopigment M and 300 by L.) From the person's perspective, these two patches of light, which are physically different, appear identical. Two stimuli that appear identical but are physically different are referred to as **metamers.**

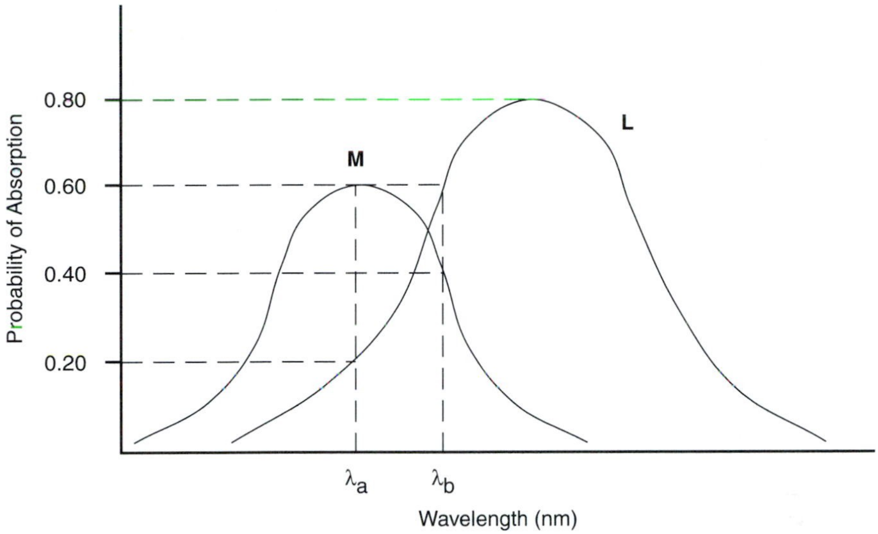

| Number of Quanta Emitted | Number of Quanta Absorbed | | Number of Quanta Emitted | Number of Quanta Absorbed | |
|---|---|---|---|---|---|
| | M | L | | M | L |
| 100 | 60 | 20 | 100 | 40 | 60 |

**FIGURE 5–4.** The two patches, $\lambda_a$ and $\lambda_b$, can be distinguished by this dichromat based on differences in wavelength. The dichromat will not be able to adjust the intensities of the two patches so that they match.

The individual just described is a **dichromat.** A dichromat has some degree of color discrimination, yet it is limited. A patch of $\lambda_a$ always looks different than a patch of $\lambda_b$; however, a patch of $\lambda_b$ may be matched by the proper combination of $\lambda_a$ and $\lambda_c$. To state this more precisely, given three wavelengths, divided into two patches, a person with dichromatic vision is able to adjust the

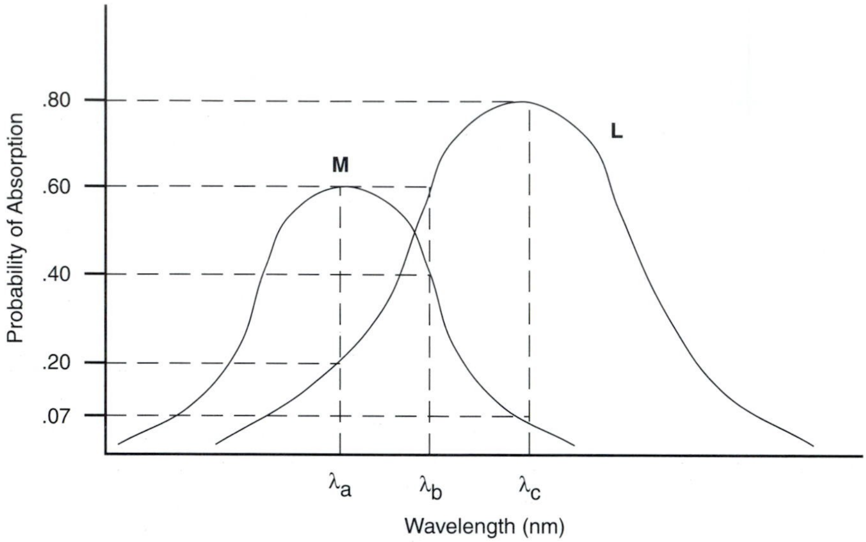


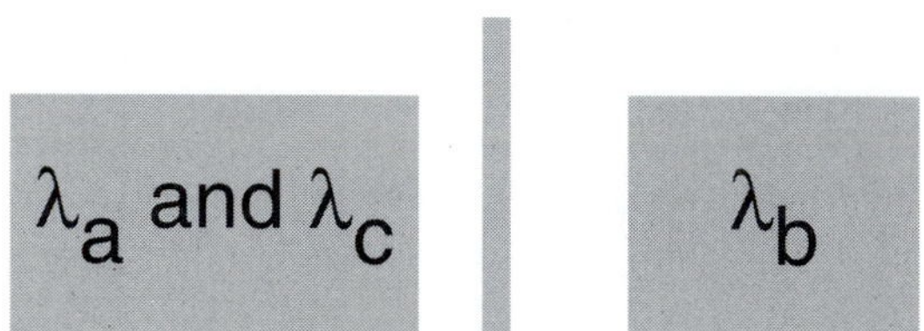


| Number of Quanta Emitted | Wavelength | Number of Quanta Absorbed M | Number of Quanta Absorbed L | Number of Quanta Emitted | Wavelength | Number of Quanta Absorbed M | Number of Quanta Absorbed L |
|---|---|---|---|---|---|---|---|
| 300 | $\lambda_a$ | 180 | 60 | 500 | $\lambda_b$ | 200 | 300 |
| 300 | $\lambda_c$ | 20 | 240 | | | | |
| TOTAL | | 200 | 300 | TOTAL | | 200 | 300 |

**FIGURE 5–5.** By proper adjustment of the intensities of $\lambda_a$, $\lambda_b$, and $\lambda_c$, the two patches will appear identical. This is because they will have the exact same effect on this dichromat's visual system. Each patch produces 200 quantal absorptions by M and 300 by L.

relative intensities of these wavelengths such that the two patches appear identical.

### Trichromacy

The concepts involved in understanding trichromacy are the same as those involved in understanding dichromacy. The only difference is that the person now has three different photopigments with overlapping absorption spectra. This is illustrated in Figure 5–6. We will not perform a detailed analysis of a trichromat's wavelength discrimination abilities. It should, however, be apparent that we can extend those principles developed during our study of dichromacy and apply them to this situation. If we do so, we find that a trichromat shows wavelength discrimination that is superior to that of a dichromat, but is still limited.

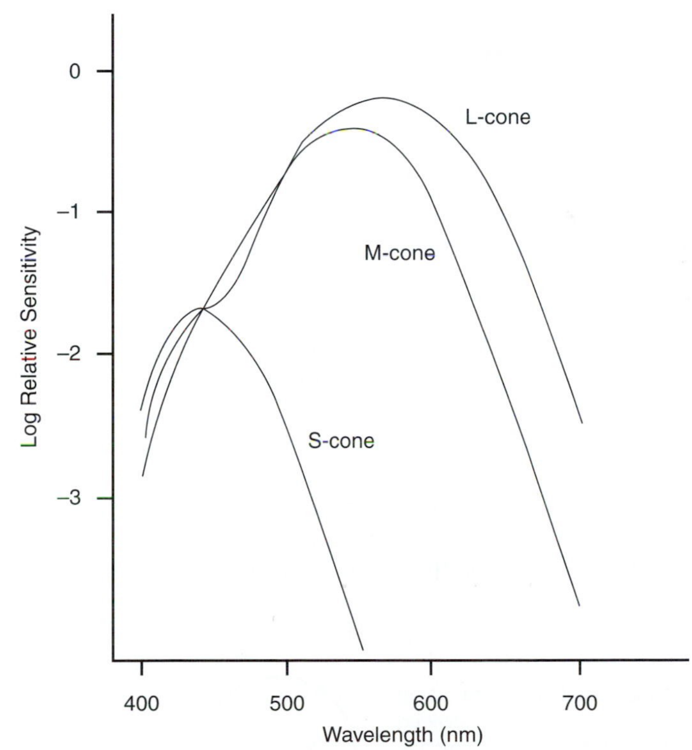


**FIGURE 5–6.** Approximations of the absorption spectra of the three human cones, based on the data of Smith and Pokorny (1975). (*From Boynton RM.* Human Color Vision. *New York: Holt, Rinehart, and Winston; 1979. Reprinted with permission of Dr. Boynton.*)

Let us formally state the definition of trichromacy. Trichromacy is the condition where given four or more wavelengths, divided into two patches, the individual is able to adjust the relative intensities of these wavelengths such that the two patches appear identical. An example is illustrated in Figure 5–7. The two patches appear identical because they result in the same number of quantal absorptions by each of the three photopigments. They are metamers.

A trichromat needs at least four wavelengths to produce a match. Given three wavelengths, as illustrated in Figure 5–5, a trichromat will not be able to create a match. Two patches that appear to be perfectly matched for a dichromat do not appear matched for a trichromat. This demonstrates that trichromats have better color discrimination than dichromats. However, given four wavelengths, the trichromat will be able to make a match, illustrating the limits of trichromacy.

## *Grassman's Laws*

Grassman's laws of metamers describe the general characteristics of trichromatic vision (Fig. 5–8) (Grassman, 1854). These three laws follow from the previous discussion of trichromatic theory.

The **additivity property** states that when the same radiation is added in an identical manner to two metamers, they remain metamers. If they were perfectly matched before we added the new light, they are still matched following this addition.

Let us examine this in more detail. Suppose that we have two identical patches of yellow light. These two yellow patches are metamers. One patch is monochromatic, say 570 nm, and the other patch is a mixture of 530, 560, and 600 nm. If we add an equal amount of 630 nm to each patch, they now both appear orange. They remain metamers because they still appear identical to each other. Think of it in the following manner. The patches were metamers to begin with and then equal amounts of 630 nm were added to each of them. Therefore, the metamerism remains unchanged.

Another of Grassman's laws concerns the **scalar property** of metamers. This law states that if the intensity of two metamers are increased (or decreased) by the same amount, they remain metamers. Consider the two patches of yellow light just discussed. Each patch produces the same number of quantal absorptions in the three cones. If the intensities of the patches are increased by

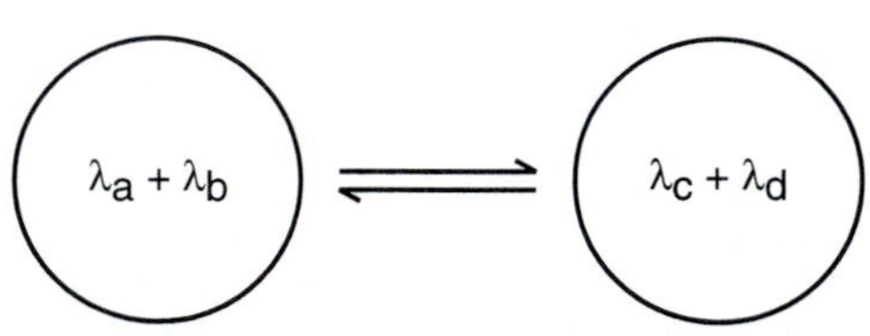


**FIGURE 5–7.** A trichromat is able to adjust the intensities of four wavelengths, divided into two patches, such that the two patches appear identical. These two patches, which are physically different but appear identical, are metamers.

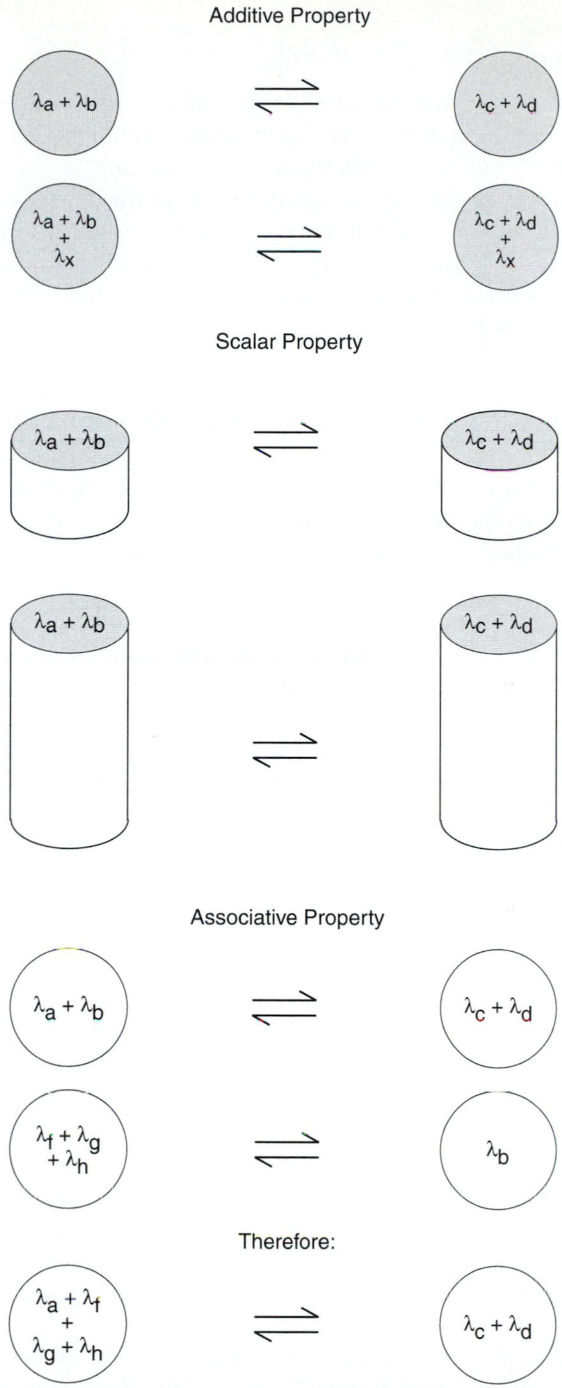


**FIGURE 5–8.** Grassman's laws of metamers. *Additive property:* The patches on the left and right side remain metamers after the addition of equal amounts of $\lambda_x$ to each side. *Scalar property:* If the intensity of each side is increased by the same amount, the metamerism holds. *Associative property:* A metamer may be substituted for $\lambda_b$ and the match will still hold; the metamerism remains unchanged.

the same amount, each patch continues to result in the same numbers of absorptions as the other patch, thereby maintaining the metamerism. The patches will appear brighter, but remain identical to one another.

Grassman's law regarding the **associative property** of metamers states that a match will be maintained if one metamer is substituted for another metamer. This makes sense when we consider that each metamer, by definition, has exactly the same effect on the visual system. Therefore, we are at liberty to substitute one metamer for another.

## *ABSORPTION SPECTRA OF THE CONE PHOTOPIGMENTS*

The basic tenets of the trichromatic theory are well established. The absorption spectra of cone spectra have been determined with a number of different experimental approaches, which are introduced in the following sections.

### *Psychophysical Color Matching Experiments*

Color matching experiments are performed in a manner very similar to the color matching examples discussed earlier in this chapter. These experiments, using observers with trichromatic and dichromatic vision, have provided scientists with excellent information regarding the cone spectra (Boynton, 1979).

### *Retinal Densitometry*

Retinal densitometry is an ingenious technique devised by W. H. Rushton in the 1960s (Rushton, 1963a, 1963b, 1965b, 1975). Others have provided lucid descriptions of this technique (Cornsweet, 1970); therefore, we discuss it only in general terms.

In retinal densitometry, a very dim measuring light is directed onto the retina. This light is reflected back from the retina and the amount of reflected light is measured. The amount of reflected light is less than the amount of incident light because of retinal absorption. If this procedure is repeated across the spectrum, it is possible to obtain absorption spectra for the retinal photoreceptors. At each wavelength, the amount of light incident on the retina is compared with the amount reflected back and, thereby, an absorption spectrum is obtained.

This procedure has been used to determine the absorption spectra for the human M and L-cone photopigments. To obtain these spectra, it is necessary to examine retinal areas that have only one cone. This is done by performing the procedure in the fovea of a red–green dichromat. (Red–green dichromats, as discussed in Chapter 6, are missing either the M or L-cone photopigment.) As the fovea does not have S-cones, the fovea of these red–green dichromats has only one cone photopigment. Retinal densitometry allows us to determine the absorption spectrum of this remaining photopigment.

Although useful, retinal densitometry is not sensitive enough to fully elucidate the cone absorption spectra. It is not sufficiently sensitive to allow determination of the photopigment absorption characteristics in the tails of the curves. As vision scientists are fond of saying, "retinal densitometry fails in the tails." This is an important consideration because the tails of the photopigment spectra are critical for predicting color matching data.

### Microspectrophotometry

Microspectrophotometry is a theoretically straightforward, yet technically difficult procedure (Liebman, 1972; Bowmaker et al, 1978). Retinal tissue (monkey or human) is back-illuminated with monochromatic light. The light beam is directed toward a single cone (Fig. 5–9). The difference between the amount of light incident on the cone and the amount of light transmitted through the cone is determined. This is repeated across the spectrum to obtain a cone absorption spectrum.

### Electrophysiologic Recordings

In the late 1980s, scientists first recorded membrane currents from the outer segments of macaque monkey and human photoreceptors (Schnapf and Baylor, 1987; Schnapf et al, 1987). These procedures are performed using an eyecup preparation. This involves removing the retina from the animal eye, or donated human eye, and bathing it in an enriched saline solution to maintain tissue viability. A cone is isolated and the retina is exposed to monochromatic light (Fig. 5–10). The amount of energy required to elicit a criterion response is determined as a function of wavelength. The reciprocal of this threshold function is the spectral sensitivity of the cone. The cone spectra obtained using this procedure are very similar to those derived through psychophysical matching experiments. These direct measurements confirm what color scientists have hypothesized for quite some time.

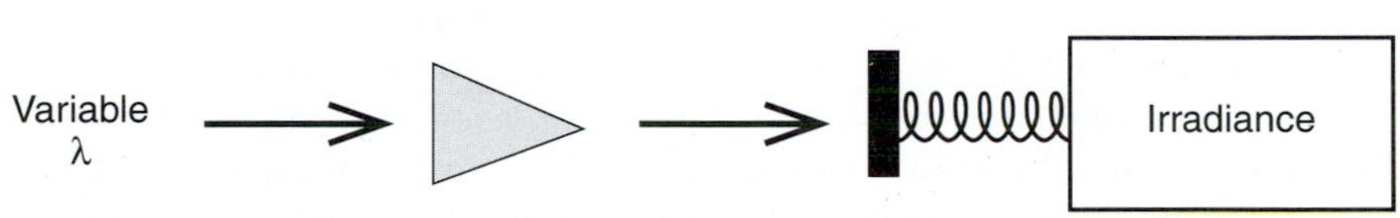


**FIGURE 5–9.** In microspectrophotometry, the amount of light transmitted by a cone is determined as a function of wavelength. This allows determination of the absorption spectrum of the cone.

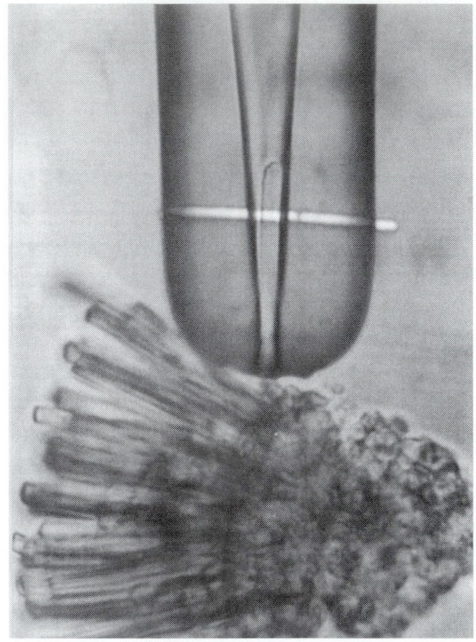

**FIGURE 5–10.** A single photoreceptor is isolated within a micropipette and exposed to monochromatic light. In this manner, the spectral sensitivity for a photoreceptor can be determined. This photograph shows the isolation of a rod, but the same principles apply to cones. (*From Schnapf JL, Baylor DA. How photoreceptors respond to light.* Sci Am. *1987;256:40–47. Reprinted with permission of authors.*)

A commonly accepted set of cone spectra are given in Figure 5–6. These curves are based on data from a number of experimental approaches.

## *THE MOLECULAR GENETICS OF CONE PHOTOPIGMENTS*

Each molecule of cone photopigment consists of the **chromophore** and an **opsin.** The chromophore, which is identical for all cone photopigments, is retinal, an aldehyde derivative of retinol (vitamin A). Light quanta are absorbed by the chromophore, initiating the series of events leading to vision (see Chap. 12). It is the opsin, a visually inert chain of amino acids that is interlaced into the disk membranes of the outer segment, that determines the absorption characteristics of the photopigment molecule. Each class of cones has a different opsin.

The genes that code for the opsins of the human photopigments have been identified and isolated with recombinant DNA techniques (Nathans et al, 1986b). The genes for the photopigments of the M and L-cones are situated on the X chromosome. This is not surprising because it has long been known that certain color vision deficiencies in which either the M or L-cone photopigment is missing or altered (i.e., red-green color anomalies) are inherited in a sex-linked manner (see Chap. 6). The gene for the S-cone photopigment is located on chromosome 7, and the gene coding rhodopsin is found on chromosome 3.

The genes for the cone photopigments are homologous to the rhodopsin gene, suggesting that all four genes evolved from the same ancestor (Fig. 5–11)

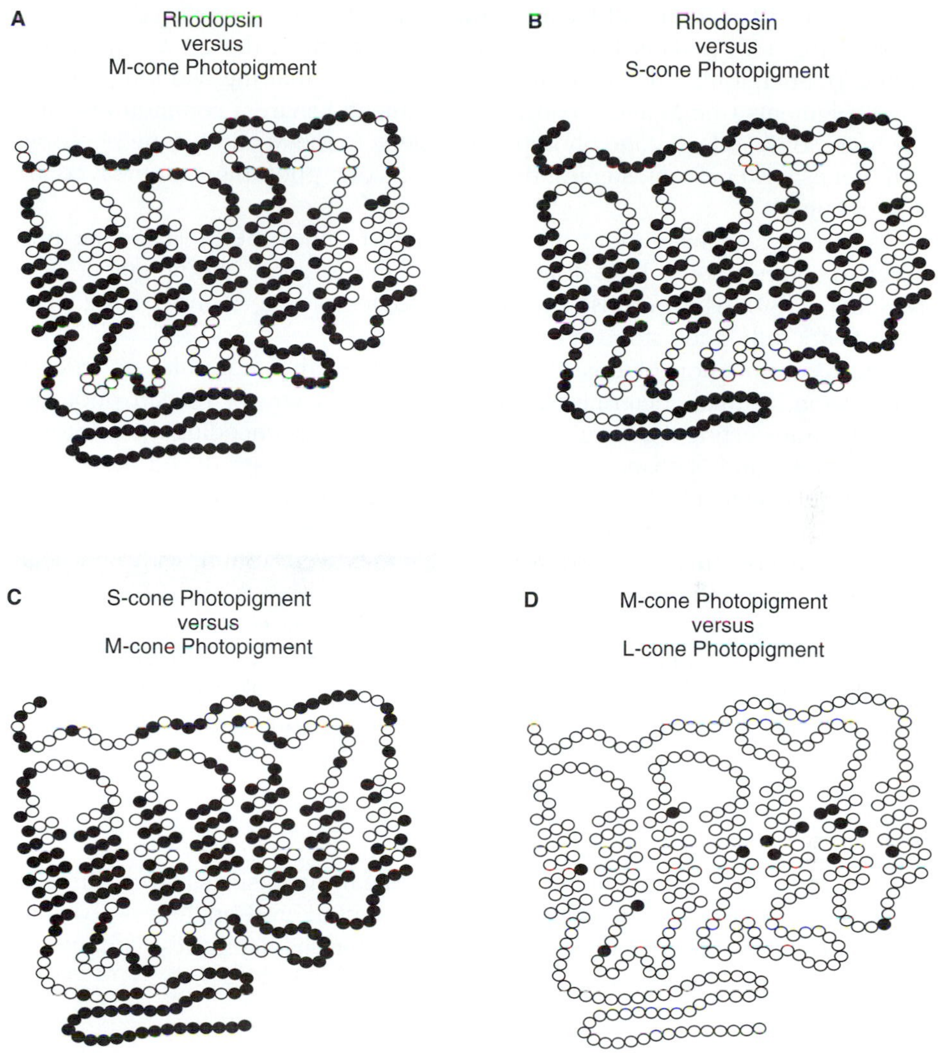


**FIGURE 5–11.** Comparison of amino acid sequences (deduced from nucleotide sequences) for **(A)** rhodopsin versus M-cone photopigment, **(B)** rhodopsin versus S-cone photopigment, **(C)** S-cone photopigment versus M-cone photopigment, and **(D)** M-cone photopigment versus L-cone photopigment. The open circles represent amino acids that are the same in both photopigments, and the solid circles represent amino acids that are different. (*Adapted from Nathans J et al. Molecular genetics of human color vision: The genes encoding blue, green, and red pigments.* Science. *1986; 232:193–202.*)

(Nathans, 1989). The M and L-cone photopigment genes are exceedingly similar, showing a 98 percent homology (i.e., 98 percent of the DNA sequence is identical). Such a high degree of homology suggests that the two longer wavelength pigments (the M and L-cone photopigments) share a common ancestor. The homology of the S-cone photopigment gene to the M and L-cone photopigment genes is 40 percent, suggesting that the S-cone photopigment evolved at a different time.

A person can have more than one copy of either the M or L-cone photopigment gene. Some have four copies of the M-cone photopigment gene (Nathans, 1989). The purpose of multiple copies of the M and L-cone opsin genes is not fully understood at this time.

In a continuation of this pioneering work on the molecular genetics of color vision, Nathans determined the absorption spectra of human photopigments by transfecting tissue culture cells with the genes encoding the photopigments (Merbs and Nathans, 1992). The transfected cells produced the various human photopigments, and the absorption spectra of these pigments were then determined. The S and M-cone photopigments peaked at 426 and 530 nm, respectively. Two variants of L-cone photopigments were found, with one peaking at 552 nm and the other at 557 nm.

The finding of two L-cone photopigments was not surprising. It has been suspected for some time that people with normal color vision do not all show the same color matching data (Neitz and Jacobs, 1986). This is apparently because some people possess a different L-cone photopigment than others.

## COLOR LABELS

Color is typically specified along three perceptual dimensions. These three dimensions, or color characteristics, are hue, saturation, and brightness. To some degree, it is possible to change one of these color characteristics without substantially altering the other two.

### *Hue*

Hue is that perception most closely associated with wavelength. A stimulus of 540 nm has a hue of green, whereas a stimulus of 570 nm has a hue of yellow. Although it is common to use the terms color and hue interchangeably, color is a much broader term that includes hue, saturation, and brightness.

### *Saturation and Desaturation*

A desaturated color appears as though it has been mixed with white. It does not seem full-bodied in its color appearance. Pastels are examples of desaturated colors. A saturated color is just the opposite. Saturated colors appear to be full of color. They do not appear washed out as do desaturated colors.

Saturation is wavelength dependent. For example, 570 nm appears less saturated than other wavelengths (Priest and Brickwedde, 1938; Kaiser et al, 1976). Keep in mind that we are referring to stimuli that have no actual white content; they are spectral hues. Nonetheless, it appears that 570 nm has white added to it, whereas other wavelengths appear more pure.

A physical attribute that is related to saturation (a perceptual attribute) is **colorimetric purity** (Pokorny et al, 1979). Colorimetric purity, *p,* is defined by the formula

$$p = \frac{L_\lambda}{L_\lambda + L_w}$$

where

$L_\lambda$ = luminance of the test wavelength
$L_w$ = luminance of the white light that is combined with the test wavelength

This relationship quantifies the amount of white that has been added to a wavelength and, therefore, gives us information regarding the saturation of the sample. If the sample is a pure spectral hue, with no white added, it has a colorimetric purity of 1.

It was previously stated that 570 nm is the least saturated spectral hue. We can quantify this by performing the experiment illustrated in Figure 5–12. A white patch is compared with an adjacent, initially white patch to which a variable amount of a wavelength is added. The participant's task is to add the least amount of the wavelength such that this adjacent patch now appears different than the white patch. The results of the experiment are typically plotted as $\log[(L_\lambda + L_w)/L_\lambda]$ as a function of wavelength (Fig. 5–12). This graph shows that to make a white patch appear colored, you need more 570 nm than, for example, 440 or 620 nm. This is consistent with 570 nm appearing less saturated (more similar to white) than other wavelengths.

### *Brightness*

As we learned in Chapters 3 and 4, brightness varies with wavelength (Wagner and Boynton, 1972). Under photopic conditions, a 555-nm stimulus is perceived as brighter than other equal energy monochromatic stimuli. Brightness sensation closely follows the photopic luminance function which, presumably, is the result of the addition of M and L-cone inputs.

It is common to interchange the terms brightness and luminance; however, these terms have different definitions and should not be used interchangeably. Brightness, as we might expect, refers to the sensation of brightness. Luminance, on the other hand, is a photometric term defined by the $V(\lambda)$ curve dis-

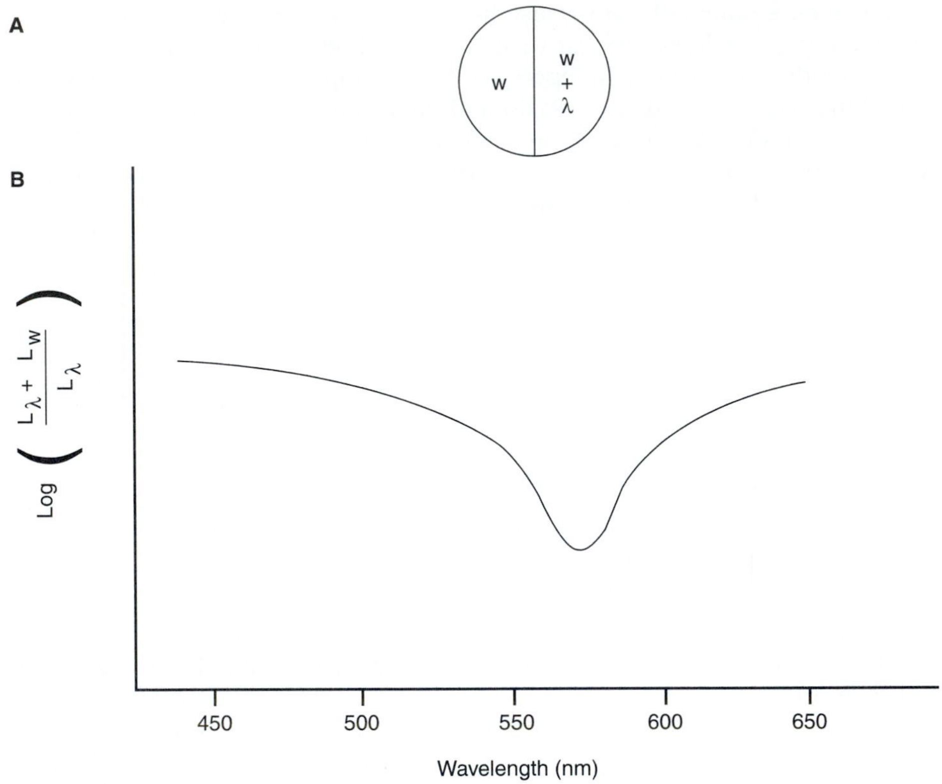


**FIGURE 5–12.** Log colorimetric purity thresholds for distinguishing a stimulus from white, as a function of wavelength. The diagram (top) schematically shows the stimulus conditions used to obtain the graph (bottom). This can be thought of as showing saturation as a function of wavelength. The curve given is an approximation. (*Adapted from Wright WD.* Researches on Normal and Defective Color Vision. *London: Henry Kimpton; 1946.*)

cussed in Chapter 4. The $V(\lambda)$ curve closely matches the sensation of brightness, but is not precisely the same function (Wagner and Boynton, 1972).

## *WAVELENGTH DISCRIMINATION*

The ability to distinguish wavelengths varies as we go across the spectrum (Wright, 1941; Pokorny and Smith, 1970). This can be demonstrated by performing the experiment depicted in Figure 5–13A, which shows a bipartite field (split field). On the left side of the field is the test wavelength $\lambda_t$. On the right side we start with the test wavelength, and we then change this wavelength by an amount $\Delta\lambda$ such that the two sides of the bipartite field no longer match in

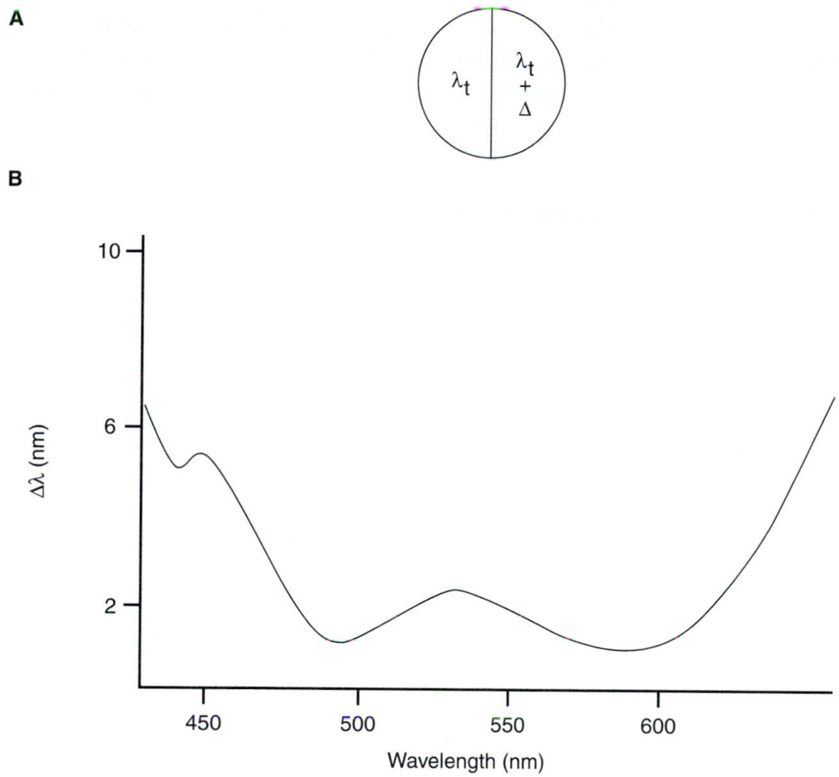


**Figure 5–13.** Wavelength discrimination (Δλ) is plotted as a function of wavelength. The upper figure **(A)** shows the stimulus conditions used to obtain the bottom graph. **B.** This graph is an approximation. (*Adapted from Pokorny J, Smith VC. Wavelength discrimination in the presence of chromatic fields.* J Opt Soc Am. *1970;60:562–569.)*

hue. In essence, we are determining how much a stimulus' wavelength must be changed so that it appears to be a different hue. (In an experiment of this nature, adjustments are made such that both sides of the bipartite field remain the same luminance. Therefore, only hue is varied as the wavelength is changed.)

The results of such an experiment, for a trichromat, are given in Figure 5–13B. This curve is often referred to as the "W curve" of color discrimination because of its W-like shape. In the regions of best discrimination—at about 495 and 590 nm—two stimuli will appear as different hues if their wavelengths are just a few nanometers different. This means that a stimulus of 490 nm will be distinguishable from one of 495 nm. However, a stimulus of 415 nm will appear the same hue as a stimulus of 410 nm because hue discrimination is relatively poor in this region of the spectrum.

Wavelength discrimination is, to some extent, predictable based on the relationship between the three cone photopigment spectral sensitivity curves (Fig. 5–6). In those areas of the spectrum where the slopes of the overlapping curves change most rapidly with respect to each other, color discrimination is best.

## BEZOLD–BRÜCKE PHENOMENON

We have previously stated that hue and brightness are, more or less, independent of each other. The qualification, more or less, is necessary because most wavelengths show a slight change in hue as the stimulus intensity is increased. This is referred to as the Bezold–Brücke phenomenon.

To demonstrate this phenomenon, an observer is presented with a bipartite field (Fig. 5–14). On the left side is the test wavelength, $\lambda_t$. The right side ($\lambda_v$) is initially identical to $\lambda_t$. During the experiment, the intensity of $\lambda_t$ is increased. The hue of the left side may change as its intensity increases. If this happens, its wavelength is adjusted so that it continues to match the hue of $\lambda_v$.

Consider the example of a greenish-yellow test wavelength of 550 nm. As the intensity of this wavelength is increased, it appears to be of a longer wavelength (i.e., it appears more yellowish). To maintain the initial hue appearance (greenish-yellow), it is necessary to reduce its wavelength. This is indicated in Figure 5–14 by the line that starts at 550 nm and tilts toward shorter wavelengths as the intensity increases. All stimuli that fall on this line, referred to as a **hue contour line,** have the same hue (greenish-yellow).

Figure 5–14 displays hue contour lines for a number of different stimuli. Note that most of the lines are tilted. This is because as the intensity of most monochromatic stimuli is increased (or decreased), the hue changes and, consequently, the wavelength must be changed to maintain a constant hue.

Curiously, three wavelengths remain a constant hue as intensity is increased (Hurvich, 1981). This is indicated by nontilted hue contour lines (Fig. 5–14). These wavelengths—478, 503, and 578 nm—are referred to as **invariant wavelengths,** or **invariant points.** The hues associated with these wavelengths—(blue at 478 nm, green at 503 nm, and yellow at 578 nm)—are called **unique hues.** These hues look pure. They do not appear to be mixed with another wavelength.

A simple rule will assist you in remembering the Bezold–Brücke phenomenon. Stimuli with a wavelength that is shorter than unique blue (i.e., the blues and violets below 478 nm) appear more blue as the intensity is increased, and stimuli longer than 478 nm appear more yellow as the intensity is increased. It is important to relate this rule to Figure 5–14. For example, a stimulus of 450 nm (initially violet) becomes more blue as we increase its intensity. To maintain its original violet hue, we need to decrease its wavelength. Therefore, the hue contour line tilts to the left. A stimulus of 585 nm (yellow-orange) will appear more yellow as its intensity is increased, requiring its wavelength to

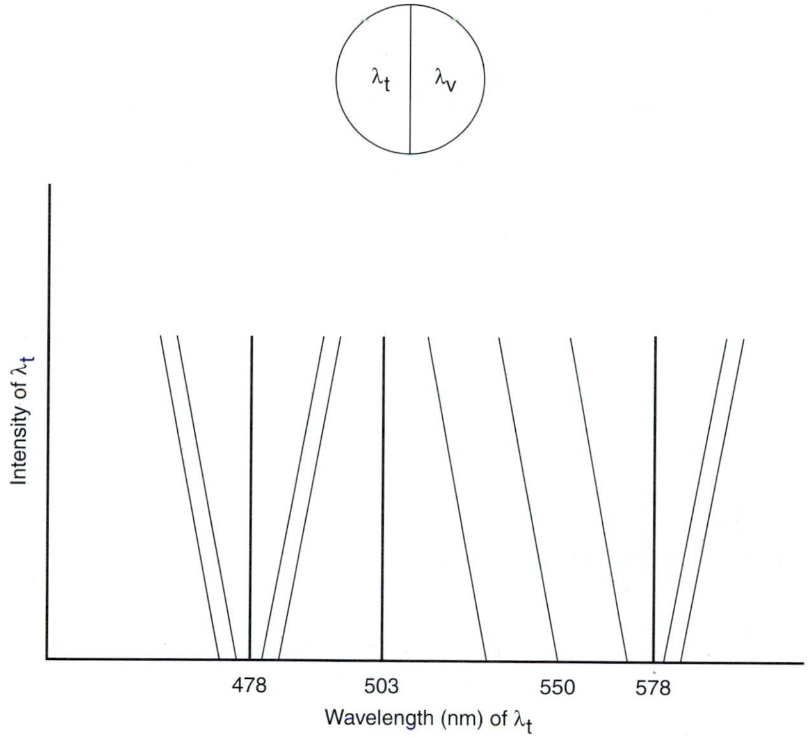


**FIGURE 5–14.** (Top) A bipartite field similar to that used to measure the Bezold-Brücke phenomenon. $\lambda_t$ and $\lambda_v$ initially have the same wavelength and equal intensity. As the intensity of $\lambda_t$ is increased, its wavelength is adjusted to maintain a hue match with $\lambda_v$. (Bottom) Approximate results of such an experiment. Along each line, hue remains constant. These lines are referred to as hue contour lines. At the three invariant wavelengths (478, 503, and 578 nm), hue does not change as intensity is increased. This graph is an approximation. (*Bottom figure adapted from Hurvich LM.* Color Vision. *Sunderland, MA: Sinauer Associates; 1981.*)

be increased to maintain the original hue. A possible physiologic basis for this phenomenon is provided by opponent color theory, which is discussed later in this chapter. (Also, see discussion question 7 in this chapter.)

## COLOR CONSTANCY

Consider a shirt with a colorful pattern. This shirt appears to consist of approximately the same colors almost regardless of the lighting conditions under which it is viewed. Whether viewed indoors under incandescent light or outdoors in natural sunlight, the shirt's colors appear almost the same. Even when viewed under a blue light, the shirt's appearance is surprisingly similar to its appearance under more natural conditions. This is an interesting phenomenon when one considers that the wavelengths reflected off the shirt are considerably different under the various lighting conditions. Color constancy refers to the approximately constant color appearance of objects as lighting conditions change (Land, 1964).

Color constancy assists us in identifying objects as lighting conditions vary. The world would be rather confusing if the color properties of objects changed dramatically as the lighting conditions varied. It is advantageous that an apricot appears approximately the same color both indoors and outdoors, and at various times of the day. The physiologic basis for color constancy has not been fully elucidated, but may be dependent on cortical processing (Zeki, 1993).

Color constancy is not absolute. As lighting conditions change, there are subtle, but important, changes in color appearance. When viewing a natural landscape, for instance, lighting conditions provide a cue that allows us to gauge the time of day (Zaidi, 1997).

## OPPONENT COLOR THEORY

### Early Formulations

Toward the end of the 19th century a German physiologist, Ewald Hering, made some astute observations regarding the perception of colors (Hering, 1920/1964). Hering noted that the colors red and green are never seen simultaneously, and the color label red–green is never used. Colors are either red or green, but not both. The same holds true for blue and yellow. These two hues are never seen in the same location and we do not use the color label blue–yellow. He also observed that a chromatic stimulus elicits an afterimage of a complementary color. A red stimulus elicits a green afterimage and a blue stimulus elicits a yellow afterimage.

These, and similar observations, led Hering to propose the opponent color vision theory. This theory proposes that color is processed by bipolar hue channels referred to as the red–green and blue–yellow channels. By bipolar we mean that, at any instant, each channel can signal only one of the two attributes it is capable of coding. For example, for a given stimulus, the red–green channel is capable of signaling only red or green but not both red and green. The same is true of the blue–yellow channel; only blueness or yellowness is encoded for any one stimulus, not both. Hering also hypothesized that brightness is coded by a separate white–black channel.

For quite some time, Hering's theory was not considered seriously. Hering incorrectly suggested that a substance is present within the visual system that could signal either green or red, and another substance that could signal either blue or yellow. Even with the primitive understanding of physiology that existed in the 19th century, this was unrealistic. In addition, the trichromatic theory was widely accepted. The trichromatic theory explained much of what was known about color perception. It certainly was sufficient to explain color matching data. Through the first half of the 20th century, many thought that the trichromatic theory and the opponent color theory were not compatible. As it turns out, both theories are true in their most fundamental aspects.

## *Modern Opponent Color Theory*

In the late 1950s, Leo Hurvich and Dorothea Jameson provided quantitative data in support of the notion that color opponency plays an important role in processing color information (Hurvich, 1981). These investigators used a hue cancellation procedure to determine the spectral sensitivities of the red–green and blue–yellow opponent channels.

For a sample wavelength, the observer adjusts the amount of red or green *and* blue or yellow that is necessary to cancel the hue sensation produced by the sample wavelength. By cancel, we mean that hue (red or green *and* blue or yellow) is added to the sample until it turns white. This procedure, when repeated for many wavelengths across the visible spectrum, can be used to derive opponent color functions similar to those in Figure 5–15, which shows the

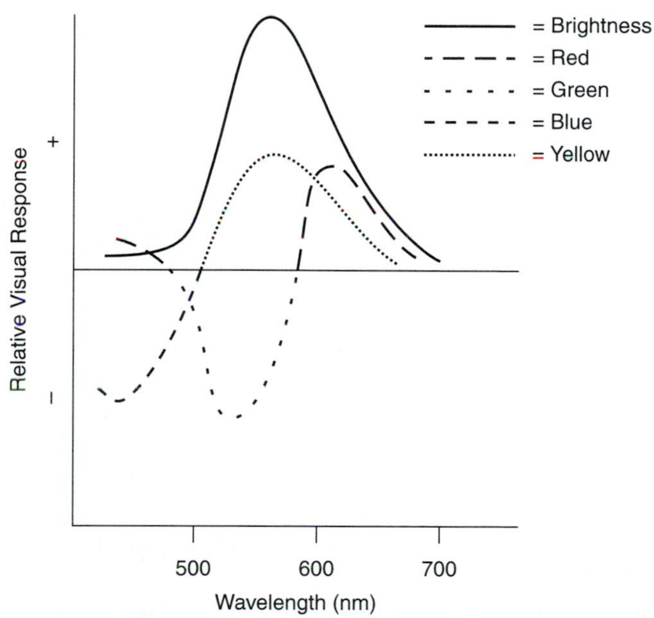


**FIGURE 5–15.** Approximations of the red–green, blue–yellow, and brightness channels proposed by Hurvich and Jameson. (*Adapted from Hurvich LM.* Color Vision. *Sunderland, MA: Sinauer Associates; 1981.)*

red–green and blue–yellow channels. Also plotted is the sensitivity of the proposed brightness channel, which has a shape very similar to the photopic luminosity function.

According to Hurvich and Jameson, all colors can be explained by the relative activity in the red–green, blue–yellow, and brightness channels. This model correctly predicts the locations of the unique hues, which are located at the crossover points of the red–green and blue–yellow channels (locate these in Fig. 5–15). At these points (e.g., 578 nm), only one of the two channels is active, resulting in the perception of a "pure" hue (yellow).

### *Electrophysiologic Evidence for Color Opponency*

Opponent color processing was placed on firm ground when Svaetichin (1956), recording from carp horizontal cells, noted that these cells were excited by some wavelengths and inhibited by others. These neurons display color opponency. A decade later, color opponent cells were found by DeValois et al (1966) and Wiesel and Hubel (1966) in the macaque dorsal lateral geniculate nucleus (dLGN).

To understand these electrophysiologic experiments, refer to Figure 5–16. The fovea of an anesthetized macaque monkey is aligned with the fixation point F on a screen. A microelectrode capable of recording action potentials is inserted into the primate's dLGN. A single cell is isolated. The neuron's receptive field is then determined. (As we will learn in Chapter 12, a neuron's receptive field is that area in visual space that influences the activity of the neuron.)

To assess this neuron's color coding capabilities, its receptive field is exposed to various spectral stimuli, all of equal energy. That is, we determine the neuron's response, as a function of wavelength, for equal-energy spectral stimuli. An example of an electrophysiologic recording from a color opponent cell is given in Figure 5–17A.

Frequency of action potentials is plotted as a function of wavelength. Note that short-wavelength stimuli (below 550 nm) cause inhibition (a decreased firing rate of the cell). In contrast, long-wavelength stimuli (longer than 550 nm) produce excitation (an increased rate of neural firing). As this cell responds to one portion of the spectrum with excitation and another portion with inhibition, it is referred to as a **color opponent,** or spectrally opponent, neuron.

This cell has color coding capabilities. If we are told that this neuron is excited by a stimulus, we would know that the stimulus is of a long wavelength. Likewise, if the cell is inhibited by a stimulus, we can assume that the stimulus is of a relatively short wavelength.

In addition to these color opponent neurons, DeValois et al (1966) found another class of neurons that were **noncolor opponent.** An example of the spectral sensitivity of such a neuron is given in Figure 5–17B. Note that this neuron responds to all spectral stimuli with excitation. It is not inhibited by any

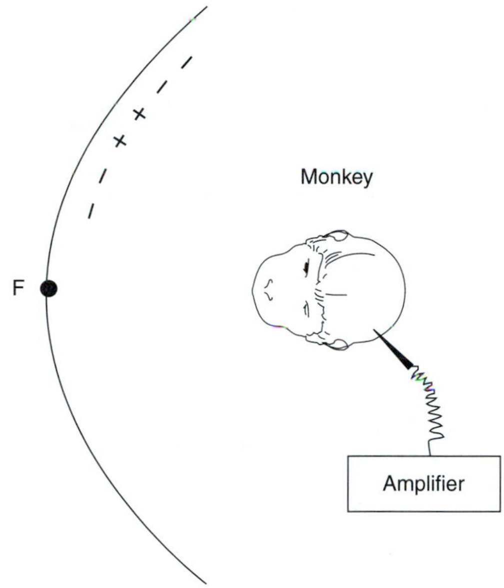


**FIGURE 5–16.** Basic setup for recording activity from an isolated neuron within the visual system. The animal's fovea is aligned with the fixation point F. A microelectrode records the electrical activity of a single neuron, and this signal is amplified and recorded.

wavelength. Consequently, this neuron does not have color coding capabilities; it is monochromatic. Recall our earlier discussion of monochromacy. A monochromat can adjust the intensity of any two wavelengths such that they appear identical. The same principle applies to this noncolor opponent neuron. Observing Figure 5–17B, we can see that a stimulus of 555 nm will produce more of an excitatory response than an equal-energy stimulus of 620 nm. If we were to increase the intensity of the 620-nm stimulus, however, we could increase the neuron's response such that it equals that produced by the 555-nm stimulus. Under these conditions, the neuron would not be able to distinguish between the two stimuli.

The spectral sensitivity function for a typical noncolor opponent neuron has a broad peak in the midspectral region, at about 555 nm. This has led some scientists to conclude that its spectral sensitivity is due to the addition of M and L-cone inputs.

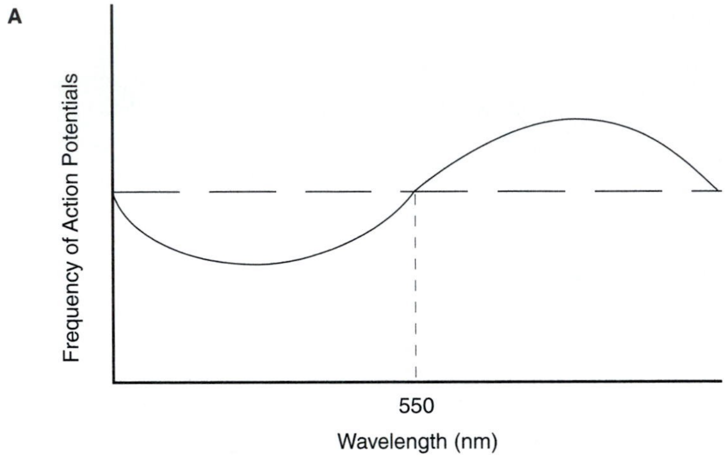


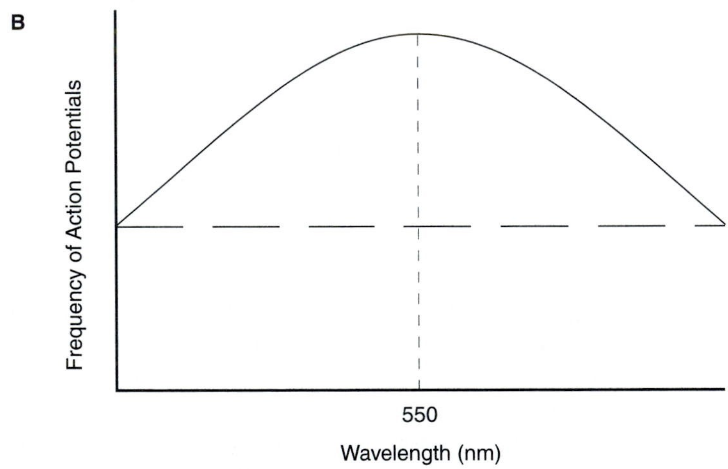


**FIGURE 5–17. A.** Frequency of action potentials as a function of wavelength for a color opponent neuron. Wavelengths below 550 nm cause a reduction in the frequency of action potentials, whereas longer wavelengths cause an increased rate of firing. **B.** Frequency of action potentials, as a function of wavelength for a noncolor opponent neuron. All wavelengths result in an increased frequency of action potentials. (These figures are schematics.)

## *Modern Models of Color Vision*

Thus far in our discussion of the physiology of color vision we have established two facts: (1) color vision is normally trichromatic, and (2) opponent processing plays a central role in coding color information. At first glance, it may appear that these two facts are incompatible. This is not the case.

Trichromacy tells us that there are three classes of cones. The presence of three classes of cones is sufficient to explain color matching data. The trichromatic theory, however, does not address the manner in which this information is handled beyond the photoreceptors at postreceptoral levels.

The finding of color opponent neurons in the visual system tells us that the receptoral information (trichromacy) is coded in an opponent fashion at postreceptoral levels. The three classes of cones are "wired" together at postreceptoral levels such that they are spectrally antagonistic. This postreceptoral antagonism occurs very early in the retina, as early as the horizontal cells. The recoding of trichromatic information in terms of color opponency is illustrated in Figure 5–18. Green and red cones oppose each other to produce a red–green opponent cells. Blue cones are opposed by an addition of red and green cones to produce a blue–yellow opponent cells.

An additional feature of the model presented in Figure 5–18 are the noncolor opponent cells. These cells are the result of the addition of red and green cone inputs. Some believe that the red–green and blue–yellow cells are exclusively devoted to coding hue, and have no role in coding brightness information. The coding of brightness is performed by the noncolor opponent cells (Lee et al, 1988; Shapley, 1990). Saturation is coded by the ratio of activity of the opponent color to noncolor opponent cells.

Others, however, believe that both hue and brightness are coded by the same cells (Ingling and Martinez-Uriegas, 1983; Kelly, 1983; Lennie, 1984; Derrington et al, 1984; Shapley, 1990). In this formulation, sometimes referred to as the "double-duty hypothesis," the red–green and blue–yellow cells do double-duty by coding both hue and brightness information.

In summary, primate color vision is trichromatic, with this trichromatic signal encoded in an opponent fashion. This opponent processing may occur very early in the visual system, at the level of the horizontal cells. Although it is established that hue information is encoded by red–green and blue–yellow neurons, it is not clear whether brightness information is encoded by these neurons or by a separate class of noncolor opponent cells.

## *Parvo and Magno Pathways*

In Chapter 13 we discuss, in detail, the roles of parvo and magno pathways in visual perception. At this time, they are briefly touched on because of their relevance to opponent color theory.

Visual information in the primate is transmitted from the retina to the visual

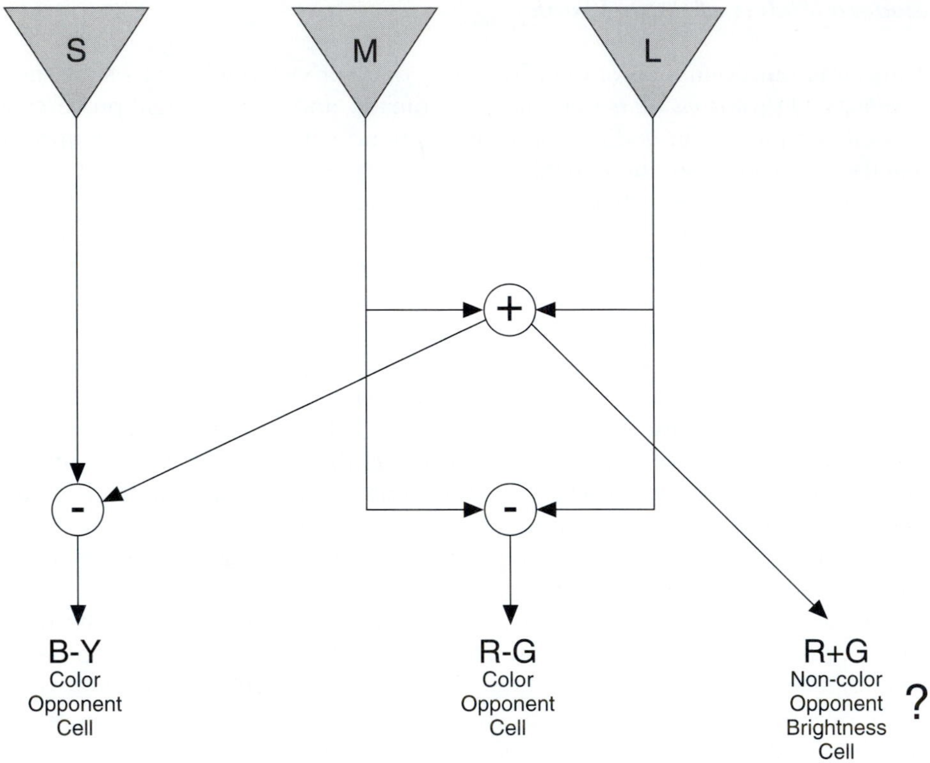


**FIGURE 5–18.** Simplified zone model of color processing. This model assumes the existence of luminance cells that are formed by the addition of M and L-cone inputs. The blue–yellow and red–green color opponent cells are formed by the subtractive (inhibitory) interaction of the various classes of cones.

cortex along two pathways, referred to as the parvo and magno pathways (Shapley, 1990). Neurons located in these two pathways manifest differences in the processing of color information, as well as detail and motion information. Parvo cells tend to be color opponent, whereas magno cells are noncolor opponent, or weakly color opponent.

Because of their color-opponency, it is thought that parvo cells are intimately involved in color perception. The role of magno cells is less clear. Some postulate that they code brightness information because their spectral sensitivity (see Fig. 5–17B) is very similar to the photopic luminance function. A similarity in the shape of the two functions, however, does not prove that magno cells code brightness information. The role of magno neurons in coding brightness is controversial and remains unresolved (Shapley, 1990).

## *THE MUNSELL COLOR APPEARANCE SYSTEM*

The ability to describe color verbally does not match the ability to perceive fine gradations in color. For example, suppose that a small area of your blue wallpaper needs to be replaced, and you would like the replacement to match the color of the original surrounding wallpaper. Although this task may seem simple, anyone who has attempted it will tell you otherwise. The problem is that because we are so good at discriminating colors, it is very difficult to find a perfect match. We could do our best to describe the color of the original wallpaper to a salesperson, but without showing her or him an actual sample, it would be virtually impossible to find an acceptable match.

There are hundreds of different colors that could be called blue. These variants of blue show differences in hue, saturation, and brightness. The Munsell color appearance system allows us to describe these colors with a great deal of specificity (Boynton, 1979; Pokorny et al, 1979; Wyszecki and Stiles, 1982). The Munsell system specifies colors along three physical dimensions: hue, chroma, and value. **Hue** is related to the wavelength of the stimulus. **Chroma** can be thought of as being akin to colorimetric purity and is related to the saturation of the color sample. **Value** refers to the reflectance of the sample and is related to brightness.

The Munsell system can be conceptualized as a cylinder containing various color samples (Fig. 5–19). Hue varies continuously along the perimeter of the cylinder, with the primary hues being red, yellow, green, blue, and purple. These are further subdivided into intermediaries. Chroma is measured as a radius from the center of the cylinder and ranges from 1 to 14, with 14 being the most saturated. Value increases along the vertical dimension, with 0 the darkest and 10 the brightest. In practical application, the Munsell system is laid out in a book, with each page containing a number of samples, all of the same hue. These samples are referred to as **Munsell chips.** The Munsell system is very useful for specifying color. For example, in the case of blue wallpaper, if we know which Munsell chip matches the wallpaper color, we can specify the wallpaper color simply by giving its hue, chroma, and value.

## *THE CIE COLOR SPECIFICATION SYSTEM*

The CIE system represents a standard manner of specifying color (Boynton, 1979; Pokorny et al, 1979; Hurvich, 1981; Wyszecki and Stiles, 1982). This is done by specifying the mixture of three primary colors required to match a given color sample. The CIE system is conceptually challenging because the CIE primaries are not real primaries, but are imaginary primaries. They represent a mathematical transformation of real primaries. This mathematical conversion to imaginary primaries is performed to avoid specifying negative quantities of primaries.

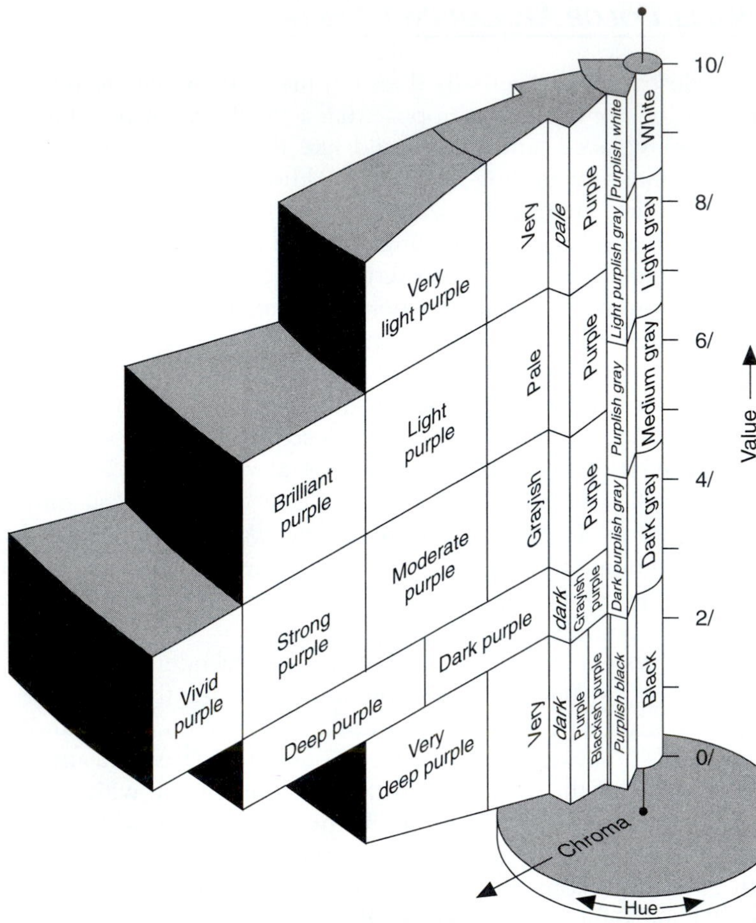


**FIGURE 5–19.** The Munsell color appearance system. Hue is specified along the perimeter of a cylinder, chroma as a radius from the center of the cylinder, and value as the vertical dimension of the cylinder. (*From Judd DB, Wyszecki G.* Color in Business, Science, and Industry. *Copyright 1963. Reprinted by permission of John Wiley & Sons, Inc.*)

## *The R,G,B System*

To understand the CIE system, first consider the **R,G,B** system of color specification. As illustrated in Figure 5–20A, the wavelength to be matched ($\lambda_v$) is placed on one side of a bipartite field. On the other side are the red, green, and blue primaries: $\lambda_r$ (645 nm), $\lambda_g$ (526 nm), and $\lambda_b$ (444 nm). The relative amounts of these three primaries are adjusted until a perfect match between the two sides of the field is obtained.

When this procedure is repeated for each wavelength, across the spectrum, we obtain **color matching functions,** which are illustrated in Figure 5–20B.

A

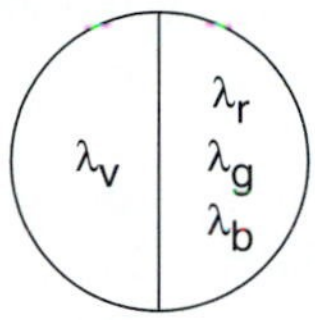


B

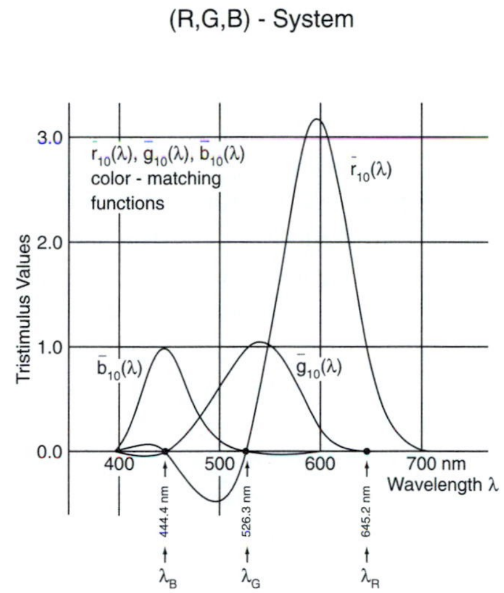


C

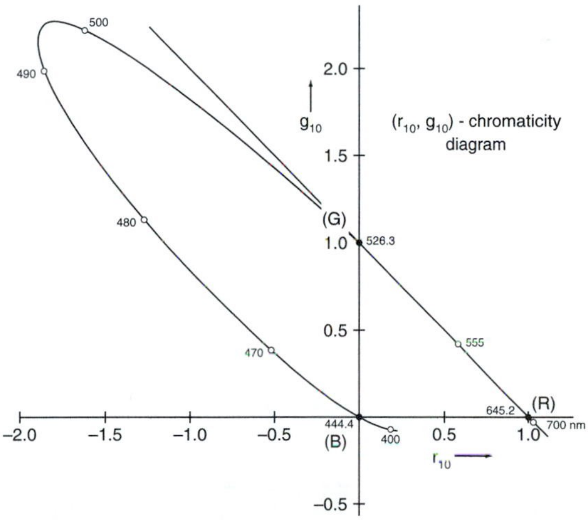


**FIGURE 5–20. A.** In the **R,G,B** system, a wavelength, $\lambda_v$, is specified by the relative amounts of the three primaries ($\lambda_r$, $\lambda_g$, $\lambda_b$) required to match it. **B.** Color matching functions for the **R,G,B** system. Note that negative quantities of the primary **R** are required over much of the spectrum. **C.** Chromaticity diagram for the **R,G,B** system. (*From Wyszecki G, Stiles WS.* Color Science: Concepts and Methods, Quantitative Data and Formulae. *Copyright 1982. Reprinted by permission of John Wiley & Sons, Inc.*)

These color matching functions show the amount of each primary required to match a given wavelength. The quantity of each primary required for a match is referred to as the **tristimulus value.**

Note that for wavelengths in the region 450 to 550 nm, negative amounts of $\lambda_r$ are required to obtain a match. This means that the required amount of $\lambda_r$ must be added to $\lambda_v$ rather than to the mixture field to obtain a match. No matter which real primaries are chosen to generate matching functions, there will always be some regions of negative quantities. The CIE system was designed to overcome this problem.

### *Imaginary Primaries*

Using matrix algebra, it is possible to transform one set of matching functions into another set of matching functions. In the CIE system, the **R,G,B** color matching functions are mathematically transformed into color matching functions for three imaginary primaries called *X, Y,* and *Z*. The color matching functions for the **X,Y,Z** primaries are given in Figure 5–21A. Note that all wavelengths can be matched with positive quantities of these primaries; it is not necessary to use negative quantities.

The **CIE chromaticity diagram** (see Fig. 5–21B) shows the relative amounts of the imaginary primaries required to match any real color. This chromaticity diagram is constructed by converting the tristimulus values to relative units, referred to as **chromaticity coordinates.**

The tristimulus values are given by uppercase letters, whereas the chromaticity coordinates are given in lowercase letters. The following equations show the relationship between the tristimulus values and the chromaticity coordinates:

$$x = \frac{X}{X + Y + Z}$$

$$y = \frac{Y}{X + Y + Z}$$

$$z = \frac{Z}{X + Y + Z}$$

where

$$x + y + z = 1$$

These equations show that the sum of the chromaticity coordinates must equal 1. Therefore, if we know two of these coordinates, we can calculate the third. The chromaticity diagram shows only the $x$ and $y$ chromaticity coordinates. Coordinate $z$ is calculated by subtracting the sum of $x$ and $y$ from 1.

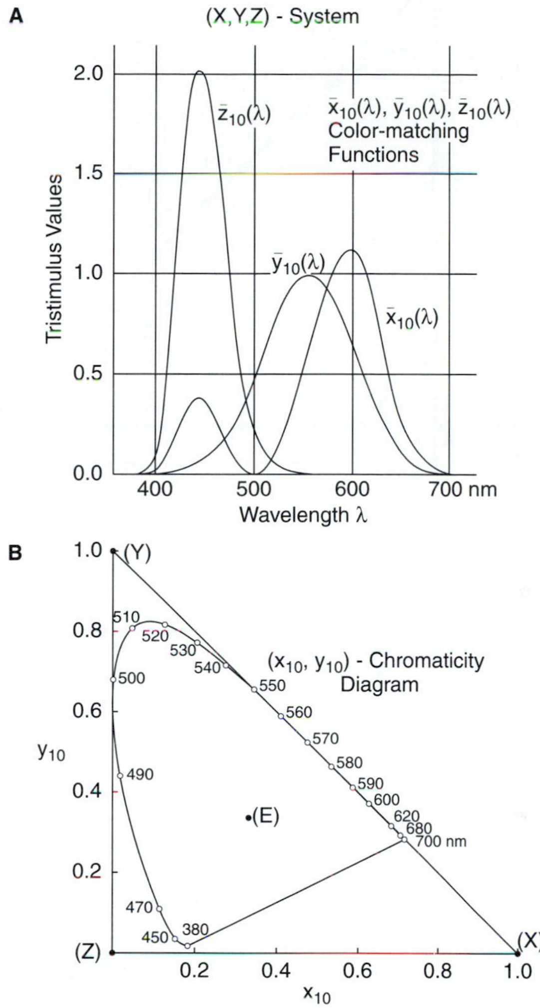


**FIGURE 5–21. A.** Color matching functions for the imaginary primaries **X,Y,Z.** These imaginary primaries are mathematical transformations of the **R,G,B** primaries. **B.** Chromaticity diagram for this system. This diagram is commonly referred to as the CIE chromaticity diagram. (*From Wyszecki G, Stiles WS.* Color Science: Concepts and Methods, Quantitative Data and Formulae. *Copyright 1982. Reprinted by permission of John Wiley & Sons, Inc.*)

## *Basic Attributes of the CIE Chromaticity Diagram*

Contained within the CIE chromaticity diagram are all physically realizable colors (Fig. 5–22). Note that the imaginary primaries themselves (points *X, Y,* and *Z*) fall outside of the diagram as they are not physically realizable.

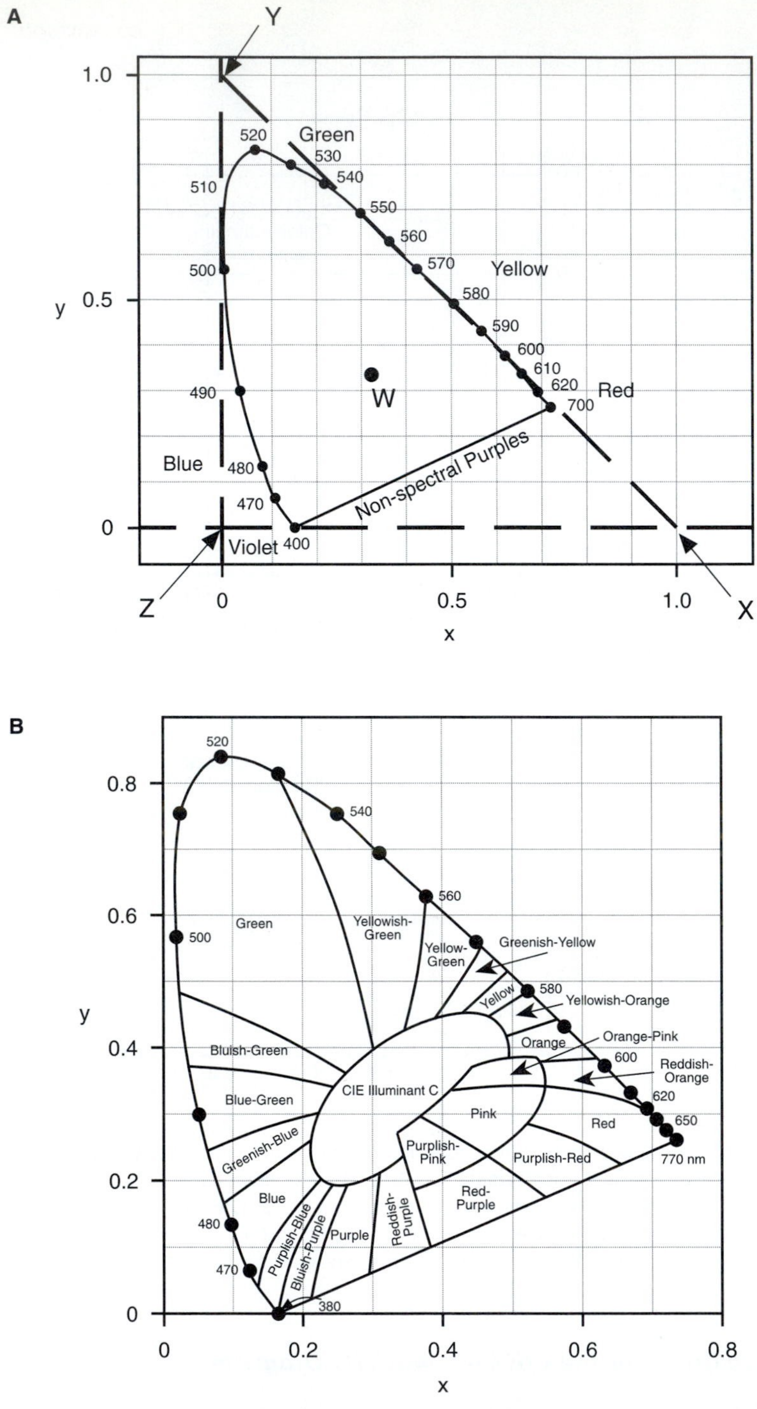


**FIGURE 5–22. A.** An approximation of the CIE chromaticity diagram. All physically realizable colors fall along the perimeter of this diagram, or within the diagram. The imaginary primaries (*X,Y,Z*) fall outside the diagram. **B.** Color labels applied to various regions of the CIE chromaticity diagram. (*From Judd DB.* Color in Business, Science, and Industry. *Copyright 1952. Reprinted by permission of John Wiley and Sons, Inc.*)

Spectral hues (monochromatic hues) are arranged along the arc of the perimeter of the diagram; this arc is referred to as the spectral locus. Nonspectral purples fall along the straight line connecting 400 and 700 nm. (Purples are not represented by a single wavelength but by mixtures of blue and red.) White falls in the center of the diagram and is indicated by *W*.

### *Calculations*

The CIE diagram has several features that make it very useful. For example, color mixtures are easily calculated on the diagram simply by joining together, with a line, the colors to be mixed. This is illustrated in Figure 5–23. If we wish to mix equal amounts of 510 and 560 nm, we connect these two points with a line. The resultant mixture falls at the midpoint of this line, represented by the letter *M*. To specify this mixture, we connect point *M* with point *W*, which represents white, and extend the line to the perimeter of the diagram. In this case, it intersects 530 nm, which is referred to as the **dominant wavelength.**

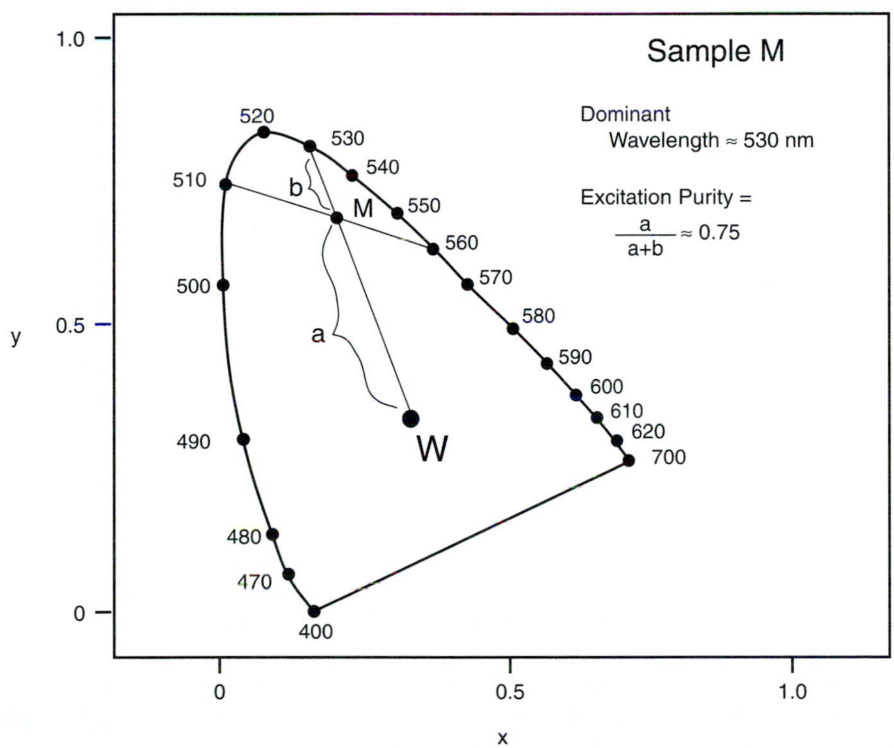


**FIGURE 5–23.** Equal amounts of 510 and 560 nm are combined to form a mixture, M. This mixture has a dominant wavelength of 530 nm and an excitation purity of 0.75.

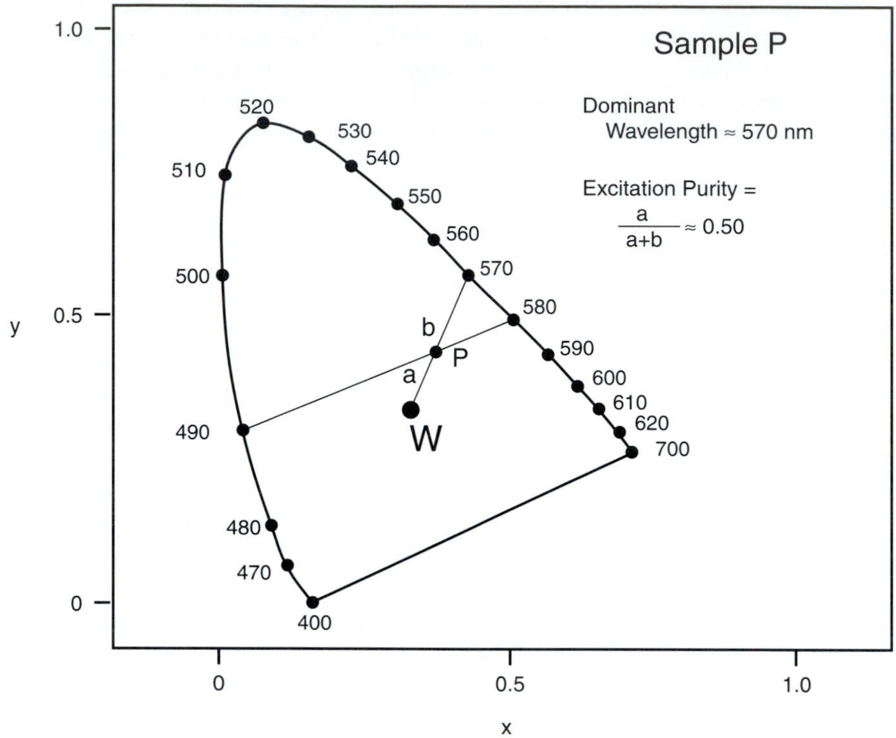


**FIGURE 5–24.** A mixture of three parts of 580 nm to one part of 490 nm produces a mixture, P. The dominant wavelength of this mixture is 570 nm, and the excitation purity is 0.50.

The relative distance of the sample from white to the perimeter of the CIE diagram is a measure of the colorimetric purity of the sample, and is referred to as the **excitation purity.** Specifically, the excitation purity of sample M is given by $a/(a + b) = 0.75$.

Take another example. In this case, we mix 490 nm with 580 nm, such that there is three times more 580 nm than 490 nm. Figure 5–24 shows the determination of the dominant wavelength and excitation purity for this mixture. The first step is to connect 490 and 580 nm. The mixture occurs at a point three fourths of the way from 490 to 580 nm because of the relative amounts of these two wavelengths contained in the mixture. Connecting this point with white gives us a dominant wavelength of 570 nm and an excitation purity of 0.50.

The CIE diagram is useful for ascertaining a color's complement. **Complementary colors,** when mixed together, produce white. To determine the complement for a given wavelength, simply connect this wavelength, through white, to the opposite side of the CIE diagram (Fig. 5–25). In this case, we

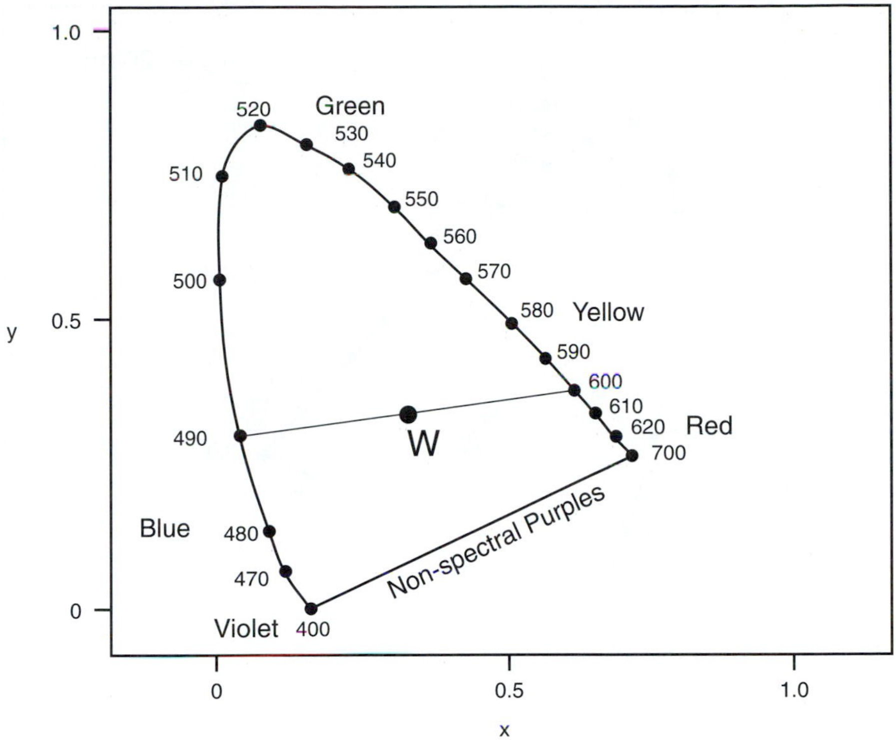


**FIGURE 5–25.** The complement of 490 nm is found by connecting 490 nm with white and extending this line to the opposite perimeter of the CIE diagram. This gives the complement of 490 nm as 600 nm.

show that the complement of 490 is 600 nm. These two wavelengths, when mixed together, produce white.

Nonspectral purples are often specified by giving their complement. For example, to specify the purple given by point *0* in Figure 5–26, we use the notation $\lambda_c$ = 520 nm. This allows us to physically locate the position of the purple on the diagram.

The CIE diagram is exceptionally valuable in specifying and understanding color vision defects. This is discussed in Chapter 6.

### *Where Is White in the CIE Chromaticity Diagram?*

Up to this point, we have assumed that white is a single point within the CIE diagram. From our discussion of color temperature in Chapter 4, however, it is clear that no single spectral distribution has exclusive claim to the label, white.

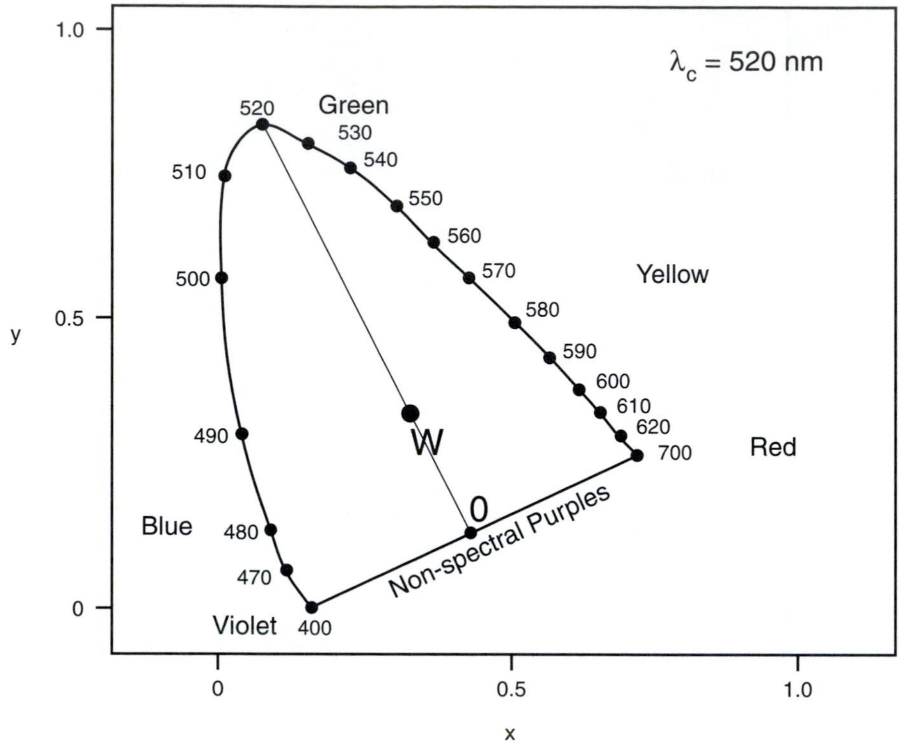


**FIGURE 5–26.** The nonspectral sample, 0, is specified by its complement. This purple is specified as $\lambda_c = 520$ nm.

Indeed, the standard illuminants A, C, $D_{65}$, and so forth are all variants of white.

Sources of various color temperatures form an arc within the CIE diagram, referred to as the **Planckian locus** (Fig. 5–27). The samples that fall on this locus, including the various standard illuminants, can be considered to be variants of white.

## *Use of the CIE System to Specify a Color Sample*

The CIE system has practical applications for specifying color samples in a manner that allows us to convey this information to others. Take, for example, sample H in Figure 5–27. This sample has chromaticity coordinates of $x = 0.2$, $y = 0.5$, and $z = 0.3$. By knowing these chromaticity coordinates and one tristimulus value, we can calculate the tristimulus values for the imaginary primaries $X$, $Y$, and $Z$. Matrix algebra can be used to convert these tristimulus values into tris-

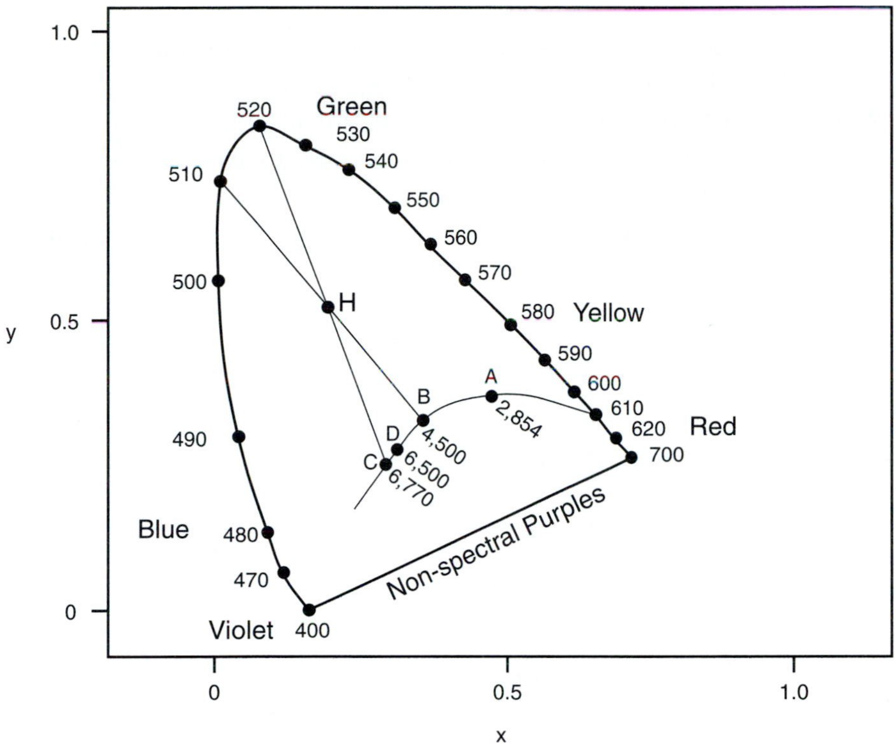


**FIGURE 5–27.** The standard illuminants fall on an arc (the Planckian locus) within the CIE diagram. The sample H can be made by combining 510 nm with illuminant B or by combining 520 nm with illuminant C.

timulus values representing real primaries. In fact, it is possible to derive an infinite number of sets of three primaries that are metamers for this sample. By specifying the chromaticity coordinates, we provide all the information required to select a combination of three primaries that will match a sample.

You may have noticed that the matching function for the primary *Y* has the same form as the photopic luminance function. This was by design and is a useful feature. The advantage is that the tristimulus value for *Y* specifies not only the amount of this primary in a sample, but also the luminance of the sample.

### *Summary of the CIE Color Specification System*

The CIE system is one of the most challenging topics in vision science. If you are having difficulty understanding this system, do not feel alone. Countless others have struggled to comprehend this highly theoretical system.

Keep in mind the following:

1. The CIE diagram specifies the relative amounts of primaries necessary to match a color sample.
2. The CIE primaries do not really exist; they are imaginary.
3. The CIE system uses these imaginary primaries to avoid the use of negative quantities.
4. Any set of color matching functions, real or imaginary, can be converted to another set of real or imaginary functions.

Now, go back to the beginning of this section on the CIE diagram and try it again. It is always easier the second time through!

## CLINICAL CONSIDERATIONS

The next chapter is devoted exclusively to the etiology of color vision defects and their diagnosis and management. In the remainder of this chapter, certain clinical considerations not covered in Chapter 6 are addressed.

### Short Wavelength Automated Perimetry

The S-cone system may be more vulnerable to certain pathologic processes than are the M and L-cone systems (Adams et al, 1990). This may be due to vulnerabilities in the S-cones themselves or the blue–yellow opponent pathway, or due to the sparse number of S-cones (which would magnify the effects of the loss of a small number of these cones).

Clinical psychophysical procedures have been developed to assess S-cone function in certain eye diseases, particularly glaucoma (Johnson et al, 1992; Johnson, 1995). The commonly used Humphrey visual field apparatus can be adapted for this function by replacing the standard white stimulus with a short-wavelength stimulus to maximize S-cone sensitivity. To suppress the M and L-cones, the background is yellow rather than the standard white. Yellow preferentially bleaches the M and L-cone photopigments and, thereby, reduces their sensitivity. The procedure is commonly referred to as short wavelength automated perimetry (SWAP).

In glaucoma, elevated (or even normal) intraocular pressure presumably leads to damage of the optic nerve with a subsequent loss of vision. The diagnosis of glaucoma is often based on visual field loss as measured with a white stimulus on a white background. This measure, however, is not very sensitive; apparently a substantial proportion of the optic nerve fibers are damaged by the time early visual field defects are first noted (Quigley et al, 1982).

Early results suggest that SWAP is a more sensitive measure of glaucomatous nerve damage than are standard, white-on-white visual fields (Johnson et al, 1995). Patients in the early stages of glaucoma are more likely to manifest S-cone field loss than standard field loss. On the basis of these encouraging results, it seems likely that SWAP, or similar procedures, will play a greater role in the future diagnosis and management of glaucoma.

### *Increment Spectral Sensitivity*

The color-opponent parvo pathway can apparently be isolated by determining threshold as a function of wavelength for spectral (monochromatic) increments presented on a white background (Fig. 5–28). If the stimulus is of a long dura-

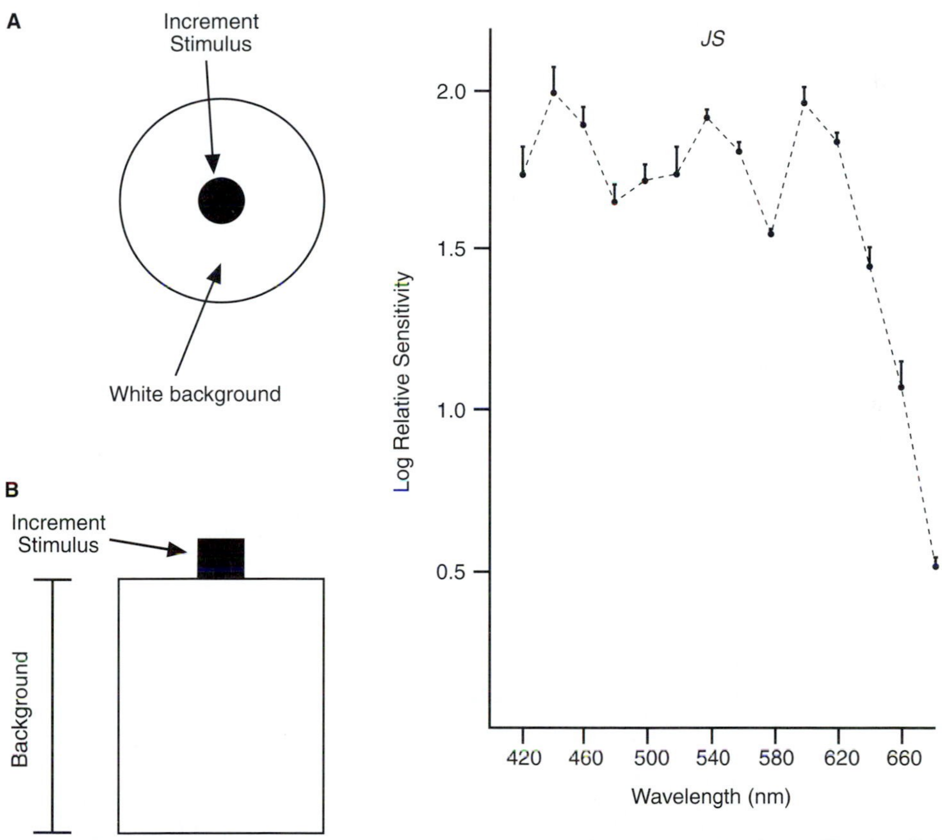


**FIGURE 5–28. A.** Stimulus configuration used for an increment threshold procedure. **B.** Intensity profile of the background and stimulus. **C.** Increment spectral sensitivity function for stimuli with a duration of 200 milliseconds. These data represent the sensitivity of the chromatic (color-opponent) system. *JS* are the initials of the experimental subject. (*Adapted from Schwartz S H. Spectral sensitivity of dichromats: Role of postreceptoral processes.* Vision Res. *1994;34:2983–2990.*)

tion (200 milliseconds), we obtain a three-peaked function. This psychophysically isolated system is referred to as the **chromatic system.**

Figure 5–29 shows spectral sensitivity functions for the chromatic system in diabetic patients (Adams et al, 1990). It is interesting to note that, as in glaucoma, the S-cone system is the most vulnerable. As was mentioned earlier, the reason for this vulnerability is not fully understood.

### *X-chrom Contact Lens*

Patients with defective color discrimination are commonly encountered in clinical practice. The X-chrom contact lens is a red contact lens, worn on one eye, that is designed to improve color discrimination.

Although this contact lens is typically prescribed for dichromats, or those with less severe color defects (anomalous trichromats, see Chap. 6), it is most easily understood in the context of monochromacy. Figure 5–30 (left) shows the absorption spectrum for a hypothetical monochromat. Next to this curve is a hy-

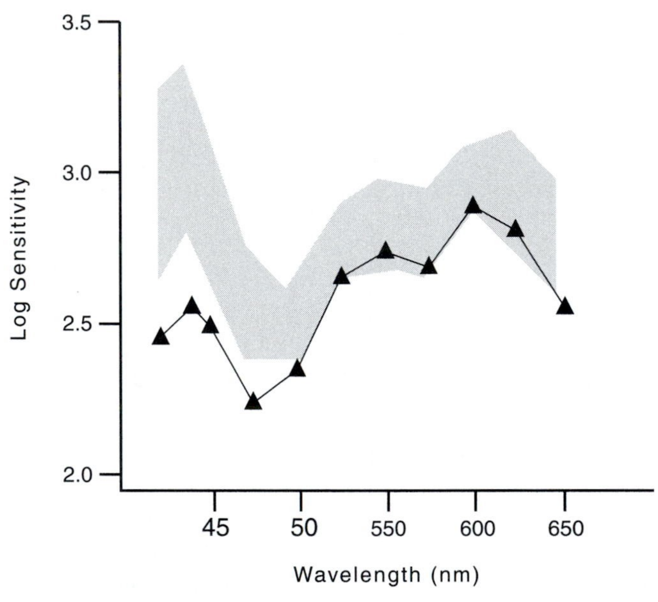


**FIGURE 5–29.** The shaded area shows the normal ranges of spectral sensitivity for the chromatic system, and the solid triangles show spectral sensitivity for the chromatic system of diabetics. Note the reduction in sensitivity at short wavelengths. (*Adapted from Adams AJ, Bodis-Wollner I, Enoch JM, et al. Normal and abnormal mechanisms of vision: Visual disorders and visual deprivation. In: Spillman L, Werner JS, eds.* Visual Perception: The Neurophysiological Foundations. *1990. Reprinted with permission of Academic Press and Dr. Anthony Adams.*)

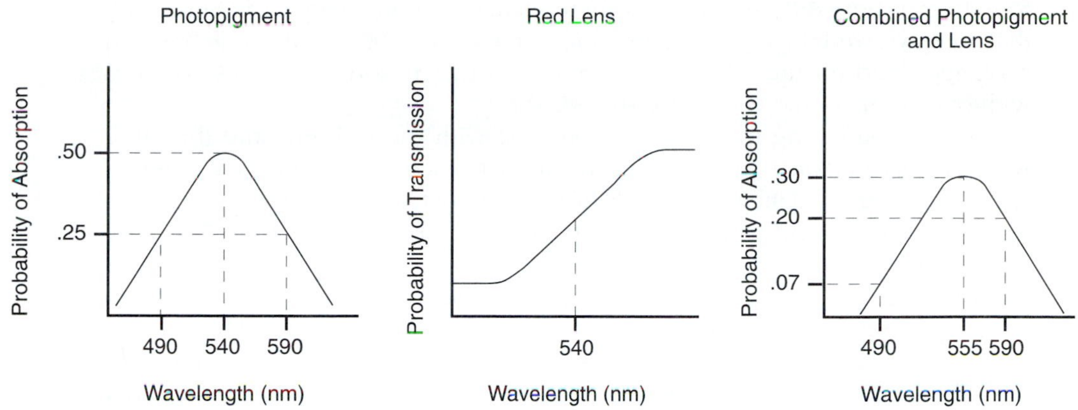


| | 490 | 590 |
|---|---|---|
| Quanta Emitted | 1000 | 1000 |
| Quanta Absorbed | 250 | 250 |

| | 490 | 590 |
|---|---|---|
| Quanta Emitted | 1000 | 1000 |
| Quanta Absorbed | 70 | 200 |

**FIGURE 5–30.** Use of a colored contact lens to improve color discrimination. The left curve shows the absorption spectrum of a hypothetical monochromat. The middle curve is the transmission curve for a red lens. This is followed by the absorption spectrum of an eye of this monochromat when wearing this lens. The lens shifts the absorption spectrum of the monochromat, and this effectively makes the individual a dichromat if he or she compares the two eyes.

pothetical spectral transmission curve for a red contact lens. Note that this lens is a long-pass lens; it blocks low wavelengths and transmits longer wavelengths.

The curve on the right is the product of the photopigment absorption spectrum and the red lens transmission curve. This final curve represents the absorption spectrum of the eye that is wearing the contact lens. Note that the contact lens has caused the original absorption curve to become displaced toward longer wavelengths.

How does this lens aid in color discrimination? Consider the two patches of light in Figure 5–30, each of which emits 1000 quanta of light. Because the photopigment is equally bleached by 490 and 590 nm, these two patches are indistinguishable when viewed with the eye that is not wearing the contact lens. When these same two patches of light are viewed by the eye wearing the red lens, however, they result in unequal numbers of quantal absorptions; therefore, they appear different. If we were to increase the intensity of 490 nm, such that when viewed through the contact lens it matched 590 nm, the match would no longer hold for the other eye. Therefore, if the person views these patches with one eye at a time, they are distinguishable.

When comparing the two eyes, one eye with the red lens and the other without, this person behaves like a dichromat. Each eye provides a different spectral sensitivity. Likewise, if a dichromat alternately views objects with this lens, he or she would behave like a tetrachromat, or as if there were four photopigments.

Although on a first analysis this approach seems useful, there are drawbacks. Some individuals suppress the eye that is wearing the red lens. Others tend to fuse the images of the two eyes rather than alternate between eyes. Consequently, these individuals act as if a red filter has been placed over both eyes. This results in a shift in spectral sensitivity for the remaining cones, but no improvement in color discrimination. Only if the person alternates viewing between the two eyes will chromatic discrimination be improved. This may not be practical and could interfere with normal binocular vision; consequently the usefulness of this lens for clinical applications is limited. In the next chapter, we discuss modifications of this filtered lens strategy.

## SUMMARY

It is firmly established that normal human vision is trichromatic. This trichromatic information is encoded in a color opponent fashion by postreceptoral visual neurons.

Color is perceived along the perceptual dimensions of hue, saturation, and brightness. Because of the ability to make fine color discriminations, sophisticated color appearance and color specification systems have been devised.

The understanding of color vision physiology has facilitated the development of psychophysical tests to aid in the diagnosis and management of certain eye diseases. The role of color vision in the assessment of eye disease is covered in more detail in the following chapter on color vision defects.

# Self-Assessment Questions

1. A monochromat puts on a pair of red sunglasses. With these glasses on, will this individual behave as a monochromat or a dichromat? Explain.

2. **A.** What is the dominant wavelength of a mixture that consists of 60 percent of 490 nm and 40 percent of 540 nm? **B.** What is the excitation purity of this mixture? **C.** What is the complement to this mixture? (When making these calculations, do so with respect to illuminant C in Figure 5–27.)

3. Answer all questions asked in question 2 for a mixture of one third of 490 nm and two thirds of 610 nm.

4. Note that illuminant $D_{65}$ lies closer to the blue corner of the CIE diagram than illuminant A, which lies closer to the red corner of the diagram. Explain this in terms of the color temperatures and chromatic appearances of these two illuminants.

5. **A.** How is it possible that a painter can match all hues with the use of only three primary colors? **B.** What is a limitation of using only three primaries for painting? Explain.

6. Hunters sometimes wear camouflaged clothing. Devise an instrument that would enable you to distinguish a camouflaged hunter from the natural background.

7. It has been mentioned that the Bezold–Brücke phenomenon could be explained by opponent color theory. Provide such an explanation. (*Hint:* Why do certain wavelengths change hue with increasing intensity, while others do not?)

# 6

# Anomalies of Color Vision

Defects of color vision are commonly encountered in clinical practice. Approximately 4.5 percent of the population manifests color vision deficiencies (Pokorny et al, 1979). Most of these defects are inherited. Although these **hereditary defects** are nonprogressive and pose no threat to vision, they may have a profound effect on the performance of visually related activities, including certain activities encountered at school and on the job.

Color vision defects that are not inherited are referred to as **acquired defects.** These defects are less common than hereditary defects. Acquired defects are typically secondary to a disease process. As such, they provide an important tool in the early and differential diagnosis of certain eye diseases.

In this chapter, we discuss the classification and characteristics of color vision defects. Clinical testing procedures are presented along with recommendations for the management of these frequently encountered conditions.

## BASIC CLASSIFICATION

Table 6–1 provides a basic classification of color vision defects. Color deficiencies can be divided into two general categories: **dichromacy** and **anomalous trichromacy.** Dichromats are missing one of the three retinal photopigments (Rushton, 1963a, b, 1965b). A **deuteranope** is missing chlorolabe, a **protanope** is missing erythrolabe, and a **tritanope** is missing cyanolabe. The missing photopigment is presumably replaced by a remaining photopigment. In the case of a deuteranope, chlorolabe is replaced by erythrolabe. In a protanope, erythrolabe is replaced by chlorolabe. This is referred to as the **replacement model** of dichromacy.

The replacement of the missing photopigment by a remaining photopigment is consistent with the normal resolution visual acuities of dichromats. If a

**TABLE 6–1. BASIC CLASSIFICATION OF COLOR VISION DEFICIENCIES**

| | Red–Green Defects | | Blue–Yellow Defects |
|---|---|---|---|
| ***Photopigment Status*** | ***Protan Defect*** | ***Deutan Defect*** | ***Tritan Defect*** |
| Dichromat | Protanope (protanopia) | Deuteranope (deuteranopia) | Tritanope (tritanopia) |
| Anomalous trichromat | Protanomalous trichromat (protanomaly) | Deuteranomalous trichromat (deuteranomaly) | Tritanomalous trichromat (tritanomaly) |

class of cones were simply missing, rather than replaced, dichromats would probably manifest clinically measurable reductions in acuity.

Anomalous trichromats have three photopigments, but the absorption spectrum of one of these photopigments is displaced to an abnormal position (Alpern and Torii, 1968a,b; Alpern and Moeller, 1977; Alpern and Wake, 1977). This is illustrated in Figure 6–1. A deuteranomalous trichromat manifests a displacement of the chlorolabe spectrum toward longer wavelengths, whereas a protanomalous trichromat shows displacement of the erythrolabe spectrum toward shorter wavelengths. These displacements of the cone photopigments from their optimal positions result in deficient color discrimination.

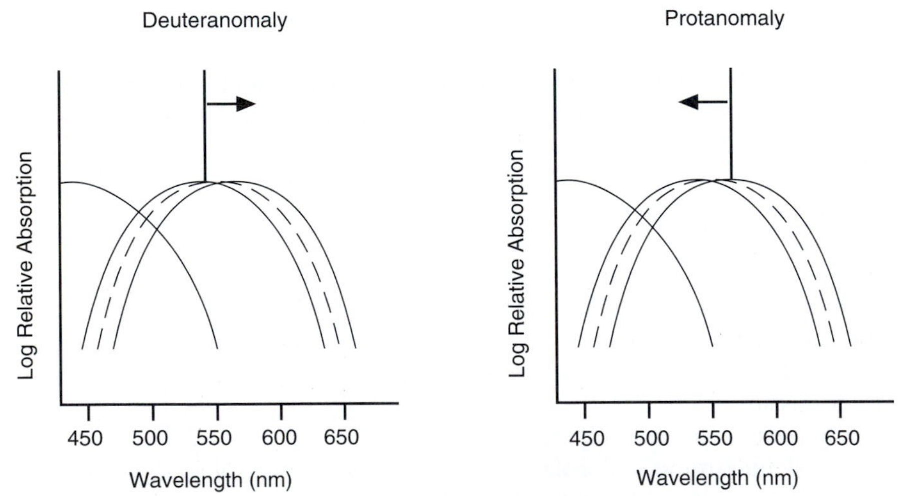


**FIGURE 6–1.** Simplified absorption spectra for anomalous trichromacy. In deuteranomaly, the M-cone spectrum is displaced toward long wavelengths, and in protanomaly the L-cone spectrum is displaced toward short wavelengths. The solid curves show the normal positions of the cone absorption spectra, and the dashed curves show the locations of the displaced spectra.

In the classification scheme in Table 6–1, the terms **protan, deutan,** and **tritan** refer to the affected photopigment. An individual who falls into one of these categories is either a dichromat or an anomalous trichromat. For instance, a protan may be either a protanope or a protanomalous trichromat. If the erythrolabe is missing, the subject is a dichromat—a protanope. If the photopigment is displaced, he or she is an anomalous trichomat—a protanomalous trichromat. Likewise, a deutan has a defect of chlorolabe such that she or he is either a deuteranope or a deuteranomalous trichromat.

Protans and deutans tend to confuse reds and greens, and are said to have a **red–green defect.** These defects are usually, but not always, inherited. Tritans, who confuse blues and yellows, are classified as having a **blue–yellow defect.** Such defects are typically acquired.

## BASIC DATA OF COLOR DEFICIENCY

People with anomalous color vision process chromatic information differently than do those with normal color vision. Among those characteristics that differentiate anomalous from normal color vision are spectral sensitivity, wavelength discrimination, color confusion lines, and the perception of saturation. The discussion that follows emphasizes data for protan and deutan defects because these defects are common and have been well documented. Tritan defects are relatively less common and, consequently, fewer data are available regarding these defects.

### *Spectral Sensitivity: Chromatic System*

In the previous chapter, we learned that the color opponent (chromatic) system can be identified by determining spectral sensitivity functions using large stimuli of long duration. In such an experiment, thresholds are determined for 200-millisecond monochromatic increments as a function of wavelength. The stimulus configuration and results of such an experiment are given in Figure 6–2.

A normal trichromat shows a color opponent spectral sensitivity function with three peaks (Sperling and Harwerth, 1971; King-Smith and Carden, 1976). The 440-nm peak corresponds to the location of the S-cone peak. The peaks at 520 and 620 nm presumably result from a subtractive, or opponent, interaction between the M and L-cones. This opponent processing causes the peaks to be displaced from the location of the peaks of the M and L-cones (535 and 565 nm, respectively).

A strikingly different result is obtained when the experiment is repeated on dichromatic subjects (Verriest and Uvijls, 1977; Schwartz, 1994). A deuteranope who is missing chlorolabe shows only two peaks. These peaks correspond to the remaining two photopigments, cyanolabe and erythrolabe. Likewise, a protanope manifests two peaks, a peak for cyanolabe and a peak for chlorolabe. These results are consistent with the replacement hypothesis of dichromacy.

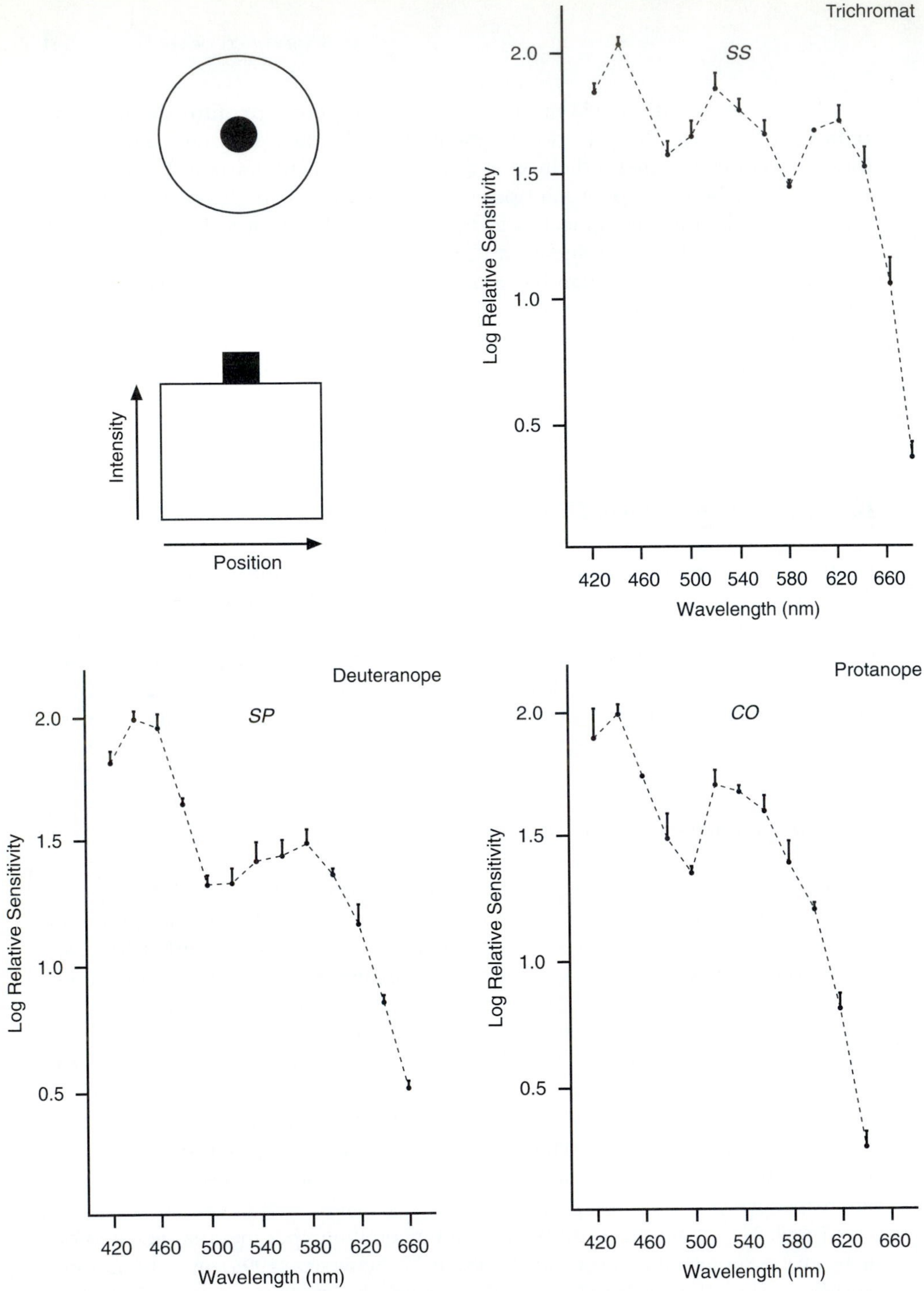


**FIGURE 6–2.** Chromatic increment spectral sensitivity functions for a normal trichromat, a deuteranope, and a protanope. Participants' initials are above each graph. Stimulus conditions are given in the upper left. (*Adapted from Schwartz SH. Spectral sensitivity of dichromats: role of postreceptoral processes.* Vision Res. *1994;34:2983–2990.*)

### *Spectral Sensitivity: Luminance Function*

Figure 6–3 shows $V(\lambda)$ (photopic luminance) functions for normal trichromacy, deuteranopia, and protanopia. As we have learned, the $V(\lambda)$ function of normal trichromats has a broad peak in the region of 555 nm. Dichromats manifest luminance functions that differ from this normal $V(\lambda)$ function (Hsia and Graham, 1957). The protanopic $V(\lambda)$ curve is substantially displaced toward shorter wavelengths, whereas the $V(\lambda)$ curve of deuteranopes shows a very slight displacement toward longer wavelengths. (The displacement of the deuteranopic luminosity function is minimal, and for clinical purposes it may be considered normal.)

The $V(\lambda)$ function of a normal trichromat is presumably due to the addition of M and L-cone inputs (see Chap. 3). Consequently, the absence of one of these cone types, as occurs in dichromacy, will produce a displacement of the

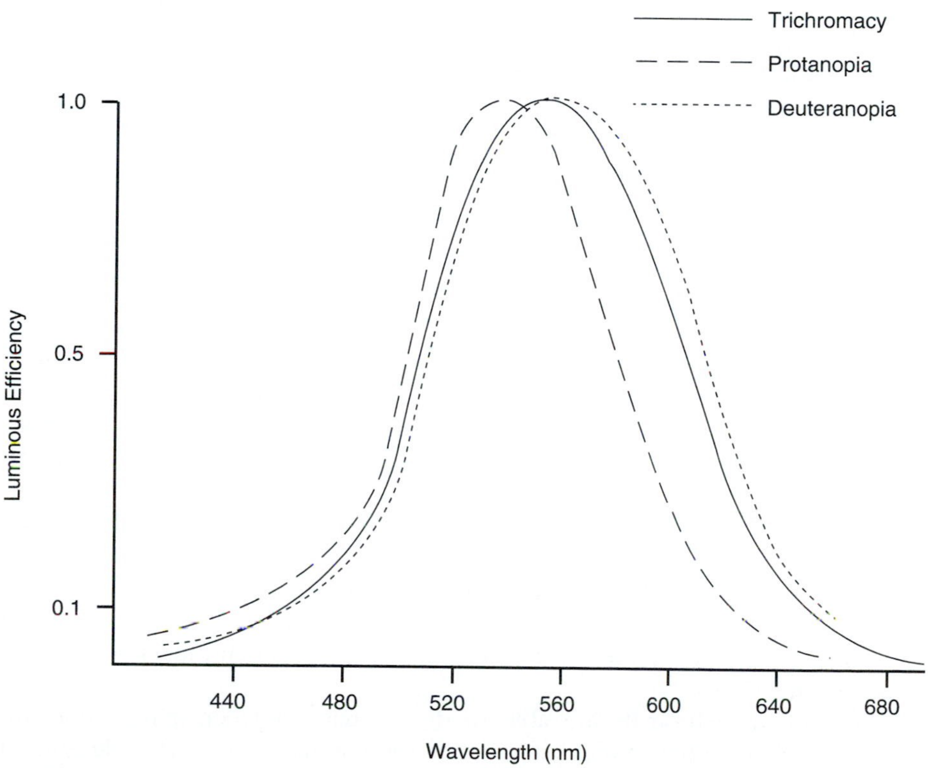


**FIGURE 6–3.** Photopic luminance functions, $V(\lambda)$, for normal trichromacy, deuteranopia, and protanopia. (*Adapted from Hsia Y, Graham CH. Spectral luminosity curves for protanopic, deuteranopic and normal subjects.* Proc Nat Acad Sci USA. *1957;43:1011–1019.*)

$V(\lambda)$ curve. For instance, a protanope is missing erythrolabe, causing the protanopic luminance curve to be displaced toward shorter wavelengths. Likewise, the missing M-cone input in deuteranopes causes their $V(\lambda)$ function to be displaced toward longer wavelengths. As the displacement that occurs in deuteranopia is less pronounced than that in protanopia, it can be concluded that M-cones play less of a role in generating the normal $V(\lambda)$ function than do L-cones.

The abnormal luminosity function found in protanopia has important clinical consequences. As a result of the displacement of the protanopic $V(\lambda)$ function toward shorter wavelengths, these individuals manifest greatly reduced sensitivity to long wavelengths. In practical terms, protanopes find it difficult to see red objects. This can be demonstrated in the laboratory by projecting a beam of 660-nm light (or a red laser) onto a screen. Whereas this stimulus is easily seen as a bright red spot by an observer with normal vision, it is invisible (or nearly invisible) to a protanope. Because the protanope is missing erythrolabe, these 660-nm quanta of light are simply not absorbed.

Anomalous trichromats also manifest abnormal luminosity functions. Their luminosity functions manifest the same general features as those of dichromats, but to a lesser degree. Protanomalous trichromats show some displacement of their luminosity function toward shorter wavelengths, but less so than protanopes. Deuteranomalous trichromats manifest a very minimal displacement of the luminosity function toward longer wavelengths; this displacement is even less than that found in deuteranopes.

### *Wavelength Discrimination*

Figure 6–4A shows wavelength discrimination as a function of wavelength for normal, deuteranopic, and protanopic observers. Note that both protanopes and deuteranopes show relatively good wavelength discrimination in the region of 490 nm, but very poor wavelength discrimination in the long-wavelength region of the spectrum (Pitt, 1935; Wright, 1946). This graph shows that beyond about 545 nm; protanopes and deuteranopes are not able to discriminate between stimuli on the basis of wavelength differences alone.

Red–green dichromats are not able to make wavelength-based discriminations for stimuli greater than 545 nm because they are essentially monochromatic in this region of the spectrum. This is illustrated in Figure 6–5. Deuteranopes and protanopes have only one cone photopigment that absorbs beyond 545 nm; consequently, these subjects behave as monochromats for stimuli greater than 545 nm.

Red–green dichromats are able to discriminate between stimuli that are longer than 545 nm only if these stimuli differ in luminance. For example, stimuli of 575 and 600 nm appear different if equated for energy. The 575-nm stimulus appears brighter because it has greater luminance. If, however, these stimuli are equated for luminance, they are indistinguishable.

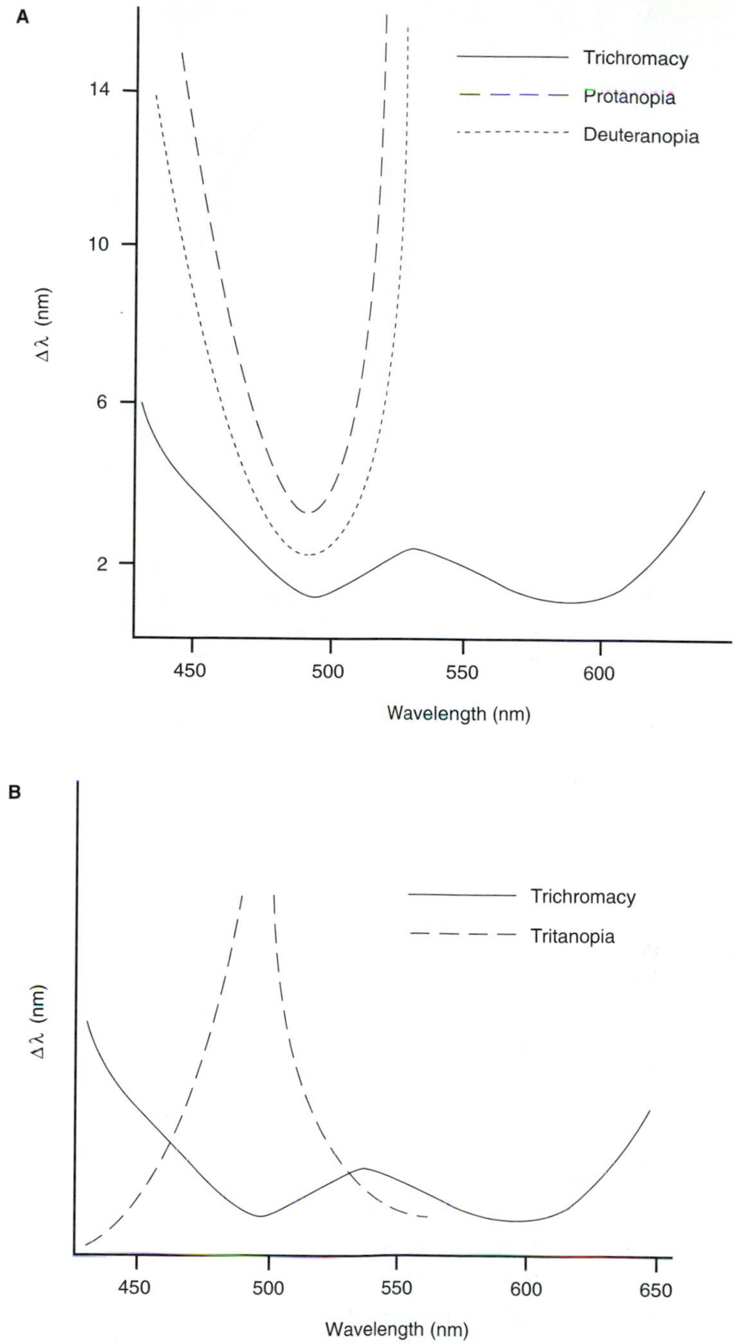


**FIGURE 6–4.** Wavelength discrimination functions for deuteranopia and protanopia **(A)** and tritanopia **(B).** The solid curves represent wavelength discrimination for a normal trichromat. (***A*** *is adapted from Pitt FHG. Characteristics of dichromatic vision with an appendix on anomalous trichromatic vision.* Great Britain Medical Report Series, *1935, No. 200.* ***B*** *is adapted from Wright WD. The characteristics of tritanopia.* J Opt Soc Am. *1952;42:509–520.*)

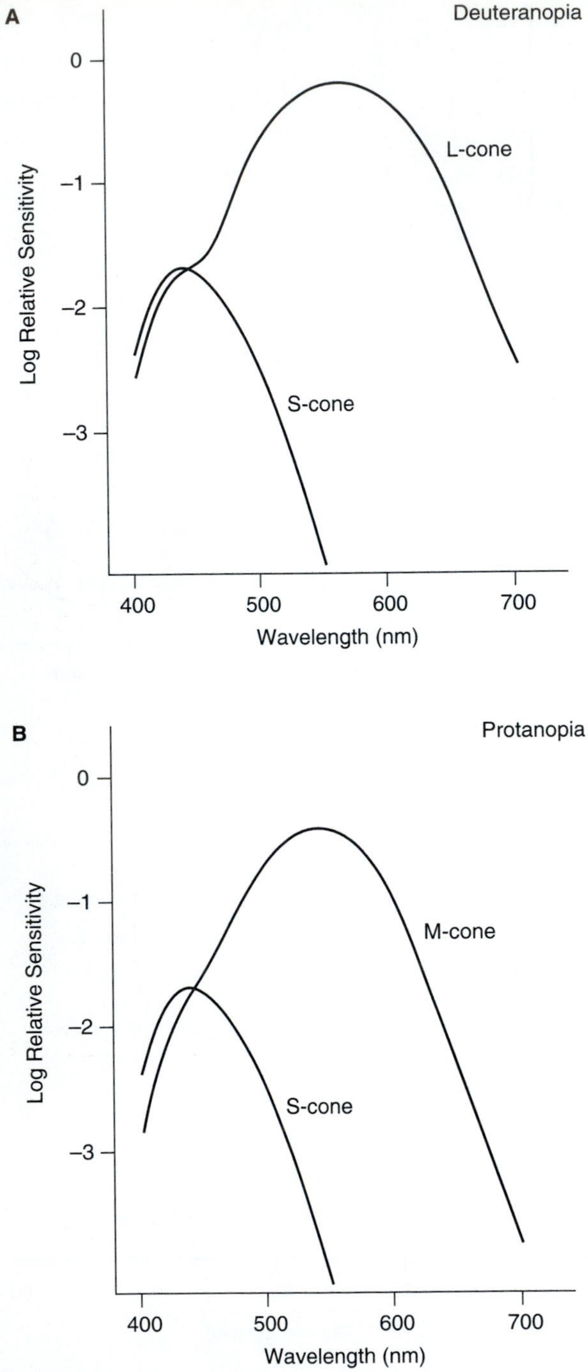


**Figure 6–5.** Approximations of the absorption spectra for the remaining photopigments in deuteranopia **(A)** and protanopia **(B).** Note that beyond about 545 nm, these dichromats are essentially monochromatic. These absorption spectra are based on the data of Smith and Pokorny (1975). (*Adapted from Boynton, 1979.*)

Figure 6–4B shows a wavelength discrimination function for tritanopia. Unlike red–green dichromats, tritanopes show good wavelength discrimination at longer wavelengths, but poor wavelength discrimination in the region of 495 nm (Wright, 1952).

### *Confusion Lines*

The color discrimination limitations of dichromats can be illustrated by plotting their color confusion lines on the CIE diagram. Confusion lines for deuteranopia, protanopia, and tritanopia are illustrated in Figure 6–6. Each of these three sets of confusion lines originate from a **copunctal point.** All colors falling along a confusion line are indistinguishable to the dichromat.

Let us take some examples. A deuteranope confuses blue-green (500 nm) with reddish purple, and a protanope confuses blue-green with red. This confusion of greens with reds is the reason that deuteranopes and protanopes are referred to as red–green dichromats. For a tritanope, stimuli of 400 nm (blue-violet) and 570 nm (yellow) are confused. Hence the term blue–yellow defect is used to describe tritanopia.

Deuteranopes and protanopes share a confusion line that is tangential to the right-side perimeter of the CIE diagram (see Fig. 6–15). This confusion line shows that red–green dichromats confuse stimuli ranging from 545 to 700 nm, and reinforces a point made in the discussion regarding wavelength discrimination. That is, red–green dichromats are monochromatic from 545 nm upward. As we will learn, this confusion line is very useful in the design of color vision tests utilized to diagnose red–green defects.

### *Saturation*

Recall from the previous chapter that not all spectral stimuli appear equally saturated. For a normal trichromat, 570 nm appears less saturated (more whitish) than do other wavelengths. The saturation function for a normal trichromat, along with those for deuteranopes and protanopes, is given in Figure 6–7A. Note that the deuteranopic function intersects the abscissa at about 498 nm, whereas the protanopic function intersects it at 492 nm. These particular wavelengths appear white, and are referred to as **neutral points.** (The neutral point for a tritanope is about 569 nm.)

The locations of the dichromatic neutral points are also given by the dichromatic confusion lines (see Fig. 6–6). All stimuli falling on a confusion line that intersects white will be confused with white. Consequently, the wavelengths that these confusion lines intersect on the CIE spectral locus are neutral points. By observation of Figure 6–6, it can be seen that the values for these neutral points are similar to those given in Figure 6–7A.

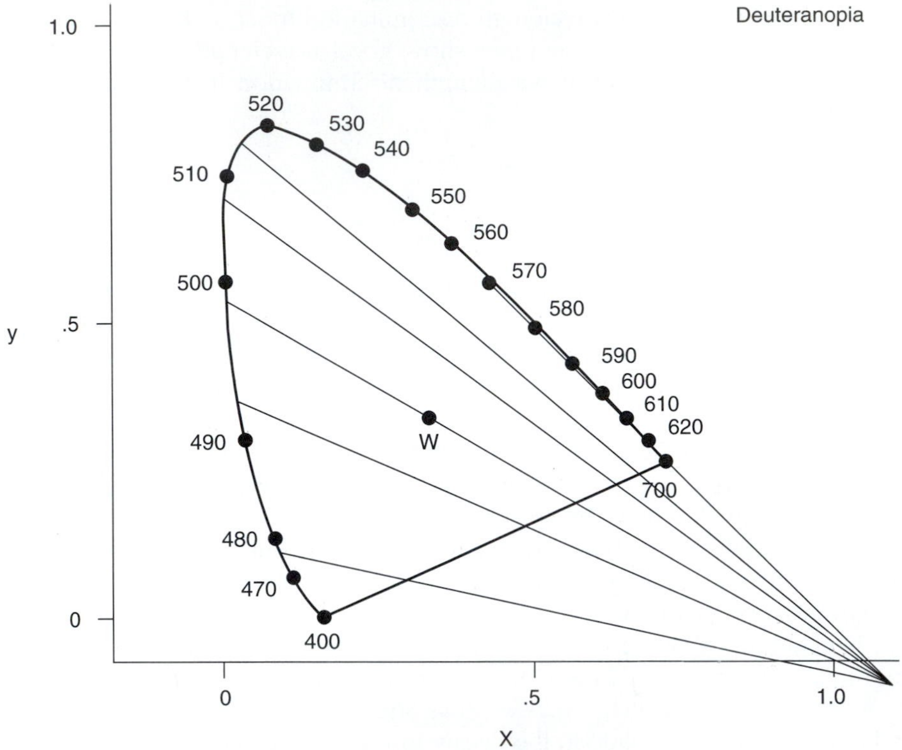


**FIGURE 6–6.** Color confusion lines for dichromats plotted on the CIE chromaticity diagram. (*Adapted from Pokorny J, Smith VC, Verriest G, Pinckers AJLG.* Congenital and Acquired Color Vision Defects. *New York: Grune and Stratton; 1979.) Continued.*

Upon questioning, dichromats often report that green traffic lights appear white (or whitish). This is because these green lights are approximate metamers for the dichromatic neutral points.

Anomalous trichromats do not manifest neutral points. They do, however, display abnormal saturation perception. This is indicated in Figure 6–7B, which shows that 498 nm is the least saturated wavelength for a deuteranomalous trichromat, whereas 492 nm is the least saturated for a protanomalous trichromat.

## COLOR LABELING

Red–green dichromats are essentially monochromatic for wavelengths beyond about 545 nm. Consequently, stimuli in this region of the spectrum are labeled on the basis of their context (apples are red) or brightness (red is perceived as dim by a protanope).

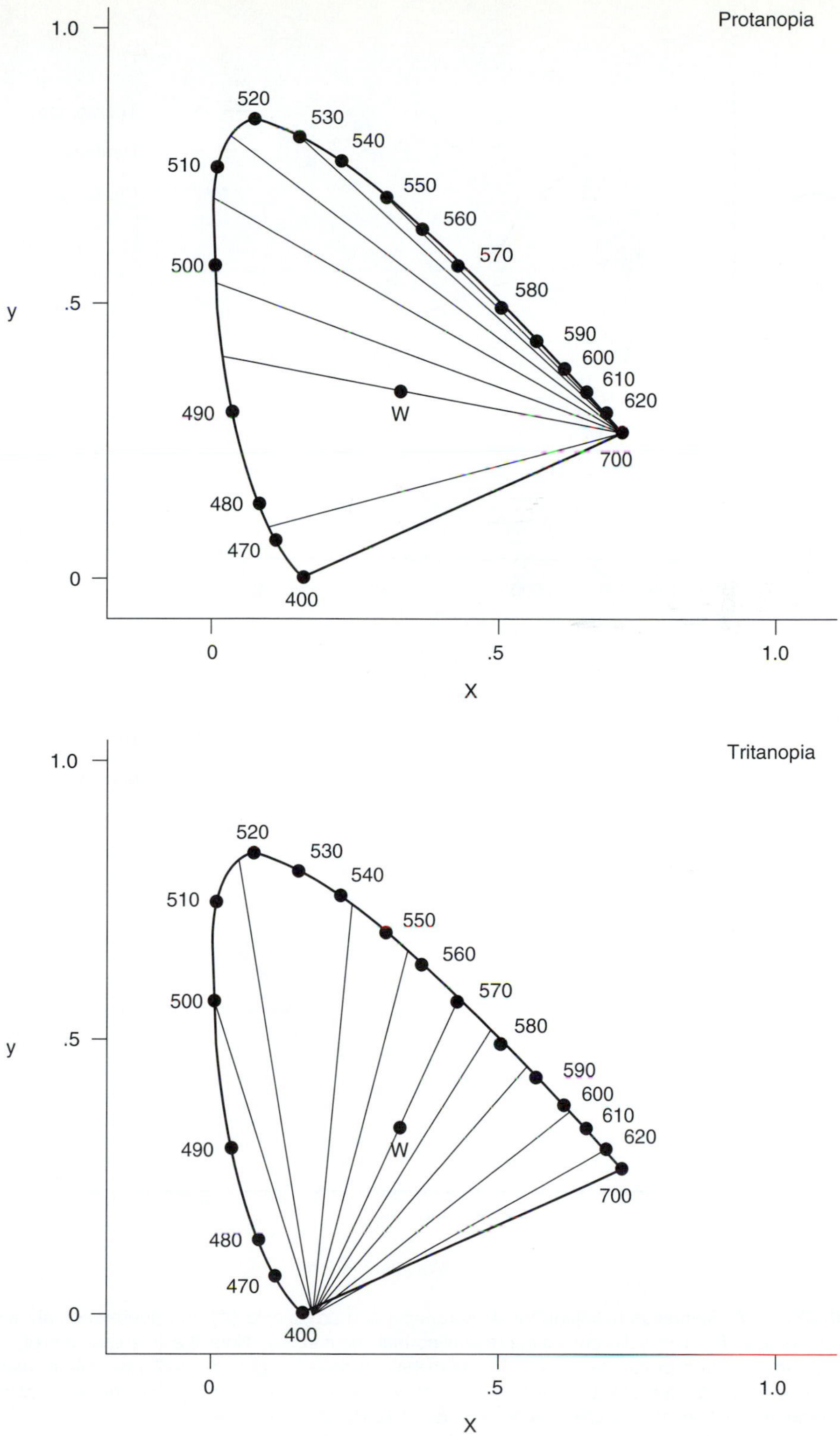


**FIGURE 6–6.** *Continued.*

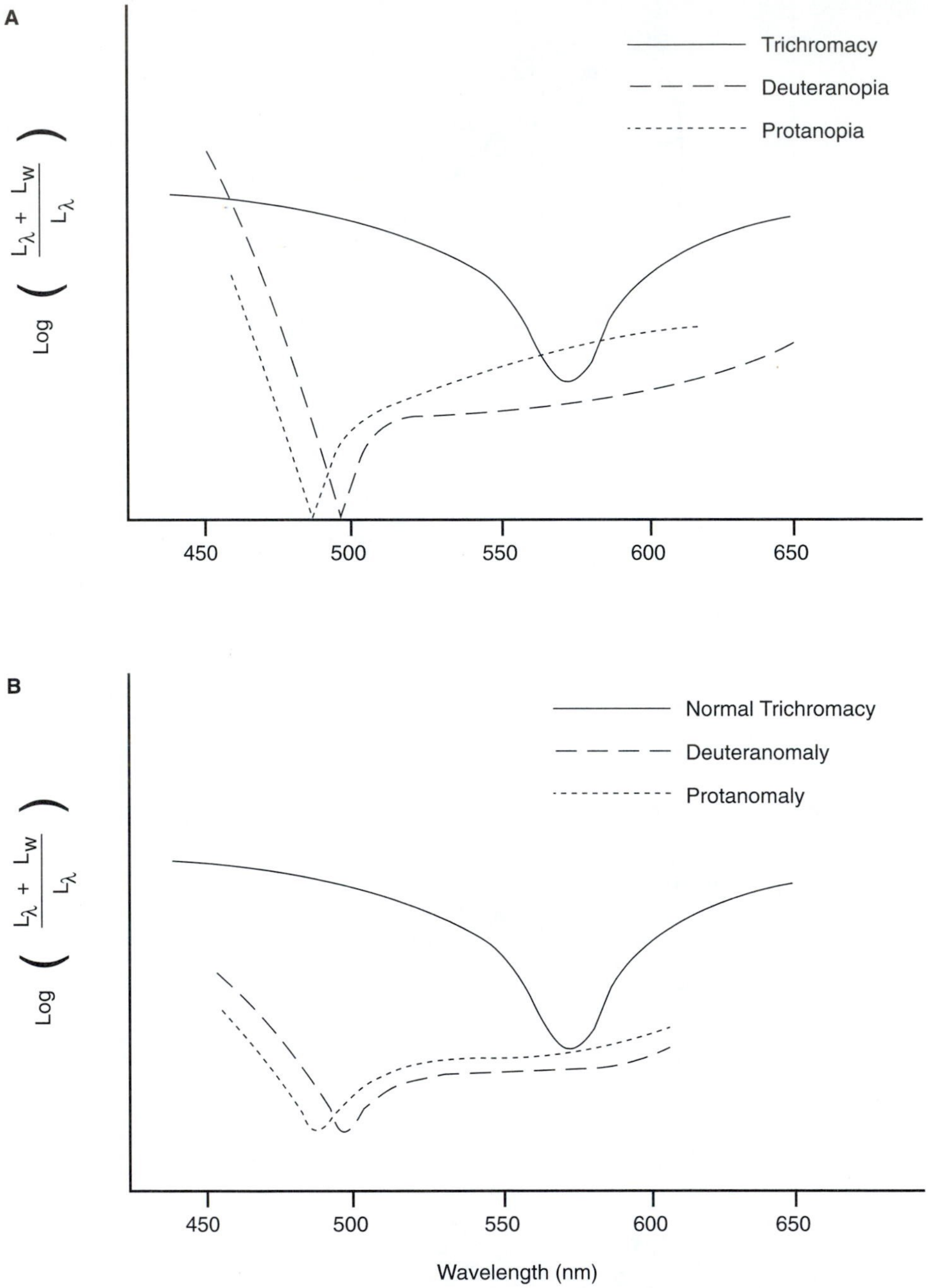


**FIGURE 6–7.** Saturation functions for deuteranopia and protanopia **(A)** and deuteranomaly and protanomaly **(B).** The solid curves represent normal trichromacy. Note the intersections of the deuteranope's and protanope's functions with the abscissa at 498 and 492 nm, respectively. These wavelengths represent the dichromatic neutral points. (*Adapted from Chapanis A. Spectral saturation and its relation to color-vision defects.* J Exp Psychol. *1944;34:24–44.*)

Color defectives, even dichromats, do remarkably well at labeling colors. This is especially true when other cues, such as context, are available. For example, a protanope has no difficulty labeling an apple as red and a banana as yellow. This is an easy task because the person has learned that others label apples as red and bananas as yellow.

Dichromats have more difficulty when labeling the colors of manufactured items, such as the pattern on a blouse or shirt. They are at a disadvantage, compared with labeling an apple, because they may not know the labels others would apply to the colors contained within the pattern. They know that others label an apple as red, but they may not know what color others label the stripes on a particular shirt. A dichromat assigns a color label to the stripes on the basis of brightness cues and, to some extent, the context in which the shirt is worn.

Consider the following example. A man is wearing a shirt with pink vertical stripes. We ask a protanope to tell us the color of the stripes. The protanope will carefully study the shirt and might label the stripes as gray. This is because the pink stripes are seen as very dim. This is interpreted by the protanope as either a red (pink) or a black (gray) color. Because a man is wearing the shirt, the protanope might assume that the stripes are gray. If, however, the context was different, the color label might well be different. For example, if a woman wore the same shirt, the protanope might label the stripes as pink.

Although a dichromat will label long-wavelength stimuli on the basis of brightness cues, we have no way of assessing what the dichromat perceives. A dichromat will label an apple as red, as will a normal color observer. We could tell the dichromat that he or she is labeling the apple as red on the basis of brightness cues, but he or she would insist that the apple appears red. Just as we cannot be certain that any two normal trichromatic individuals are experiencing the same perception when viewing a red object, we cannot be certain of what a dichromat perceives when viewing the same object.

Figure 6–8 shows how the spectrum might appear to individuals with normal color vision and various color-defective observers. The density of the vertical bars indicates wavelength discrimination; the more dense the bars, the better the wavelength discrimination. The color labels (V, B, G, Y, O, R) show the approximate regions of the spectrum that are assigned these color labels.

Consider the diagram for normal color vision. The bars are most dense in the regions of 490 and 590 nm, indicating best wavelength discrimination in these regions of the spectrum. Compare this with the diagrams for the protanopic and deuteranopic individuals. For these dichromats, the spectrum is essentially divided into two regions: a blue region and a long-wavelength "variable" region. These two regions are separated by the neutral point wavelength, which is perceived as white. The "variable" region represents that area of the spectrum over which these dichromats are monochromatic. As discussed, stimuli within this region are discriminated largely on the basis of brightness differences.

Note that the protanopic visible spectrum ends prior to that of the other individuals. This is because protanopes, who are missing erythrolabe, are unable

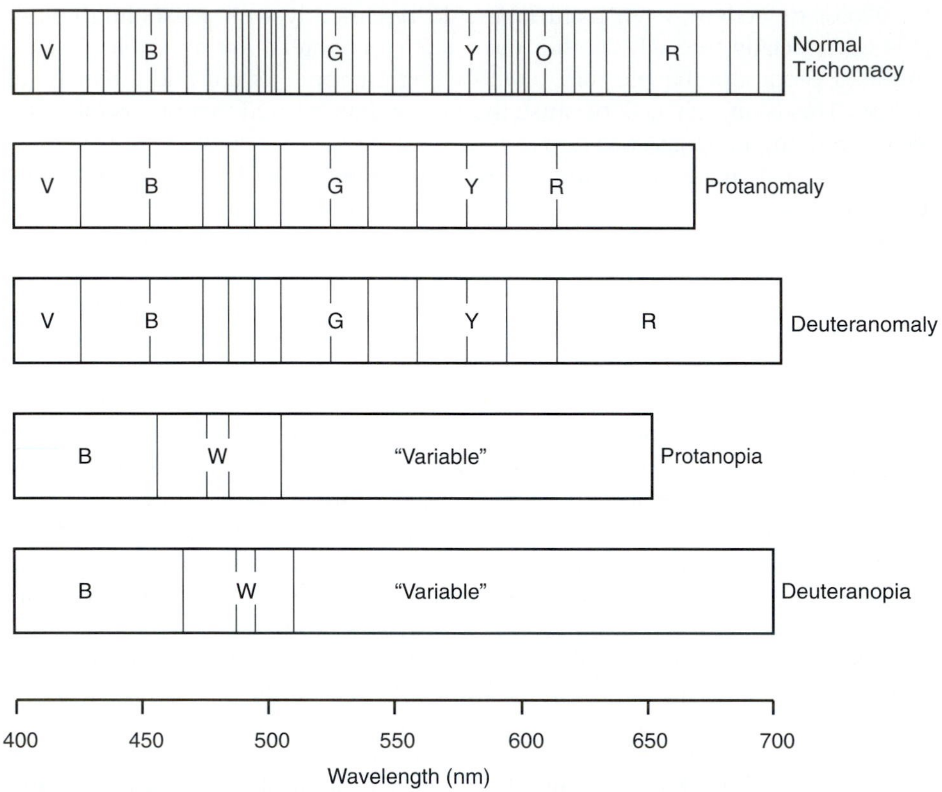


**FIGURE 6–8.** Color discrimination and color labeling by normal trichromats and the various classes of red–green color defectives. The density of the vertical lines is reflective of the individual's ability to discriminate wavelengths. Note that the spectrum for dichromats (protanopes and deuteranopes) is divided into a blue and "variable" region separated by the white neutral point. The term *variable* indicates that the subject labels these wavelengths on the basis of brightness and context cues. (*Adapted from Heath GG. Color vision. In: Wick R, Hirsch MJ (eds).* Children's Vision. *Philadelphia: Chilton; 1963.*)

to perceive longer wavelengths. These individuals (and those with severe protanomalous defects) may have difficulty seeing red tail and brake lights and red traffic lights.

Also given in Figure 6–8 are the visible spectra for protanomalous and deuteranomalous observers. These subjects display wavelength discrimination considerably superior to that of dichromats, but less developed than that of normal trichromats.

## *HEREDITARY COLOR VISION ANOMALIES*

The vast majority of red–green color defects are inherited. These defects are inherited in a sex-linked, X-linked recessive fashion (Nathans et al, 1986a; Nathans, 1989). The prevalence and inheritance of the various color deficiencies are given in Table 6–2. Note that inherited tritan defects are rare and are transmitted in an autosomal dominant fashion (Kalmus, 1955).

Because of their sex-linked inheritance, red–green defects are considerably more common in men than women. Whereas the prevalence in men is about 8 percent, only about 0.40 percent of women manifest hereditary color defects (Pokorny et al, 1979).

Figure 6–9 shows several examples of the transmission of red–green defects from parents to their offspring. When reviewing this figure, it is important to keep in mind that a heterozygous female ($\bar{X}X$) is a carrier, whereas a male with the defective gene is color defective ($\bar{X}Y$). Because the gene is recessive, a female must be homozygous ($\bar{X}\bar{X}$) to express the defect. Note that a color-defective boy always receives the defective gene from the mother. Patients often assume that color defects are transmitted from father to son.

## *THE MOLECULAR GENETICS OF RED–GREEN COLOR VISION ANOMALIES*

Recent work on the molecular genetics of color vision may explain how color vision anomalies originated in our ancestors (Nathans et al, 1986a; Nathans, 1989; Neitz and Neitz, 1994). The highly homologous genes for the M and L-cone photopigments are positioned on the X chromosome in a head-to-tail tandem array (Figure 6–10A). This arrangement suggests that erroneous crossover of genetic

**TABLE 6–2. PREVALENCE AND INHERITANCE OF THE MOST COMMON COLOR VISION DEFECTS[a]**

| Classification | Prevalence in Males (%) | Inheritance |
|---|---|---|
| Deuteranopia | 1 | X-linked recessive |
| Protanopia | 1 | X-linked recessive |
| Deuteranomaly | 5 | X-linked recessive |
| Protanomaly | 1 | X-linked recessive |
| Tritanopia and tritanomaly | 0.005 | Autosomal dominant |

[a]Note that figures given are for males.

Adapted from Krill AE. Congenital color defects. In: Krill AR, Archer DB (eds). *Krill's Hereditary Retinal and Choroidal Diseases.* Vol. II. *Clinical Characteristics.* Hagerstown, MD: Harper and Row, 1977.

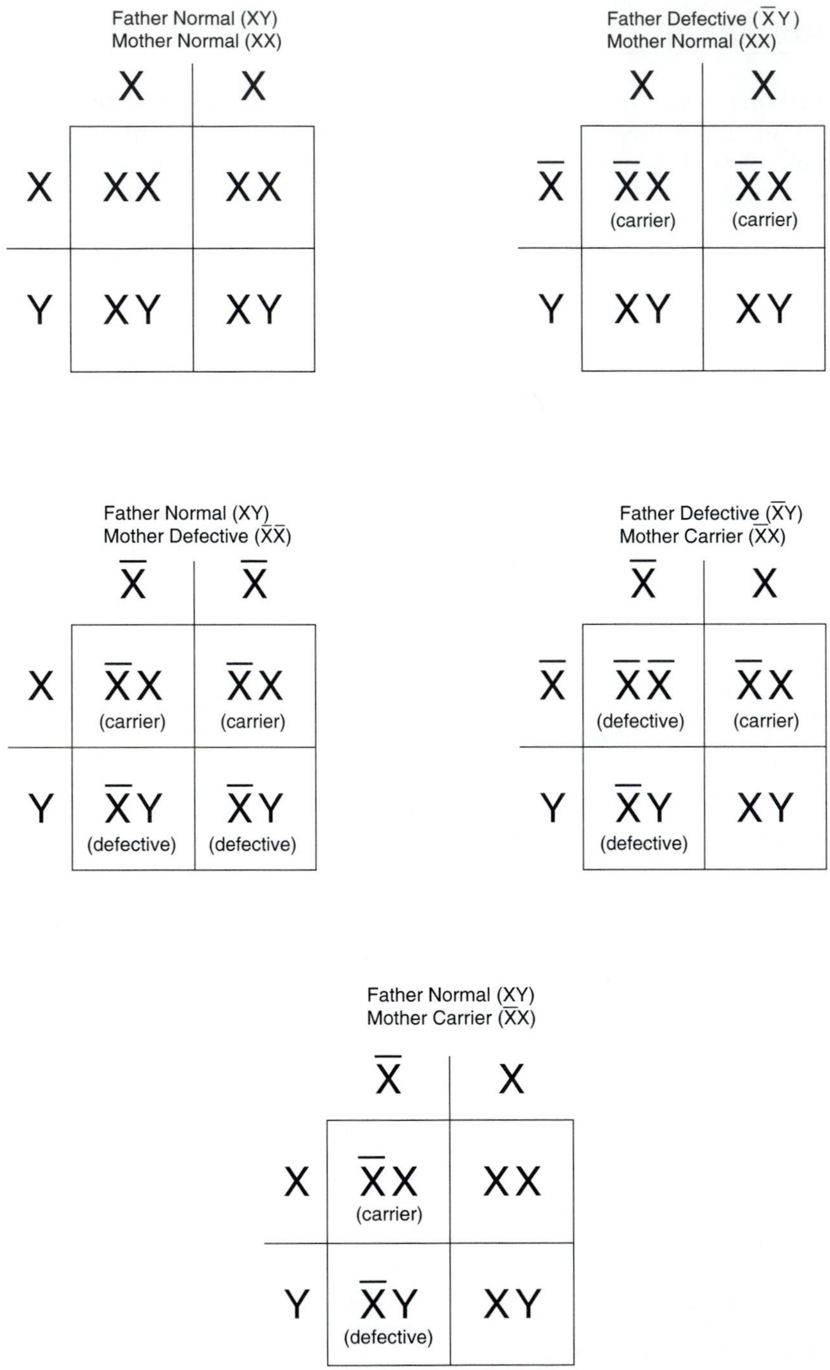


**FIGURE 6–9.** Examples of the transmission of X-linked, red–green defects from parents to offspring.

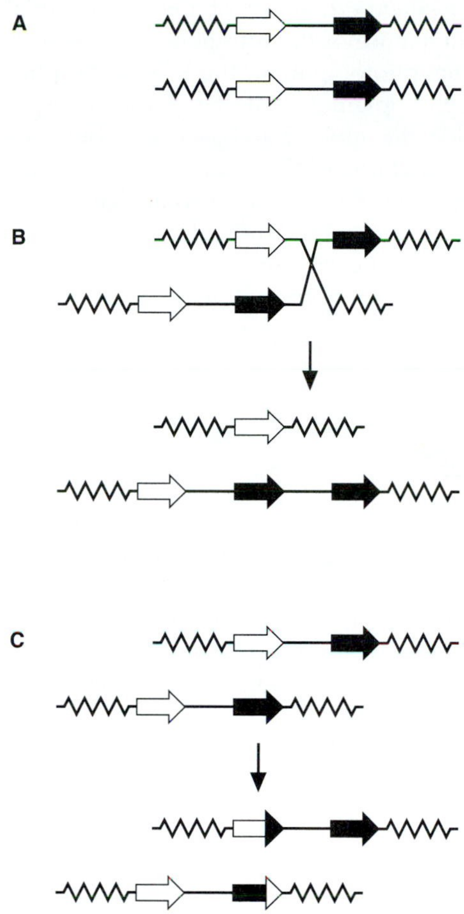


**Figure 6–10. A.** During meiosis, the L-cone photopigment and M-cone photopigment genes (white and black arrows, respectively) on one chromosome normally align the L-cone and M-cone photopigment genes on the paired chromosome **B.** Dichromacy could result when the L-cone photopigment gene erroneously aligns with the highly homologous M-cone photopigment gene, leading to the *intergenetic* crossover of the M-cone photopigment gene. As a result, one chromosome has no M-cone photopigment genes; the offspring who inherit this chromosome will be deuteranopes. The paired chromosome has one copy of the L-cone photopigment gene and two copies of the M-cone photopigment gene; the offspring who inherit this chromosome will have normal color vision. **C.** *Intragenetic* crossover results in hybrid genes (black and white arrows). Depending on the specific nature of the crossover, a hybrid gene may result in a normal photopigment, the loss of a photopigment (dichromacy), or a photopigment with an absorption spectra that is displaced from its normal location (anomalous trichromacy). (*Adapted from Nathans J. The genes for color vision.* Sci Am. *1989;260(2): 42–49.*)

information could occur when the pair of X chromosomes align and exchange genetic information during meiosis (i.e., unequal homologous recombination). For instance, the gene coding for the M-cone photopigment could mistakenly align with the gene coding for the L-cone photopigment leading to an unequal exchange of genetic information. As a result, one of the chromosomes could lose a photopigment gene. The absence of such a gene results in dichromacy.

Figure 6–10B provides an example where the gene coding for the M-cone photopigment crosses over during meiosis (*intergenetic* crossover). As a result, one of the X chromosomes does not have the gene coding for the M-cone photopigment, and the offspring that inherit this chromosome will be deuteranopes. The other chromosome has multiple copies of the gene coding for the M-cone photopigment. Offspring inheriting this chromosome will have normal color vision.

Hybrid genes result from the *intragenetic* crossover of genetic material (Figure 6–10C). Depending on the specific nature of the intragenetic crossover, the resultant hybrid gene leads to a normal photopigment, the loss of the photopigment (dichromacy), or an aberrant photopigment. The latter case is especially interesting because it could provide the molecular basis of anomalous trichromacy, where the absorption spectrum of one of the photopigments is displaced from its normal location (see Fig. 6–1). Recent data reveal that hybrid genes differing greatly from normal genes lead to severe anomalous trichromacy (the M and L-cone photopigment absorption spectra almost completely overlap), whereas hybrid genes that are more similar to normal genes lead to mild forms of anomalous trichromacy (the M or L-cone photopigment is only slightly displaced from its normal location) (Neitz et al, 1996).

## *ACQUIRED COLOR VISION ANOMALIES*

Acquired color defects are not inherited but develop secondary to a disease process or toxicity. These color vision defects may be either red–green or blue–yellow in nature. As we have learned, hereditary red–green defects are very common. Therefore, the presumption is that a clinically encountered red–green defect is inherited. However, as hereditary blue–yellow defects are so rare, it must be assumed that a blue–yellow defect is acquired until proven otherwise.

Table 6–3 summarizes the major differences between hereditary and acquired defects. These distinctions are explained by differences in the basic processes that produce hereditary and acquired defects. Hereditary defects, because they are secondary to stable physiologic variations, produce clear-cut

**TABLE 6–3. DISTINCTIONS BETWEEN HEREDITARY AND ACQUIRED DEFECTS**

| Hereditary Defects | Acquired Defects |
|---|---|
| Typically red–green | Often blue–yellow |
| More prevalent in males | Equally prevalent in males and females |
| Symmetric: same in each eye | Asymmetric: often a difference in severity between the eyes |
| Color naming errors rare | Recent history of color naming errors |
| Defect is stable with time | Defect is unstable and changes over time |
| Easily classified with standard clinical color tests | Classification often not straightforward with standard clinical color tests |
| Not associated with disease or toxicity | Associated with ocular or systemic disease or toxicity |

Adapted from Adams AJ, Haegerstrom-Portnoy G. Color deficiency. In: Amos JF (ed). *Diagnosis and Management in Vision Care.* Boston: Butterworths; 1987.

results on color vision tests and remain stable throughout life. In comparison, the pathologic processes that produce acquired defects are not stable and are variable in their course. Consequently, acquired color vision defects do not produce clean results on testing and often follow an unpredictable course.

### *Laterality*

An important distinction between hereditary and acquired defects concerns the laterality of the defect. Hereditary defects are bilateral and symmetric in their presentation. Acquired defects, however, are often present in only one eye or are asymmetric (Adams and Haegerstrom-Portnoy, 1987). Consequently, any difference in the color vision of the two eyes, as demonstrated on a color vision test, must be assumed to reflect an acquired color vision defect.

Because acquired color vision defects are asymmetric, it is important to perform color vision tests under monocular conditions. If a person is tested binocularly, a unilateral acquired defect will be missed because the test results will reflect the performance of the unaffected eye. This is an important clinical consideration.

It is best to develop the habit of performing all color vision tests under monocular conditions. The test should be first administered to the eye that is most likely to be affected by a disease process (Adams and Haegerstrom-Portnoy, 1987). A simple rule is to first test the eye with the worst corrected acuity. For instance, if the corrected visual acuities are OD 20/20 and OS 20/25, the color vision test should be first administered to the left eye. If the acuities are normal and equal, the choice of eye is generally not critical. When a color vision defect is found using this procedure, the other eye should then be tested. In this manner, it can be determined whether the defect is symmetric or asymmetric.

### *Köllner's Rule*

Köllner's rule states that those color vision defects produced by outer retinal disease and media changes will be blue–yellow defects, whereas defects secondary to disease of the inner retina, optic nerve, visual pathways, or visual cortex will be of a red–green nature (Kollner, 1912). This rule serves as a general guideline when assessing acquired defects. It is, however, not correct in every instance and important exceptions have been reported (Schneck and Haegerstrom-Portnoy, 1997). Table 6–4 provides examples of the application of Köllner's rule.

It is not uncommon for a blue–yellow defect to be present in the early stages of an eye disease, and for this blue–yellow defect to change into a red–green defect as the disease progresses. In many instances, patients with acquired color vision loss manifest both blue–yellow and red–green defects, some-

**TABLE 6–4. COLOR VISION DEFECTS PREDICTED BY KÖLLNER'S RULE ALONG WITH EXAMPLES OF CONDITIONS EXPECTED TO PRODUCE THESE DEFECTS**

| Location | Defect | Condition |
|---|---|---|
| Media | Blue–Yellow | Nuclear sclerosis |
| Outer retina | Blue–Yellow | ARMD[a] |
| | | Diabetic retinopathy |
| Inner retina | Red–Green | Leber's optic atrophy |
| | | Toxic amblyopia |
| Pathways | Red–Green | Lesions |

[a]Age-related macular degeneration

times referred to as a nonselective loss. Although Köllner's rule predicts red–green deficiencies in optic neuritis, it has recently been demonstrated that this condition is associated with nonselective defects (Schneck and Haegerstrom, 1997).

## *ACHROMATOPSIAS*

Achromatopsias are rare conditions in which the patient behaves largely as a monochromat (Pokorny et al, 1979; Adams and Haegerstrom-Portnoy, 1987). These patients typically manifest other serious visual symptoms including nystagmus, photophobia, and reduced visual acuity.

The most common achromatopsia is **rod monochromacy (typical achromacy).** The label rod monochromacy is a misnomer because these patients may have M and L-cones, but in greatly reduced numbers (Haegerstrom-Portnoy, 1991). These patients demonstrate very poor color discrimination, nystagmus, photophobia, and visual acuity of about 20/200. This condition is inherited in an autosomal recessive fashion.

Rod monochromacy is fully expressed at birth, differentiating this condition from rod–cone degenerations, such as retinitis pigmentosa, which typically develop later in life and are progressive.

Other achromatopsias include **blue cone monochromacy** and **cone monochromacy.** Blue cone monochromacy (also called incomplete congenital cone dysfunction or monocone monochromacy) is a condition in which only rods and S-cones are present. It is inherited in an X-linked recessive fashion. Symptoms and signs are similar to those of rod monochromacy. This condition is very rare.

Cone monochromacy is an exceedingly rare condition in which visual acuity is normal, yet the patient behaves as a monochromat. Although this condition is too rare to have been extensively studied, it appears to involve a defect in postreceptoral processing of color information.

## CHROMATOPSIAS

Chromatopsias are not true color vision defects since they typically do not produce a decreased ability to discriminate colors. Rather, they represent a distortion of color vision, similar to looking through a colored filter. Patients report that objects have a colored tinge or halo.

Chromatopsia frequently follows cataract extraction. A nuclear cataract acts as a yellow filter, absorbing blue light. The patient has experienced this yellow filter effect, in all likelihood, for several years. Removal of the cataract allows the retina to be exposed to considerably more blue light than it has experienced in some time. This results in the perception of blueness **(cyanopsia).** As the visual system adapts to the new distribution of radiant energy, the effect wanes.

Chromatopsias can occur secondary to various medications. For example, digitalis may produce **xanthopsia** (yellow vision). Fluorescein, used in fluorescein angiography, can also produce xanthopsia.

## STANDARD COLOR VISION TESTS

### Pseudoisochromatic Plate Tests

Pseudoisochromatic plate tests are the most commonly used color vision tests. They offer the advantages of being easy and quick to administer and comparatively inexpensive to purchase.

The tests consist of a number of plates arranged into a booklet. Vanishing plates are the most common; these plates consist of a figure that must be distinguished from the background (Fig. 6–11). Patients with normal color vision can easily distinguish the figure from the background based on chromatic differences. Patients with anomalies of color vision, however, have difficulty distinguishing the figure from the background. This is because both the colors that make up the figure and the colors that constitute the background fall on a common dichromatic confusion line (see Figs. 6–6 and 6–15). The colors are indistinguishable to color defectives; consequently, they do not see the figure that is embedded in the surround.

Pseudoisochromatic plate tests are useful for detecting red–green color vision defects. These tests, however, do not distinguish between dichromats and anomalous trichromats. In addition, they may not be reliable for differentiating protan and deutan defects, although some tests have plates designed for this purpose. For routine clinical practice, however, these limitations are of little importance.

A limitation of typical pseudoisochromatic plate tests, which is of clinical concern, is the lack of plates to test for blue–yellow defects. Although some of these tests do have tritan plates, they are the exception rather than the rule. This is an important clinical consideration because acquired color vision defects are frequently of a tritan nature.

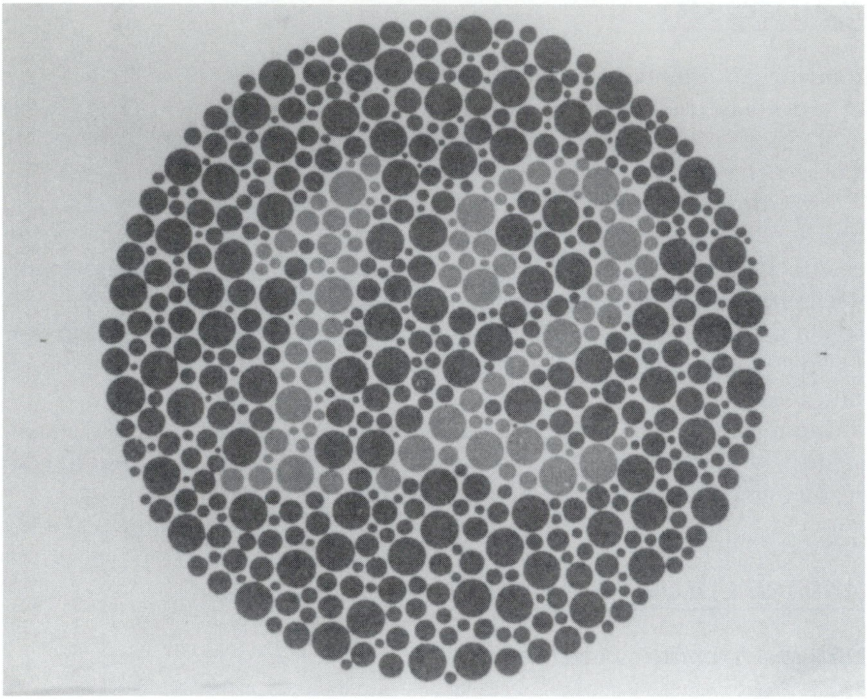

**FIGURE 6–11.** Black and white photograph of a plate used in the Ishihara pseudoisochromatic plate test.

### *Farnsworth Dichotomous Test*

The Farnsworth dichotomous test (Panel D-15) test consists of 15 colored caps (or chips) that form a hue circle within the CIE diagram (Figs. 6–12 and 6–13). The patient arranges the colored caps such that they follow an orderly progression of color. To start, the examiner asks the patient to choose the colored cap that looks most like the affixed reference cap. The selected cap is placed next to the reference, and the procedure is repeated using the selected cap as the new reference. The process continues until all caps are arranged in an orderly sequence of color. Like the desaturated D-15 test and the 100-hue test, which are described later, the Farnsworth D-15 test is referred to as an **arrangement test.**

The test is scored by connecting the cap numbers in the sequence arranged by the patient (Fig. 6–13). A color-defective individual arranges the caps such that there are crossovers on the hue circle. The axis of these crossovers will typically follow the confusion lines for either a protan, deutan, or tritan defect. Therefore, by determining the axis of the crossovers, one may determine the nature of the defect.

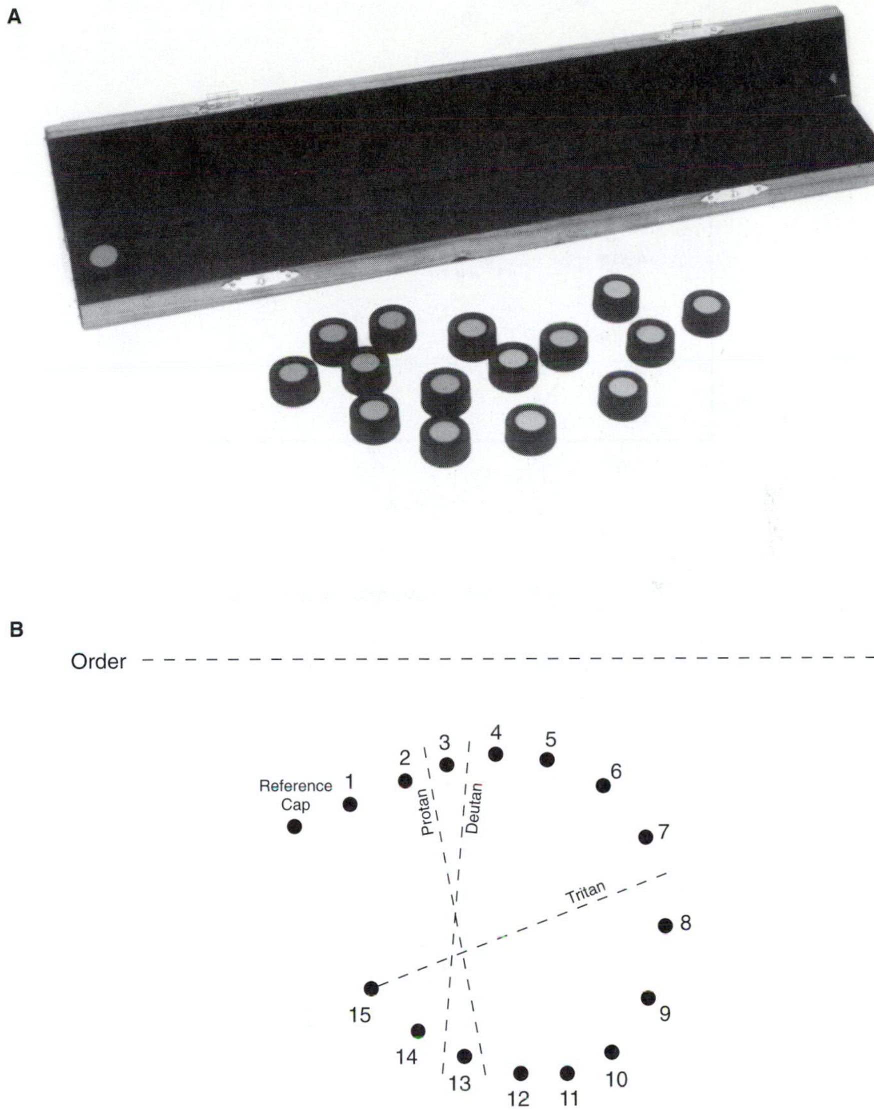


**FIGURE 6–12. A.** Black and white photograph of the Farnsworth D-15 color vision test. Note the reference cap that is affixed to the tray. **B.** Score sheet used to grade the Farnsworth D-15 test. Points are connected in a sequence corresponding to the arrangement of caps by the patient. When a defect is present, crossovers typically fall along the protan, deutan, or tritan axis.

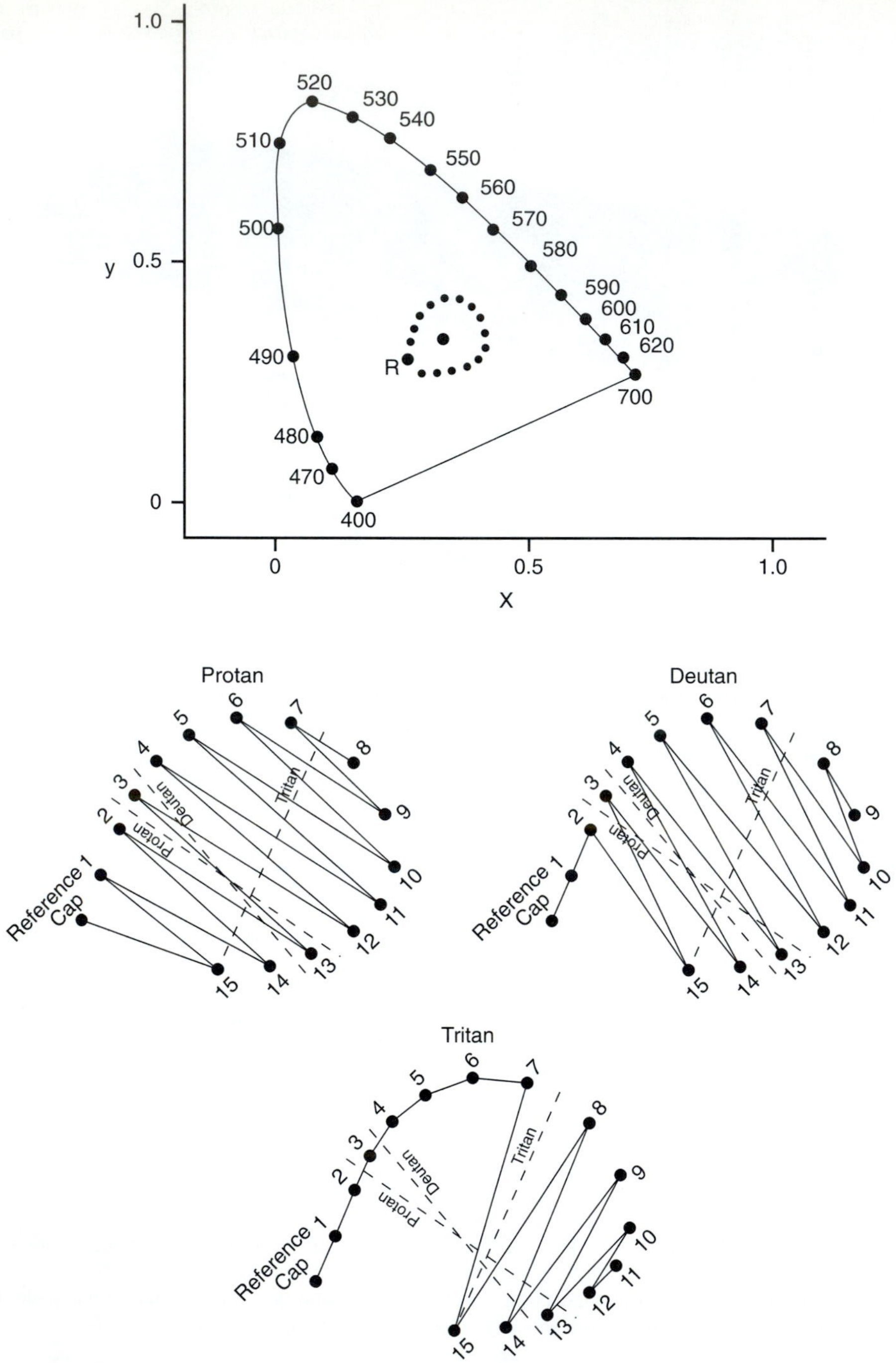


**FIGURE 6–13.** The top diagram shows the locations of the chips used for the D-15 test plotted on the CIE chromaticity diagram. These chips form a hue circle. "R" is the reference cap. The bottom three diagrams show the arrangement of caps expected by protans, deutans, and tritans. Diagnosis of the defect is made by noting the axis of the crossovers. This axis typically corresponds to the color confusion lines for protan, deutan, or tritan defects (see Fig. 6–6).

Although the Farnsworth D-15 test does allow the differentiation of protan, deutan, and tritan defects, it does not allow the differentiation of dichromats from anomalous trichromats. The anomaloscope, which is discussed later in this chapter, is the only clinical instrument that allows this diagnosis. The Farnsworth D-15 test does not detect minor defects. Certain anomalous trichromats pass the test. This is not a serious disadvantage because these minor defects are unlikely to have practical consequences for the patient. A distinct advantage of the Farnsworth D-15 test is its capacity to detect tritan defects. It is important to test for these defects because they are typically associated with eye disease or drug toxicity.

### *Desaturated D-15 Test*

The desaturated D-15 test is the same as the standard D-15 test, except that the chips are desaturated. (The chips form a hue circle with a radius that is shorter than that formed by the chips of the standard D-15 test.) Because the chips are desaturated, the task is more difficult. The desaturated test offers the advantage of detecting minor defects that would be missed by the standard test. It is especially useful in the detection of early defects that occur in certain eye diseases, such as glaucoma (Adams et al, 1982).

### *Farnsworth–Munsell 100-Hue Test*

Despite its name, the 100-hue test consists of only 85 color chips. These chips, which form a hue circle in the CIE diagram, are divided among four separate trays. The patient arranges, according to color, the chips contained within each tray. The test is scored by plotting the data on a scoring sheet and calculating a total error score. When the total error score is greater than the norms provided by the manufacturer, a diagnosis of a color anomaly is made. The axis indicates whether it is a protan, deutan, or tritan defect. Although the error score indicates the severity of the anomaly, this test does not distinguish dichromacy from anomalous trichromacy.

The 100-hue test is time consuming and expensive to purchase. For these reasons, it is rarely used in routine clinical practice. On occasion, it has industrial application for the screening of employees for color aptitude.

## THE NAGEL ANOMALOSCOPE

The Nagel anomaloscope allows the complete diagnosis of red–green defects. It is the only clinical instrument that can be used to differentiate dichromacy from anomalous trichromacy. The anomaloscope is a wonderful teaching tool. If you understand its use for the diagnosis of color anomalies, you have mastered the fundamentals of color vision.

The patient views a bipartite field through the eyepiece of the instrument (Fig. 6–14). The bipartite field is composed of an upper mixture field and a lower test field (Pokorny et al, 1979). The task is to match the mixture field to the test field.

The mixture field consists of variable amounts of 546 nm (green) and 670 nm (red). The relative amounts of 546 and 670 nm are controlled by turning a knob. If the mixture knob scale is set at zero, the mixture field consists of only 546 nm. When the mixture scale is set at 73, the mixture field consists exclusively of 670 nm. Mixture scale settings between 0 and 73 represent various combinations 546 and 670 nm. An important feature of the mixture field is that the luminance of this field, measured for a normal trichromat, does not change. Whether the mixture field consists of pure 546 nm, pure 670 nm, or any combination thereof, the luminance is the same.

The lower test field consists of 590 nm (yellow) of variable radiance. The radiance is controlled by turning a knob. A test knob scale setting of 0 represents very dim yellow, and a test scale reading of 87 represents bright yellow.

None of the Nagel anomaloscope's three primaries are absorbed by the S-cones (see Fig. 5–6). Therefore, for the region of the spectrum covered by these three primaries, normal trichromats use only two of their cones; they are dichromatic. The primaries fall along the shared deutan and protan confusion line (Fig. 6–15) and constitute what is referred to as the **Rayleigh equation** (Rayleigh, 1881).

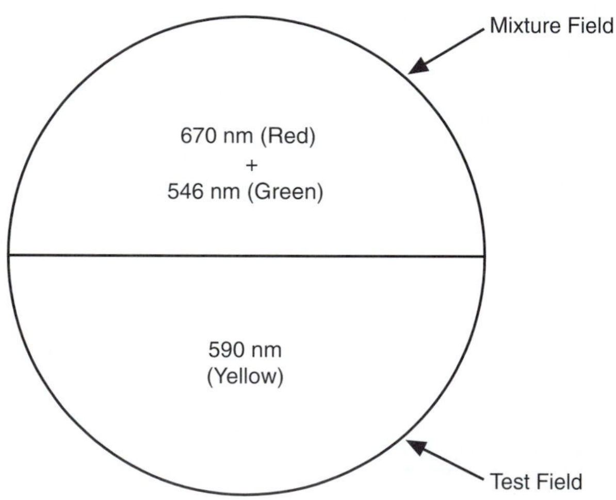


**FIGURE 6–14.** Bipartite field of the Nagel anomaloscope. The top field (mixture field) consists of 670 nm, 546 nm, or any combination of these two wavelengths. The luminance of this field, measured for a normal trichromat, does not change as the wavelength mixture is varied. The bottom field (test field) consists of 590 nm. This test field's radiance can be adjusted from a very low (dim) to a very high (bright) setting.

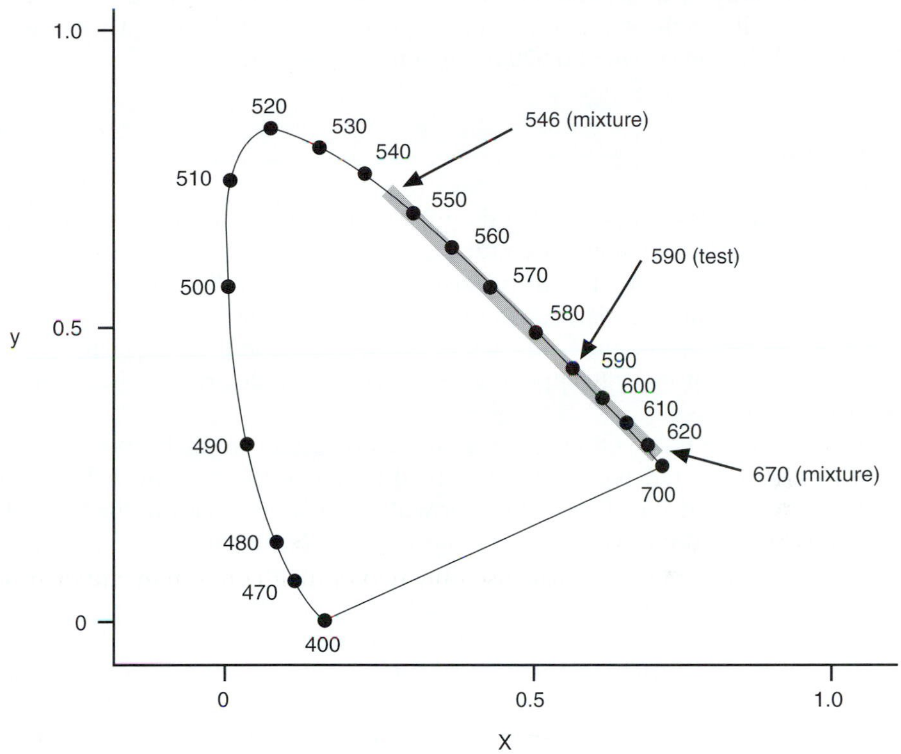


**FIGURE 6–15.** The three primaries of the Nagel anomaloscope plotted on the CIE chromaticity diagram. The line formed by connecting these three primaries corresponds to a color confusion line shared by deuteranopes and protanopes. (*Adapted from Pokorny J, Smith VC, Verriest G, Pinckers AJLG.* Congenital and Acquired Color Vision Defects. *New York: Grune and Stratton; 1979.*)

### *Normal Trichromats*

When asked to match the mixture and test fields so that they appear identical, a normal trichromat adjusts the mixture field such that it appears yellow. He or she then adjusts the radiance of the test field to match this mixture field. Normal trichromats will generally set the mixture scale to a value of about 45 and the test scale to about 17. Although there is some variability between individuals with normal color vision, the variability is not very large.

This is a simple color matching procedure, similar to those discussed in the previous chapter. As a normal trichromat is dichromatic from about 545 to 700 nm, he or she is able to match any single wavelength (in this case 590 nm) by combining two other wavelengths (546 and 670 nm).

Another way of understanding this match is to examine Figure 6–15. Note that 590 nm falls on the straight line that connects 546 and 670 nm. Therefore, a proper combination of 546 and 670 nm will match 590 nm.

### Dichromats

***General Principles.*** Suppose that the mixture field is set to pure 546 nm, and a dichromat is asked to adjust the radiance of the 590-nm test field such that it matches the mixture field. The dichromat will be able to adjust the radiance of the test field such that it matches the mixture field. When viewed by a person with normal color vision, the fields will not appear matched; the top will appear green and the bottom will appear yellow. Yet, to a dichromat they appear matched.

If the mixture field is then set at pure 670 nm, and the dichromat is again asked to adjust the radiance of the test field to match the mixture field, he or she will be able to do so. To an observer with normal color vision, the top field will appear red and the bottom field yellow, but to the dichromat, they appear matched. In fact, no matter what combination of 546 and 670 nm is present in the mixture field, the dichromat will be able to adjust the radiance of the 590-nm test field such that it matches the mixture field.

The preceding matching behavior occurs because all three anomaloscope primaries fall upon a shared protan and deutan confusion line (see Fig. 6–15). The three primaries appear identical to a red–green dichromat when their radiances are properly adjusted. Another way to understand this is to remember that, for the wavelengths used, dichromats behave as monochromats. From about 545 to 700 nm, dichromats have only one responsive photopigment (see Fig. 6–5). In this region of the spectrum, any two wavelengths can be matched by adjusting their relative radiances. Therefore, a stimulus of 546 nm, 670 nm, or any combination thereof will match 590 nm of the proper radiance.

***Deuteranopes Versus Protanopes.*** A deuteranope will match any mixture field setting with a test field setting of about 17. This occurs because the luminosity function of a deuteranope (see Fig. 6–3) is similar to that of a normal subject. Since the luminance of the mixture field is designed to remain constant for a person with normal color vision as the field is adjusted from 546 to 670 nm, a deuteranope (with a similar luminosity function) does not perceive a change in brightness. Consequently, the deuteranope does not need to change the radiance of the test field to maintain a match.

A protanope has a luminance function very different than that of a person with normal color vision. Observing Figure 6–3, we see that the protanopic luminosity function is displaced toward shorter wavelengths. Consequently, the 546 and 670-nm mixture field stimuli will not have the same luminance. The 670-nm stimulus appears very dim, whereas the 546-nm stimulus appears bright. Therefore, a protanope adjusts the 590-nm test field to a very low radiance when matching 670 nm and to a relatively high radiance when matching 546 nm.

In summary, both deuteranopes and protanopes are able to adjust the radiance of the test field such that it matches any mixture field (546 nm, 670 nm, or any combination of these two wavelengths). Deuteranopes keep the radiance of the test field constant for all mixture field combinations. This is because the luminance of the mixture field remains approximately constant for deuteranopes. Protanopes, however, find it necessary to reduce the radiance of the test field when matching 670 nm and to increase it when matching 546 nm. This is because the protanopic luminance function is displaced toward shorter wavelengths relative to a normal (or deuteranopic) observer's luminance function.

### *Anomalous Trichromats*

***General Principles.*** If asked to adjust the mixture field so that it has the same color as the test field, anomalous trichromats generally select a mixture scale setting different than that selected by normal trichromats. For example, a deuteranomalous trichromat may set the mixture scale at 20, rather than the normal 45. The deuteranomalous trichromat must add more 546 nm than a normal trichromat because of his or her displaced M-cone phototpigment spectrum (see Fig. 6–1). In comparison, a protanomalous trichromat may set the mixture scale at 60. This mixture field has more 670 nm than is required by a person with normal color vision because of the displacement of the L-cone photopigment spectrum in protanomaly.

A normal trichromat sets the mixture scale at about 45. If we were to adjust the mixture field to 50 and ask the individual (a normal trichromat) to adjust the yellow test field to obtain a match, he or she would not be able to do so. To this individual, the top would appear reddish and the bottom yellow. He or she would be unable to adjust the radiance of the yellow test field such that it matches the reddish mixture field.

Anomalous trichromats are less specific in their matches. Consider, for example, a protanomalous trichromat who matches the yellow test field by adjusting the mixture scale to 55. If we were to readjust the mixture scale to 70, the subject might still be able to adjust the test field so that it matches the mixture field. This protanomalous trichromat would, however, manifest more specificity in his or her match than a protanope. If the mixture field was adjusted to pure 546 nm, the protanomalous individual would not be able to match the test field to the mixture field, whereas a protanope would be able to do so.

***Deuteranomaly Versus Protanomaly.*** We have discussed one important feature that allows the differentiation of deuteranomaly and protanomaly, the mixture scale setting. Deuteranomalous trichromats add extra amounts of 546 nm to the mixture field. This is reflected by mixture scale settings typically between 0 and 40. Protanomalous trichromats, on the other hand, add more 670 nm to the mixture field. This results in mixture scale readings that range from about 50 to 73.

The test field setting is also useful in distinguishing deuteranomaly from protanomaly. A deuteranomalous person manifests essentially the same luminosity function as an individual with normal color vision. Consequently, he or she adjusts the test scale to a normal setting, about 17. A protanomalous observer, however, has a luminance function similar to that of a protanope; it is displaced toward shorter wavelengths. Because a protanomalous trichromat adds much 670 nm to the mixture field to match the yellow test field, the mixture field appears dim. To match this dim mixture field, the protanomalous trichromat sets the test field radiance to a low value, less than 15.

The anomaloscope results expected for various classes of color-defective observers are summarized in Table 6–5. Figure 6–16 presents these results graphically. These results are predictable based on an understanding of the principles of normal color vision and the anomalies of color vision.

## *ADDITIONAL CLINICAL CONSIDERATIONS*

### *Inherited Defects*

Although hereditary color vision defects remain stable throughout life and pose no threat to vision, they can interfere with the performance of many visually related activities. Of particular concern is the effect that hereditary color vision anomalies may have on the performance of elementary school children. School lessons, in the elementary grades, are sometimes taught through the use of color-

**TABLE 6–5. SUMMARY OF EXPECTED RESULTS USING THE NAGEL ANOMALOSCOPE TO DIAGNOSE RED–GREEN COLOR DEFECTIVES[a]**

| | Mixture Field | | Test Field | |
|---|---|---|---|---|
| *Condition* | *Setting* | *Appearance to a Normal Trichromat* | *Setting* | *Appearance to a Normal Trichromat* |
| Normal trichromat | 45 | Yellow | 17 | Yellow |
| Deuteranope | Any setting from 0 to 73 will be matched | Green (0) to yellow (45) to red (73) | 17 | Yellow |
| Protanope | Any setting from 0 to 73 will be matched | Green (0) to yellow (45) to red (73) | 35–5 | Bright to dim yellow |
| Deuteranomaly | 0–45 | Greenish | 17 | Yellow |
| Protanomaly | 45–73 | Reddish | 10 | Dim yellow |

[a]The appearances given are those reported by a normal observer, not a color defective. Values given are approximations.

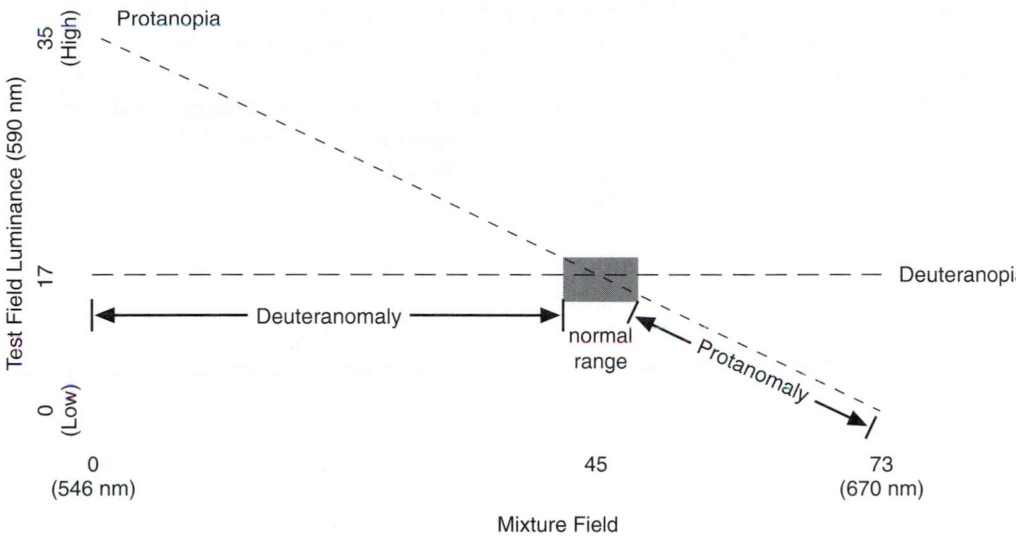


**FIGURE 6–16.** Anomaloscope results presented graphically. As indicated by the dashed line, a deuteranope matches all mixture fields with a constant test field luminance. The protanope is also able to match all mixture fields; however, he or she must adjust the luminance of the test field. The protanope increases the luminance of the test field when matching 546 nm, and decreases it when matching 670 nm. Anomalous trichromats reject the normal match and add either 546 nm (deuteranomaly) or 670 nm (protanomaly). The protanomalous observer needs to reduce the luminance of the test field as he or she adds 670 nm. The deuteranomalous observer does not need to adjust the luminance of the test field as he or she adds 546 nm.

coded visual aids. A color-deficient child may be at a serious disadvantage when such teaching methods are used. Occasionally, a child with a color vision anomaly is labeled as a slow learner. This label could produce psychological trauma that lasts a lifetime.

For this reason, it is important that all school-age children be screened for color deficiencies. A pseudoisochromatic plate test or the D-15 should be administered at the child's first eye examination. Because these defects remain stable, it is typically not necessary to repeat the test on subsequent visits. The parents should be reassured that color vision defects are common, stable, and pose no threat to vision. Parents should be encouraged to have their other children tested because of the hereditary nature of color vision deficiencies. The child's teacher and the school administration should be notified of the color deficiency. They should be informed that color-coded learning tasks may pose an undue burden for the child.

Parents often ask if a color vision defect will limit their child's occupational options. Certain occupations related to public safety (e.g., airline pilot, firefighter) may have specific color vision standards that would be difficult for individuals with color vision defects to meet. For other professions, including electrical engineering, pharmacy, optometry, ophthalmology, dentistry, and surgery, normal color discrimination can be an advantage.

Individuals with red–green defects may have difficulty distinguishing between colors that are dark (e.g., socks) or desaturated (pastels) if these colors fall along the red–green confusion lines (Table 6–6). The ability of protans and deutans to discriminate and name colors is improved by increasing the level of illumination (Adams and Haegerstom-Portnoy, 1987).

Protan defects have been associated with an increased frequency of rear-end automobile accidents due to the diminished abilty to see red tail and brake lights (Birch, 1993). Protans may also have difficulty seeing red traffic lights.

### *Acquired Defects*

It is best to screen adults with a test that detects acquired defects, which are often blue–yellow in nature. The D-15 test is suitable for this purpose.

It is recommended that all patients be screened on their first visit to an office. This establishes baseline information that can serve as a reference. As was discussed previously, testing should be performed monocularly, first testing the eye with the worst corrected visual acuity or the eye suspected of manifesting a disease process. When a defect is found, the other eye should be tested to determine if the defect is symmetric or asymmetric.

**TABLE 6–6. COLORS FREQUENTLY CONFUSED BY DEUTANS AND PROTANS**

| |
|---|
| Light grayish purple (mauve)—Gray |
| Pink—Gray |
| Green—White |
| Green—Gray |
| Light yellowish brown (beige)—Green |
| Dark purplish red (maroon)—Brown |
| Olive—Brown |
| Light green—Light yellow |
| Light green—Light orange |
| Light yellow—Light orange |
| Light yellowish green (chartreuse)—Pink |
| Light purple—Light blue |
| Light orange—Light red |

Adapted from Adams AJ, Haegerstrom-Portnoy G. Color deficiency. In: Amos JF (ed). *Diagnosis and Management in Vision Care.* Boston: Butterworths; 1987.

### *Lighting Conditions for Color Vision Testing*

Commonly used color vision tests are designed to be administered under standard illuminant C lighting conditions. The **MacBeth lamp** provides illumination very similar to that provided by illuminant C and serves as an excellent light source for administering color vision tests. Unfortunately, this lamp is expensive and not readily available.

If an unfiltered incandescent source is used, it is likely that the patient will perform better than if the proper illumination were utilized. Because of its uneven wavelength profile, standard fluorescent lighting is generally not advisable (Adams and Haegerstrom-Portnoy, 1987).

Several practical lighting options are available for routine clinical practice. A nonstandard fluorescent tube, the Varilux F15T8/VLX, appears to provide appropriate illumination for color vision testing (Rodenstock and Swick, 1974). If an incandescent source is used, the patient should view the test through an appropriately colored filter that renders the lighting conditions suitable (Higgins et al, 1978). Alternatively, color vision testing can be performed using (indirect) sunlight (Adams and Haegerstrom-Portnoy, 1987).

### *X-chrom Lens and Colored Filters*

The X-chrom lens is a tinted contact lens that is worn on one eye. This colored lens changes the absorption spectrum of the eye on which it is worn. Consequently, alternately viewing objects with the eye that is wearing the filter and the other eye essentially doubles the effective number of retinal photopigments. The result is that a dichromat behaves as a tetrachromat.

The details of this lens were discussed in Chapter 5. It was pointed out that a disadvantage of this contact lens is that patients do not routinely view objects alternately with their two eyes. Rather, they view objects with both eyes simultaneously. This can result in a fused image that provides no advantage in color discrimination. It is equivalent to viewing an object with both eyes simultaneously through a large colored filter.

It has been claimed that the X-chrom lens improves color vision. These claims are often based on improved performance on pseudoisochromatic plate tests. The same claim has also been made for binocular viewing through a large colored filter. Although it is true that a patient wearing an X-chrom lens, or viewing binocularly through a large colored filter, may perform better on a plate test, this does not indicate improved color discrimination. It does show that these filters shift the dichromatic confusion lines to a new location. The patient is still a dichromat, but the standard plate test is not designed for this "new" type of dichromat. An appropriately redesigned plate test could, however, detect this individual's dichromacy.

Color-defective patients occasionally come to an eye exam carrying a filter, typically a red filter. The patient claims that this filter assists them in making color discriminations. If used properly, this red lens can indeed be useful. The patient uses the red filter to distinguish objects that they cannot normally distinguish. For example, an electrical technician may have difficulty distinguishing two color-coded wires; however, when viewed through the red filter, these wires are more easily differentiated.

For those patients for whom color discrimination is important, it is appropriate to recommend a colored filter. Proper use of the filter should be demonstrated in the office. It is critical that the patient understand that the filter will be useful only if objects are alternatively viewed with and without the filter. The comparison between the filtered and unfiltered views is the key element.

Spectacles with colored lenses are generally not recommended. As improvement in color discrimination using colored filters is due to a comparison of the filtered with the nonfiltered condition, the patient would need to compare his or her vision with and without the spectacles. This is inconvenient, and there is a tendency for these patients to leave the glasses on; this generally offers no advantage.

## SUMMARY

Color vision defects are frequently encountered in clinical practice. These defects are detectable with available clinical tests.

Patients with hereditary defects should receive counseling with respect to the nature of their defect. This involves reassurance and practical suggestions that may be of use in a school or work setting.

Acquired defects are typically secondary to eye disease. The detection of such defects during routine screening should alert the clinician to the possibility of ocular pathology. In those instances where pathology is already suspected, the finding of an acquired defect may prove useful in confirming a diagnosis.

# Self-Assessment Questions

1. A color-defective patient is unable to read the numbers given in a pseudoisochromatic plate test. **A.** Will he or she be able to read these numbers when viewing them through a red filter? **B.** Explain your answer.

2. A normal trichromat matches the mixture and test fields in the Nagel anomaloscope. **A.** Will the two fields appear matched when they are viewed through a red filter? **B.** Describe the appearance of the mixture and test fields when viewed through this red filter. **C.** Explain these results.

3. A normal trichromat matches the mixture and test fields in the Nagel anomaloscope. He or she then observes a large, bright red, adapting light for several minutes. Following this red adaptation, he or she observes the original match. **A.** Does the match between the mixture and test field still hold? **B.** Describe the appearance of the mixture and test fields. **C.** Provide an explanation.

4. A rod monochromat is tested on a Nagel anomaloscope. **A.** Describe the test field settings that are expected to match 546 and 670 nm. **B.** Explain your answer.

# 7

# Spatial Vision

When we speak of spatial vision, we refer to the visual system's ability to detect and analyze changes in brightness across space. The perception of borders, lines, and edges are all examples of spatial vision tasks. Indeed, spatial vision is so central to our visual experience, it is hard to conceive of meaningful vision without it.

The clinical measurement of spatial vision is of fundamental importance in routine eye care. Virtually all patient visits include the determination of visual acuity, a spatial vision task. Visual acuity is a highly sensitive measure of visual function; one of the first signs of many disorders and diseases of the visual system is a reduction in visual acuity.

## *How Do We Study Spatial Vision?*

Spatial vision is exceedingly complex. How do we study such a complex process? The key is to choose the proper stimuli. These stimuli must be simple and capable of serving as building blocks to construct more complex stimuli. The stimuli that scientists have chosen to study spatial vision are sine wave gratings.

A photograph of a sine wave grating is given in Figure 7–1 along with its luminance profile. The grating consists of alternating bright bars and dark bars. Note that the peak of the luminance profile corresponds to a bright bar of the grating, whereas the trough of the profile corresponds to a dark bar. The transition from bright to dark bars is a gradual (sinusoidal) transition, not an abrupt transition.

## *Characteristics of a Sine Wave Grating*

To fully describe a sine wave grating, it is necessary to specify four attributes of the grating. These four attributes are frequency, contrast, phase, and orientation.

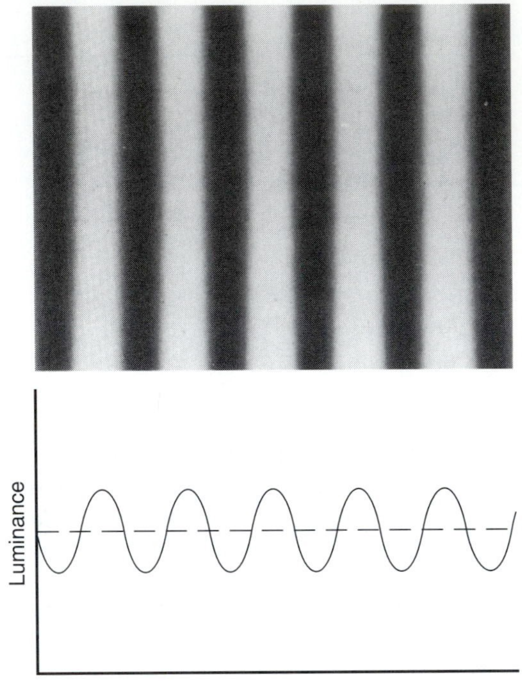


**FIGURE 7–1.** A sine wave spatial grating (top) and its luminance profile (bottom).

### *Frequency*

Compare the two gratings in Figure 7–2. In the space taken up by the photograph, there are more alterations, or cycles, in the bottom grating. Therefore, this bottom grating is said to have a high spatial frequency, while the top grating has a low spatial frequency.

The spatial frequency of a grating can be specified by giving the number of cycles per degree of visual angle (e.g., 30 cycles per degree) or the number of cycles per unit of space (e.g., 4 cycles per centimeter). As we shall see, the specification of spatial frequency in terms of cycles per degree offers many practical advantages.

### *Contrast*

The top of Figure 7–3 shows a grating of low contrast along with its luminance profile. The bottom of this figure shows a grating of the same spatial frequency, but of a higher contrast. The dashed line across the luminance profiles represents the average luminance of the gratings (the average of the peaks and troughs). Note that the average luminance ($l_{ave}$) is the same for both gratings.

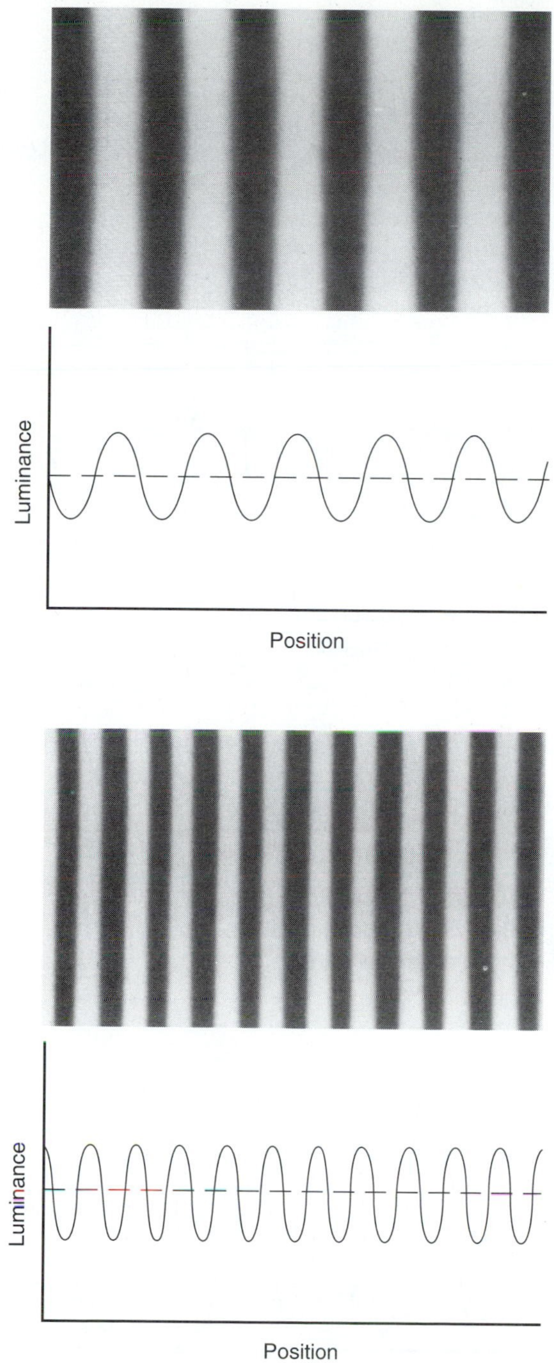


**FIGURE 7–2.** A low-frequency spatial grating (top) and a higher-frequency grating (bottom). Both gratings have the same contrast.

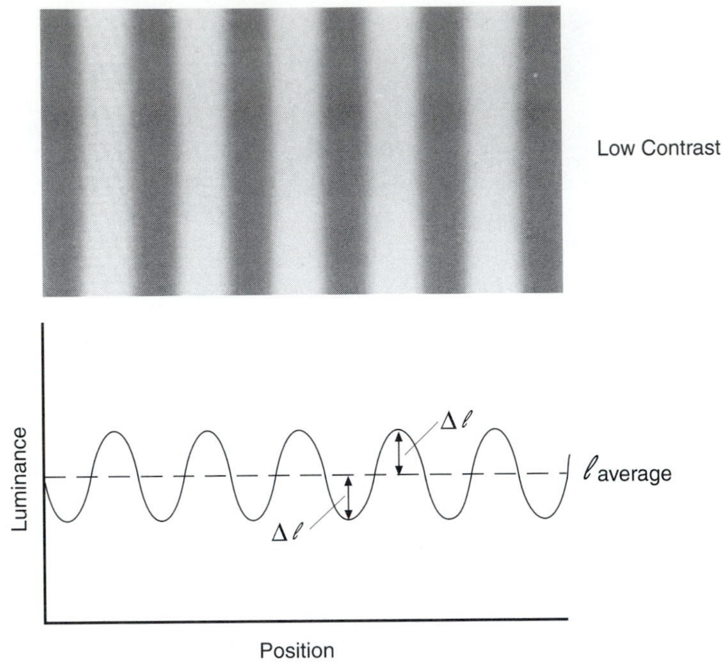


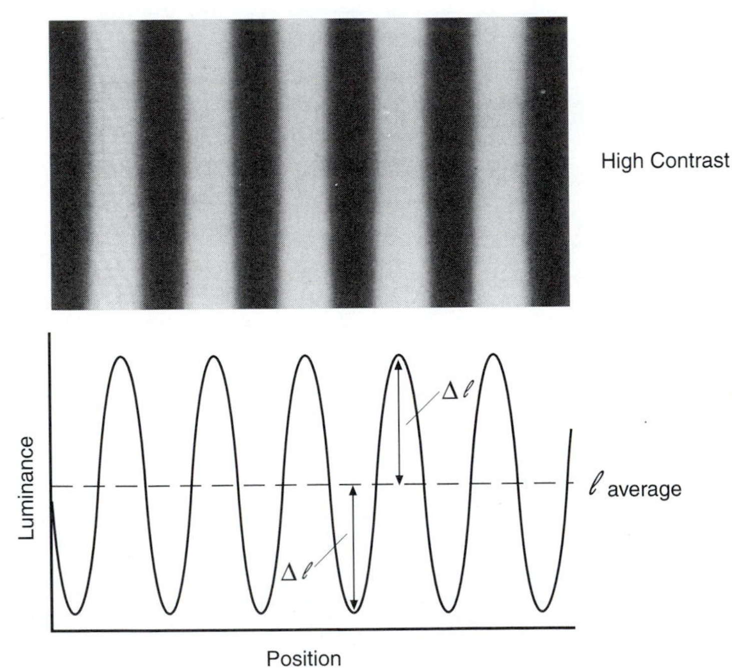


**FIGURE 7–3.** A low-contrast spatial grating (top) and a higher-contrast grating (bottom). Both gratings are of the same spatial frequency.

The grating on the bottom, however, has a larger difference between its peak and the average luminance value, giving it a higher contrast.

Contrast is often defined by way of a formula:

$$\text{contrast} = \frac{\Delta l}{l_{ave}} \qquad (7\text{–}1)$$

where

$\Delta l$ = the difference in luminance between the peak (or trough) and the average luminance ($l_{ave}$)

$l_{ave}$ = the average luminance of the grating (the average of the light peaks and dark troughs)

This formula states that contrast is the ratio of the difference between the peak luminance and average luminance to the average luminance. Although this formula is useful in defining and understanding contrast, it is not very practical for the measurement of contrast. In the laboratory, the scientist may find it easiest to measure the peak luminance ($l_{max}$) and the minimum luminance ($l_{min}$) and, from these values, calculate the contrast. The formula used is

$$\text{contrast} = \frac{l_{max} - l_{min}}{l_{max} + l_{min}} \qquad (7\text{–}2)$$

where

$$l_{max} = l_{ave} + \Delta l$$
$$l_{min} = l_{ave} - \Delta l$$

It can be demonstrated that Formula 7–2 provides the same result as Formula 7–1. Substituting for $l_{max}$ and $l_{min}$ we have

$$\frac{(l_{ave} + \Delta l) - (l_{ave} - \Delta l)}{(l_{ave} + \Delta l) + (l_{ave} - \Delta l)} = \frac{\Delta l}{l_{ave}}$$

It should be clear from examining Figure 7–3 and the preceding formulas, that contrast ranges between 0 percent and 100 percent. Contrast cannot be greater than 100 percent because of the physical impossibility of making $\Delta l$ greater than $l_{ave}$. (The trough of the luminance profile is at zero luminance when $\Delta l = l_{ave}$. It is not possible to have less than zero luminance.)

### *Phase and Orientation*

Phase refers to the position of a sine wave grating with respect to another sine wave grating. For instance, if two gratings are in phase, the peaks and troughs of their luminance profiles will be in alignment. If two gratings are 180 degrees out of phase, the peak of one luminance profile will be aligned with the trough of the other profile.

Orientation describes the angle made by a grating with respect to a reference, such as the horizontal. For the purposes of this chapter, only examples where all gratings are of the same orientation are presented.

## FOURIER ANALYSIS: BASIC INTRODUCTION

Sine wave gratings offer a unique advantage to the scientist interested in spatial vision. This advantage is that sine waves of the proper frequency, contrast, phase, and orientation can be used to construct any other spatial stimulus. This process is referred to as **Fourier analysis** or **linear system analysis.**

Although it may not be intuitively obvious, any black and white scene can be constructed of sine waves. A black and white photograph of a house, forest, or face can be thought of as consisting of sine waves of the appropriate frequency, contrast, phase, and orientation. To construct a complex visual stimulus, such as a face, from sine waves is complicated, and we will not attempt to do so in this text. Using the same principles, however, we can use sine waves as building blocks to construct relatively simple objects.

Consider the grating in Figure 7–4. This is a square wave grating. The luminance profile for this grating shows that there is an abrupt change in luminance between bright and dark bars. (This is sometimes referred to as a "step" change in luminance.) The appearance and the luminance profile of this square wave grating are very different from those of a sine wave grating. It turns out, however, that like any other complex spatial stimuli, a square wave can be constructed by adding together appropriate sine waves.

Figure 7–5 shows how this is done. We see that the progressive addition of appropriate sine waves produces a spatial profile that looks like a square wave. The primary sine wave, which is of the same frequency as the square wave, is referred to as the fundamental sine wave. The low contrast sine waves are referred to as harmonics. (The third harmonic has three times the frequency of the fundamental and one third of its contrast, the fifth harmonic has five times the fundamental frequency and one fifth of its contrast, and so on.) The addition of the fundamental sine wave, and just a couple of odd numbered harmonics (third and fifth), produces a wave that is almost indistinguishable from a square wave. (An exact square wave could be produced by adding up the fundamental and all odd numbered harmonics out to infinity.) Constructing a square wave is a far cry from constructing a face. The same principles, however, apply in both cases.

## SPATIAL MODULATION TRANSFER FUNCTION OF A LENS

A spatial modulation transfer function (SMTF) tells us how well an optical lens (or system) transfers information; it describes the quality of the optical image produced by the lens. In this section, we learn how a SMTF is determined for a lens, such as a spectacle lens. In the next section we see how these same principles can be applied to the visual system as a whole.

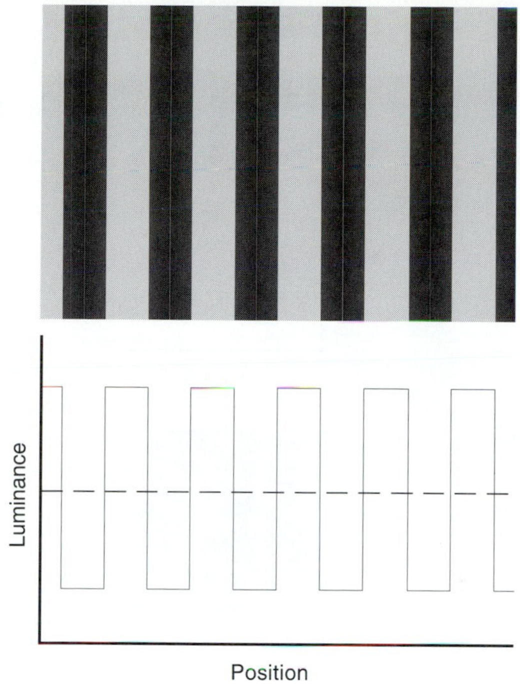


**FIGURE 7–4.** A square wave grating and its luminance profile.

Figure 7–6 schematically illustrates how we would go about determining the SMTF for a lens. A grating of a specified spatial frequency serves as the object. This grating has a known contrast. An image of this grating is produced by the lens and its contrast is measured. (This image is in perfect focus.) The ratio of the image contrast to the object contrast is then calculated. This ratio tells us how well the lens transfers the information (contrast) contained in the object. If the lens were perfect (and no lens is perfect) the image contrast would equal the object contrast; there would be no loss of information. In reality there is some image degradation, and this results in the image contrast being less than the object contrast.

This procedure is repeated for a spectrum of spatial frequencies ranging from low spatial frequencies to high spatial frequencies. The result is a SMTF such as is represented by the solid line in Figure 7–7. You may think of this function as representing the quality of the reproduction of the image as a function of spatial frequency.

The form of the SMTF given in Figure 7–7 is characteristic of an optical lens. The optical image is transferred with good fidelity (little image degradation) at low and moderate spatial frequencies. At high frequencies, however, the image becomes more degraded. This is due to the aberrations inherent in

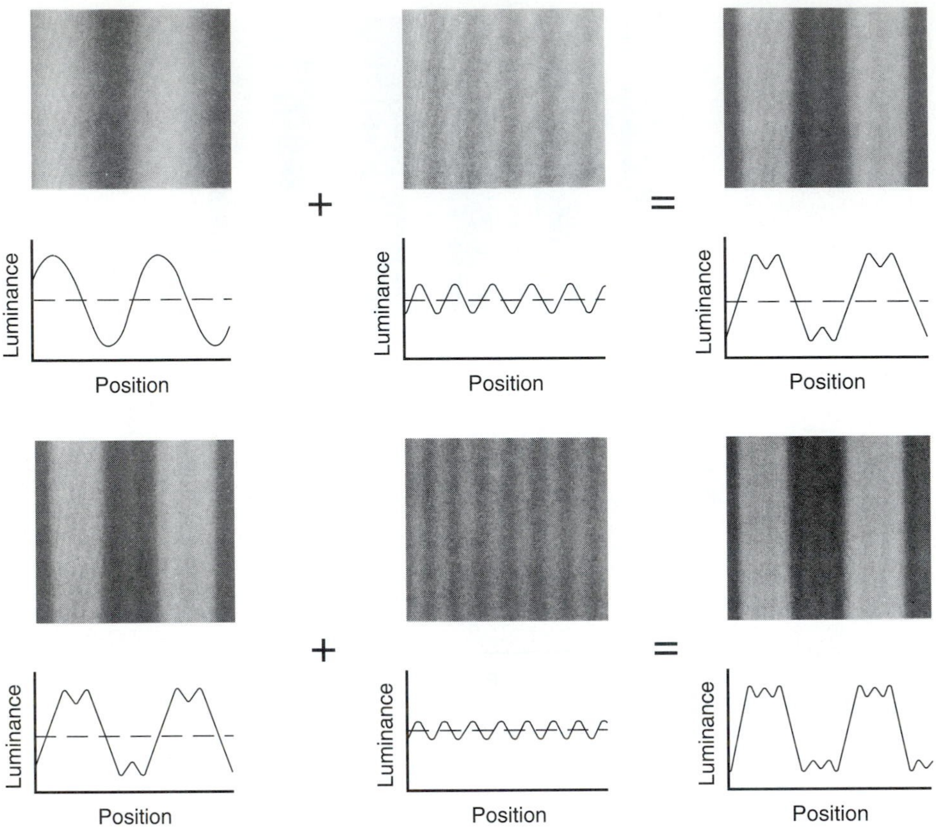


**FIGURE 7–5.** Construction of a square wave grating from the appropriate combination of sine wave gratings. (*Adapted from Levine MW, Shefner JM,* Fundamentals of Sensation and Perception. *2nd ed. Pacific Grove, CA: Brooks/Cole; 1991.*)

any optical system. These same aberrations have comparatively little effect on optical image quality at low and moderate spatial frequencies.

An important clinical consideration concerns the effect of optical defocus on the SMTF. The solid line in Figure 7–7 shows the SMTF for a lens in perfect focus. The dashed curve shows the SMTF for the same lens when the image is out of focus. (For example, the image screen is moved away from the plane of focus.) Note that this results in a reduction in image quality primarily at high spatial frequencies; the low and moderate frequencies are less affected. A key point

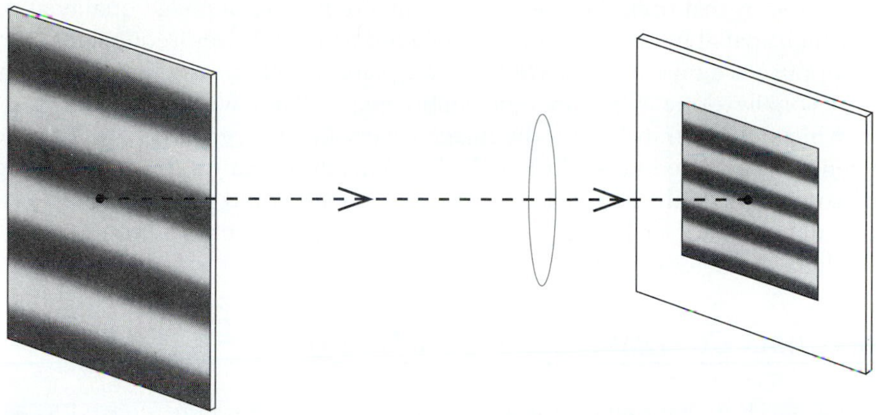

**FIGURE 7–6.** A spatial grating is focused by an optical lens to determine the spatial modulation transfer function for the lens. (*Adapted from Cornsweet T.* Visual Perception. *New York: Academic Press; 1970.*)

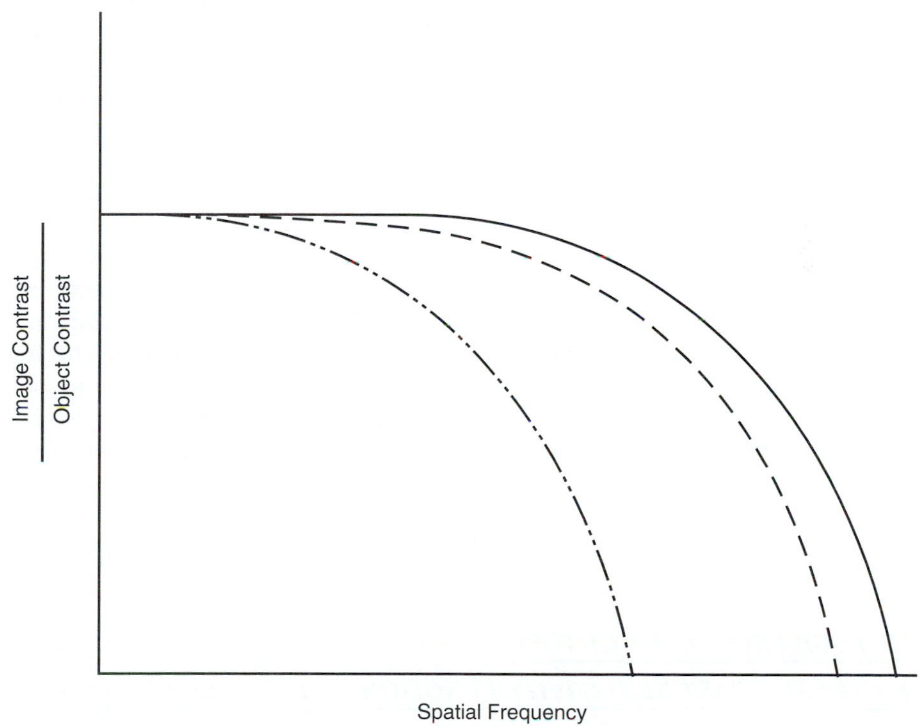


**FIGURE 7–7.** The solid line represents the spatial modulation transfer function (SMTF) for an optical lens in focus. The dashed line is for the same lens when out of focus. The dash-dotted line represents the SMTF for a translucent lens.

to remember is that optical defocus results in a reduction of image quality at primarily high spatial frequencies and less of a reduction at lower frequencies.

Suppose we take a spectacle lens and paint it with clear nail polish. (This is occasionally done when treating amblyopia.) When we look through this lens, which is now translucent, the image is very much degraded. The SMTF for this lens (dash-dotted curve in Fig. 7–7) reveals an overall reduction in image contrast at all spatial frequencies. This effect, which could also be obtained by roughening the surface of the lens with sandpaper, is largely due to the scattering of light at the lens surfaces.

## THE HUMAN CONTRAST SENSITIVITY FUNCTION

When a SMTF is determined for a human observer, it is often referred to as a contrast sensitivity function (CSF) rather than a SMTF. This is because the test involves a psychophysical determination of contrast sensitivity for sine wave gratings rather than the objective measurement of the physical contrast of gratings.

To determine a CSF, an individual is presented with a sine wave grating (on a computer screen) of a given spatial frequency. Initially this grating is below threshold. It has such a low contrast that the person does not see a grating. Instead, he or she sees a screen of even luminance across its surface. The examiner increases the contrast of the grating until a point is reached where the individual reports seeing the grating. The grating appears to emerge out of the background. This represents the contrast threshold for this grating. (The contrast sensitivity is the reciprocal of this threshold value.) This procedure is repeated for a large number of different spatial frequencies. The result is a graph that shows contrast sensitivity as a function of spatial frequency, a CSF.

A typical CSF is shown in Figure 7–8. (Note that the coordinates are plotted in log units.) The human CSF is a band-pass function; it shows a distinct peak sensitivity and decreasing sensitivity on either side of this peak (Campbell and Robson, 1968). A typical CSF peaks in the region of 4 cycles/degree. The human visual system is most sensitive to this frequency; it will detect a grating of 4 cycles/degree at a contrast lower than that required for the detection of other frequencies. This can be visualized by observing Figure 7–9 which shows, from left to right, gratings of increasing spatial frequency. From bottom to top, the contrast increases. Note that gratings of moderate frequencies are seen at lower contrast levels (lower on the diagram) than are other frequencies.

## THE HIGH-FREQUENCY CUTOFF OF THE CONTRAST SENSITIVITY FUNCTION

The CSF shows a reduction in sensitivity for both low and high spatial frequencies. The origins of these reductions in sensitivity tell us a great deal about the operation of the visual system.

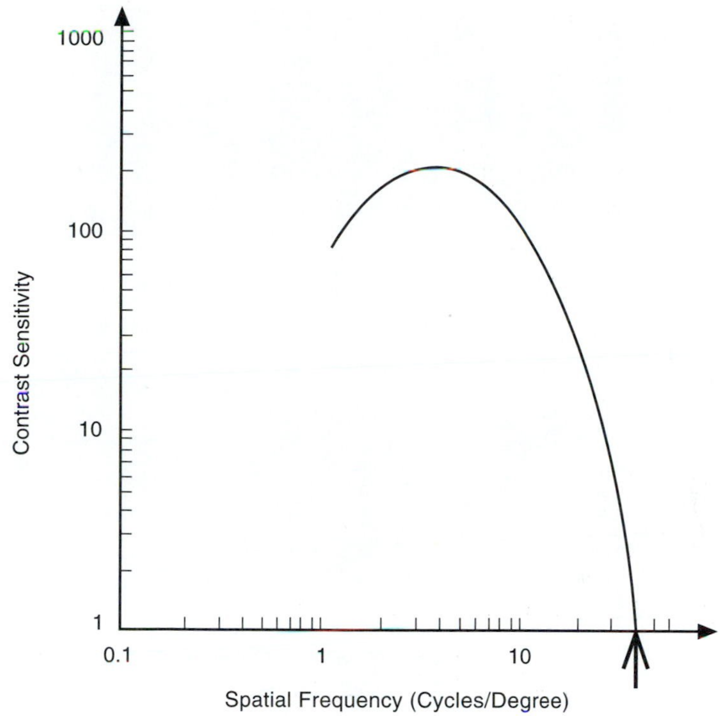


**FIGURE 7–8.** Typical human contrast sensitivity function. The arrow points to the high-frequency cutoff. The abscissa represents 100 percent contrast. (Contrast sensitivity is the reciprocal of percent contrast.)

The high-frequency cutoff in sensitivity reveals that there is a finite limit to the visual system's ability to resolve detail. As a spatial grating is made of a higher and higher frequency (the grating becomes finer), a point is reached where the grating can no longer be resolved, even at 100 percent contrast. For a young, healthy adult, the high-frequency cutoff can be about 60 cycles/degree. (This is represented by the arrow in Fig. 7–8.)

This high-frequency limitation is equivalent to the patient's clinically measured visual acuity. Visual acuity is determined by requiring a patient to resolve the details of special visual characters (optotypes), such as stylized letters of the alphabet. The optotypes on an eye acuity chart (Fig. 7–10) are presented at a very high contrast. Even with this high-contrast eye chart, there is a limit to the patient's ability to see small (high-frequency) letters. In this acuity task we are, essentially, determining the high-frequency cutoff of the patient using a 100 percent contrast target. (As we will learn later in this chapter, there are several forms of visual acuity; the form of acuity measured with a standard eye chart is referred to as recognition acuity.)

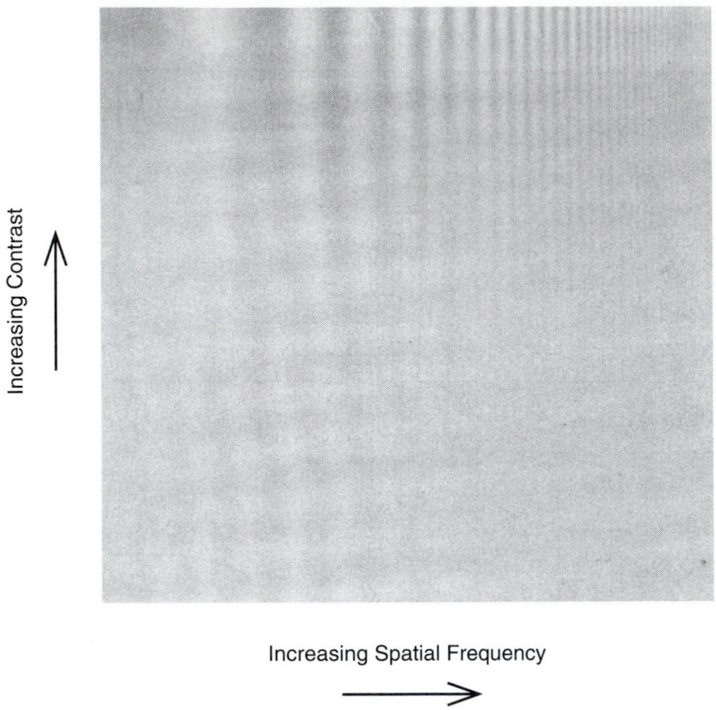


**FIGURE 7–9.** A plate that demonstrates the contrast sensitivity function. Note that when held at arm's length, moderate spatial frequencies are seen at lower contrasts than low or high spatial frequencies. (*Adapted from Cornsweet T.* Visual Perception. *New York: Academic Press; 1970.*)

Figure 7–11 illustrates the relationship between visual acuity, as measured in a standard eye exam, and the CSF. The gratings are at 100 percent contrast. Directly above these gratings is a horizontal row of optotypes at 100 percent contrast. These letters diminish in contrast as they approach the envelope of the CSF. In a typical acuity measurement, all letters would be at 100 percent contrast (or close to it). The patient would be instructed to read the smallest letter (of 100 percent contrast) that he or she can resolve.

This illustration demonstrates a limitation of typical acuity measurements; only a small portion of the patient's CSF is examined. A typical acuity task does not assess the patient's ability to detect moderate spatial frequencies even though we are most sensitive to these frequencies. (That is, we are able to see a moderate frequency of 4 cycles/degree at a lower contrast than a high-frequency acuity target of 30 cycles/degree.) This is an important concept and we return to it later in this chapter.

Why does the visual system show this high-frequency reduction in sensitivity? We have already discussed one reason, optical limitations. Any optical system,

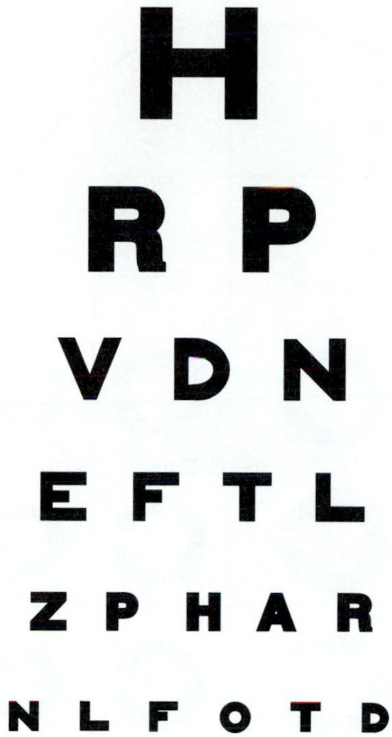


**FIGURE 7–10.** Acuity chart.

including the eye, will show a high-frequency limitation because of inherent optical aberrations. This is the case even when the eye is in perfect focus.

Another factor that plays a role in the high spatial frequency cutoff is the packing density of retinal photoreceptors. Consider the schematic illustrations of photoreceptors packed at low and high densities in Figure 7–12. A grating is superimposed on each of these matrices of photoreceptors. If it is assumed that each photoreceptor sums up all the light that falls on it, it is hard to imagine how the coarse matrix given on the left could resolve this grating. The finer matrix of photoreceptors could, however, resolve this grating. This is because the photoreceptors are packed sufficiently dense to allow bright bars to fall on alternate rows of photoreceptors. When stated more formally, this is referred to as the **Nyquist theorem** (Williams, 1986).

### *The CSF in Uncorrected Refractive Errors*

What happens to the high-frequency cutoff in the case of an eye that is out of focus, such as an uncorrected myopic eye? The result is predictable based on the earlier discussion regarding the effect of defocus on the SMTF of a lens;

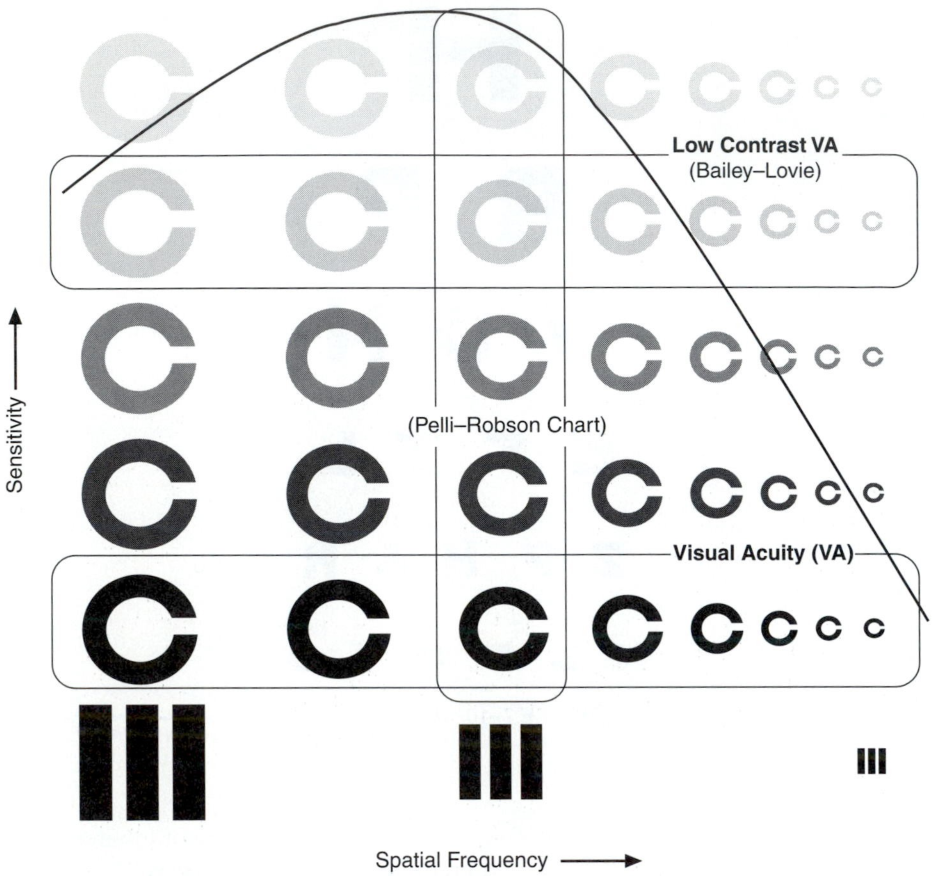


**FIGURE 7–11.** The contrast sensitivity function (CSF) forms an envelope for optotypes (letters) of various contrast and size. The optotype **C** and the spatial gratings, along the bottom, are at 100 percent contrast. Contrast decreases as the envelope of the CSF is approached. Note that a horizontal array of low-contrast optotypes, of diminishing size, serve as the stimuli for the Bailey–Lovie chart. For the Pelli–Robson chart, all stimuli are the same size, but of diminishing contrast. This is represented by a vertical column of optotypes. (*Reproduced with permission from Adams AJ, Impact of emerging instrumentation on optometry.* Optom Vis Sci. *1993;70:272–278.*)

there is a reduction in high-frequency sensitivity. The solid curve in Figure 7–13 shows the CSF for a myope who is fully corrected, and the dashed curve shows the CSF for the same myope without spectacles. Note that the uncorrected condition results in the CSF intersecting the abscissa of the graph, which represents 100 percent contrast, at a lower frequency than when corrected. This is consistent with our common sense understanding that an uncorrected myope has reduced visual acuity.

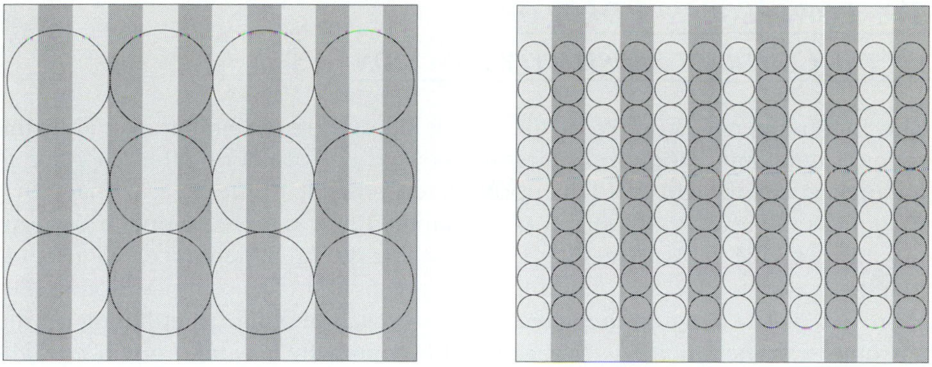

**FIGURE 7–12.** A spatial frequency grating projected on a coarse photoreceptor matrix (left) and on a finer photoreceptor matrix (right). The finer matrix would enable resolution of the grating because the bright bars of the grating fall on every other row of photoreceptors.

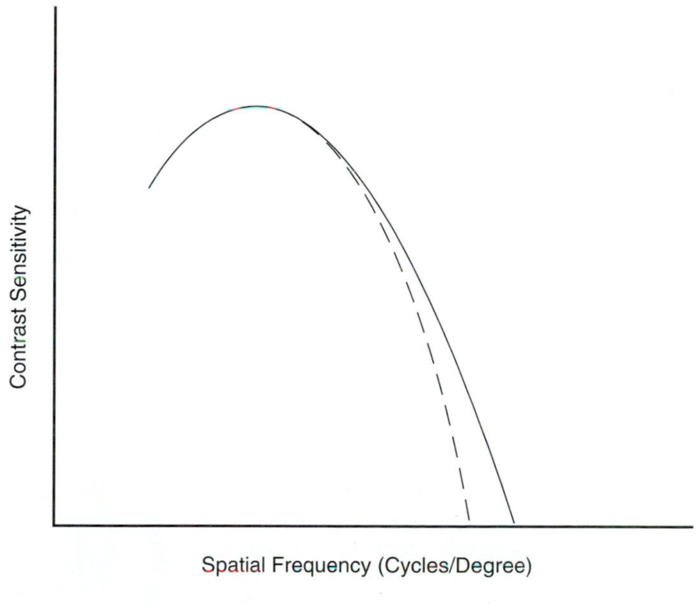


**FIGURE 7–13.** Contrast sensitivity functions for an eye in focus (solid line) and an eye out of focus (dashed line).

## *THE LOW-FREQUENCY DROP-OFF OF THE CONTRAST SENSITIVITY FUNCTION*

The low-frequency drop-off of the CSF is due to lateral inhibition within the retina. Lateral inhibition can best be understood by considering the response of a ganglion cell to light that falls upon its receptive field, the area in space that influences the activity of the cell (see Chapter 12 for a more complete description of receptive fields). The receptive field of a typical ganglion cell (Fig. 7–14) manifests a center and surround region that respond in opposing fashion to illumination. Light falling on the center causes excitation, while light falling on the surround causes inhibition. This cell will be optimally activated when a bright bar falls on the center of its receptive field and a dark bar on its surround, as depicted in the top panel of Figure 7–14. A lower spatial frequency, as seen on the bottom, will result in less of a response because the bright bar falls on both the receptive field's center and surround. Lateral inhibition results in a decreased sensitivity to this lower spatial frequency and accounts for the reduction in sensitivity to low frequencies displayed by the CSF.

## *THE VISUAL SYSTEM AS A FOURIER ANALYZER*

In the 1970s, it became common to think of the visual system as acting as a Fourier analyzer. That is, the visual system was thought to break the visual world down into its various spatial frequency components and reassemble these

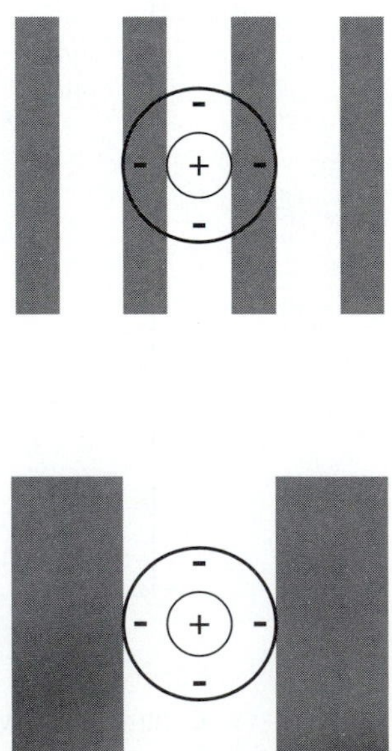

**FIGURE 7–14.** The spatial frequency grating on the top is a more optimal stimulus for this ganglion cell than the lower spatial frequency grating on the bottom. This is because the large bright bar of the low-frequency grating falls on both the receptive field's center and surround. This results in lateral inhibition, which reduces the neuron's response.

components to produce a unified spatial percept. (This is also referred to as linear system analysis.)

This view is supported by the existence of independent spatial frequency channels within the visual system. Figure 7–15 illustrates this concept. Rather than consisting of a single channel that is maximally sensitive to 4 cycles/degree, we can think of the CSF as forming an envelope that encompasses several more narrow channels. Each of these channels is presumably independent.

An experiment that supports the preceding view was conducted by Blakemore and Campbell (1969). After determining an observer's normal CSF, these investigators adapted the observer to a specific spatial frequency and redetermined the CSF. This means that the individual viewed a specific adapting grating for a period prior to the redetermination of the CSF. (The adapting grating drifted across the computer screen to prevent the formation of a retinal afterimage.)

The results of this experiment are given in Figure 7–16A. Note that there is a discrete reduction in sensitivity at the specific frequency to which the observer was adapted. This is the result predicted by the multiple-channel hypothesis. What would we expect if there was only a single channel? In this case, there would be an overall reduction in the CSF across all frequencies. Moreover, if there was only a single channel, adaptation to any spatial frequency would have the same effect; it would produce a reduction in sensitivity for all frequencies.

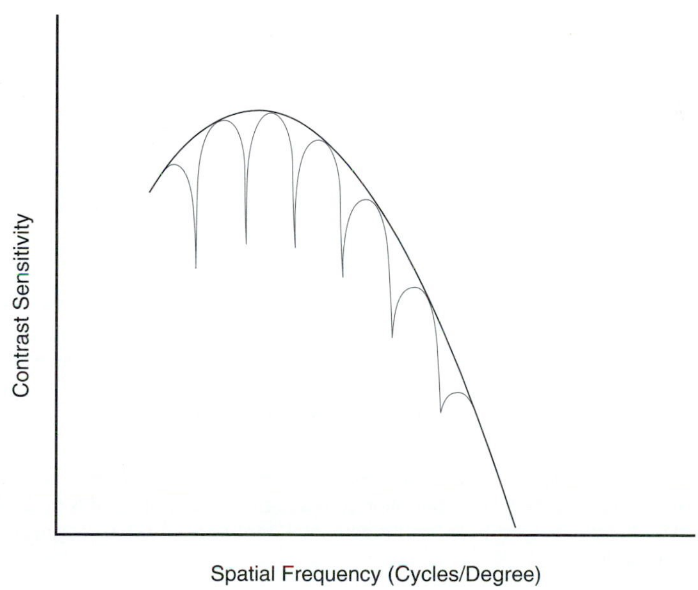


**FIGURE 7–15.** The contrast sensitivity function can be thought of as forming an envelope for a number of independent narrow spatial frequency channels.

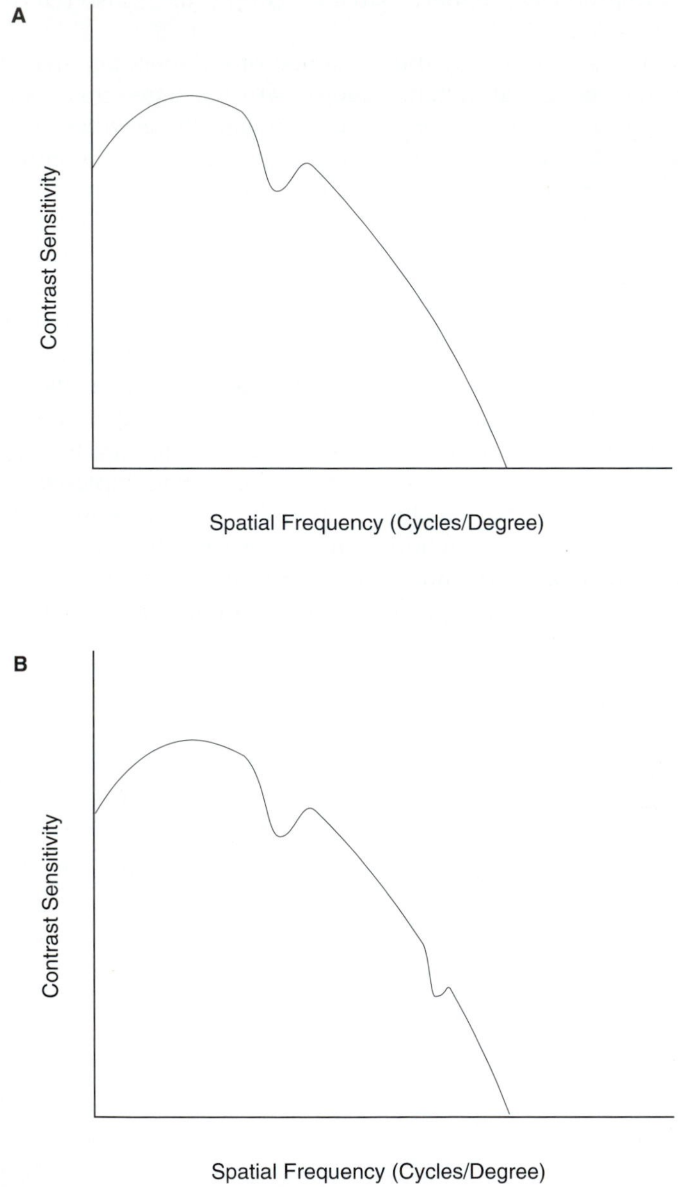


**FIGURE 7–16. A.** Prior adaptation to a sine wave grating of 6 cycles/degree results in reduced sensitivity at this frequency. **B.** Prior adaptation to a square wave grating of 6 cycles/degree produces a reduction in sensitivity at both the fundamental frequency (6 cycles/degree) and the third harmonic (18 cycles/degree).

Further support for the visual system performing a Fourier analysis comes from an ingenious experiment in which the observer adapts to a square wave grating rather than a sine wave grating (Blakemore and Campbell, 1969). The results of an experiment in which an observer adapts to a square wave grating of 6 cycles/degree are given in Figure 7–16B. As we expect, there is a reduction in sensitivity at the fundamental frequency of the square wave, 6 cycles/degree; however, note that there is a secondary reduction in sensitivity at 18 cycles/degree. We can account for this reduction at 18 cycles/degree by recalling that a square wave is composed of a fundamental sine wave of the same frequency and harmonic sine waves of odd multiples of this fundamental frequency. The secondary reduction in sensitivity represents adaptation to the third harmonic, which has a frequency of 18 cycles/degree. (A reduction in sensitivity to the fifth, seventh, and other odd harmonics is not noted because of the low contrast of these harmonics.) In this experiment, it appears as though a complex stimulus, the square wave, is broken down by the visual system into its components (a fundamental and its harmonics). This has been interpreted to represent a form of Fourier analysis by the visual system.

**Mach bands** also demonstrate the usefulness of considering the visual system as a Fourier analyzer. The transition between the bright and dark regions in Figure 7–17A is a gradual transition; this is indicated by the luminance profile of the stimulus (Fig. 7–17B). This gradual transition is not, however, perceived as such. Instead, observers typically report bright and dark bands at the junctions of the bright and dark regions. These perceived bands, which do not actually exist, are referred to as Mach bands.

Mach bands can be explained by assuming that the visual system performs a Fourier analysis of the stimulus. The gradual transition between the bright and dark regions consists of low spatial frequencies. As the CSF manifests low sensitivity to low frequencies, these low frequencies are not perceived. (Recall that this reduced sensitivity to low frequencies is due to lateral inhibition within the retina.) The result is a relative enhancement of high spatial frequencies. This relative enhancement of high spatial frequencies results in the perception of enhanced boundaries, represented by the Mach bands, at the borders of the gradual physical transition.

Single-unit electrophysiologic data from the primate visual cortex are consistent with the notion that the visual system could act as a Fourier analyzer (see Chap. 14). Single neurons in visual area 1 appear to be finely tuned to specific spatial frequencies (DeValois et al, 1982). A collection of such neurons could form the physiologic basis for the spatial frequency channels we have discussed.

Does the visual system really act as a Fourier analyzer? The jury is still out on this question. Although the preceding experimental evidence is consistent with this model, it does not prove that this model is correct. Nonetheless, the CSF is a useful tool for understanding how the visual system processes certain information.

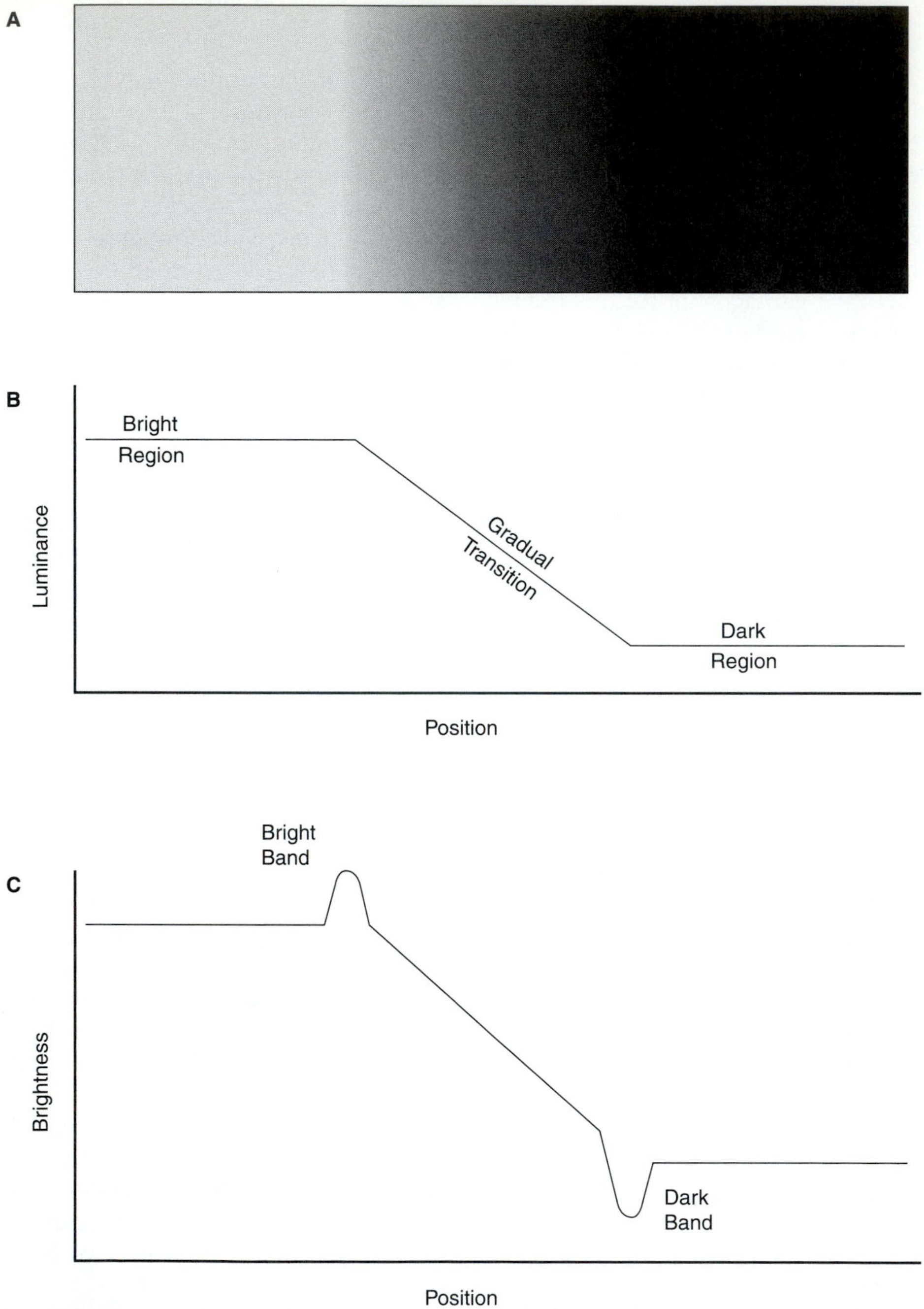


**FIGURE 7–17. A.** Observe the borders at the bright and dark regions of this pattern. Note the bright and dark bands at these borders. These bands, which are not physically present, are referred to as Mach bands. They represent a perceptual enhancement of the borders. **B.** Luminance profile for the pattern in A. Note the gradual transition between the bright and dark regions of the pattern. **C.** Brightness of the pattern as perceived by a typical observer. The bright and dark bands, which are not physically present, are Mach bands.

## RELATIONSHIP OF THE CONTRAST SENSITIVITY FUNCTION TO SNELLEN ACUITY

One of the first procedures in an eye examination is the determination of the patient's visual acuity. The patient is directed to read the smallest optotypes (e.g., a row of letters) he or she can resolve on a high-contrast chart. In the typical office, the familiar Snellen acuity chart (or a derivative) is used (see Fig. 7–10).

Determination of visual acuity is, essentially, a measurement of the high-frequency cutoff of the patient's CSF. Consider the optotype **E** as diagramed in Figure 7–18. The legs of the letter **E** can be thought of as being bars of a spatial grating. For the patient to read the **E,** he or she must be able to resolve the bars (or gaps between the bars) that make up the **E.** The angle that *just resolvable* bars (or gaps) represent at the eye is called the **minimum angle of resolution (MAR).**

A typical optotype is designed such that its overall size is five times the size of its detail (Fig. 7–19). The optotype **E** may be thought of as consisting of five details that must be resolved, the legs and gaps of the **E.**

Visual acuity is typically recorded in the form of the Snellen fraction. The numerator represents the distance at which the measurement is taken, for example, 20 ft. The denominator (sometimes referred to as foot-size) represents the distance at which the smallest resolvable optotype subtends an overall angular subtense of 5′ arc at the eye. At this same distance, the detail of the optotype subtends one fifth of this value (1′ arc).

A very important advantage of the Snellen fraction is that it allows easy calculation of the patient's MAR. The MAR is simply the reciprocal of the Snellen fraction. Consider an example. What information does a Snellen fraction of 20/20 provide? It tells us that the measurement was taken at 20 ft; the smallest letter the patient can read subtends 5′ arc, overall, at 20 ft (i.e., it has a foot-size

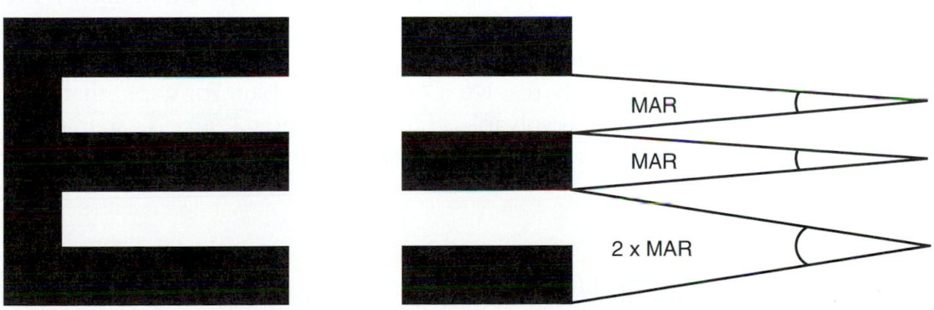


**FIGURE 7–18.** The optotype **E** may be thought of as consisting of the bright and dark bars of a grating. The smallest resolvable bar (or gap) subtends the minimum angle of resolution (MAR) at the eye. The combination of the bar and a gap represents twice the MAR, or one complete cycle of an equivalent grating.

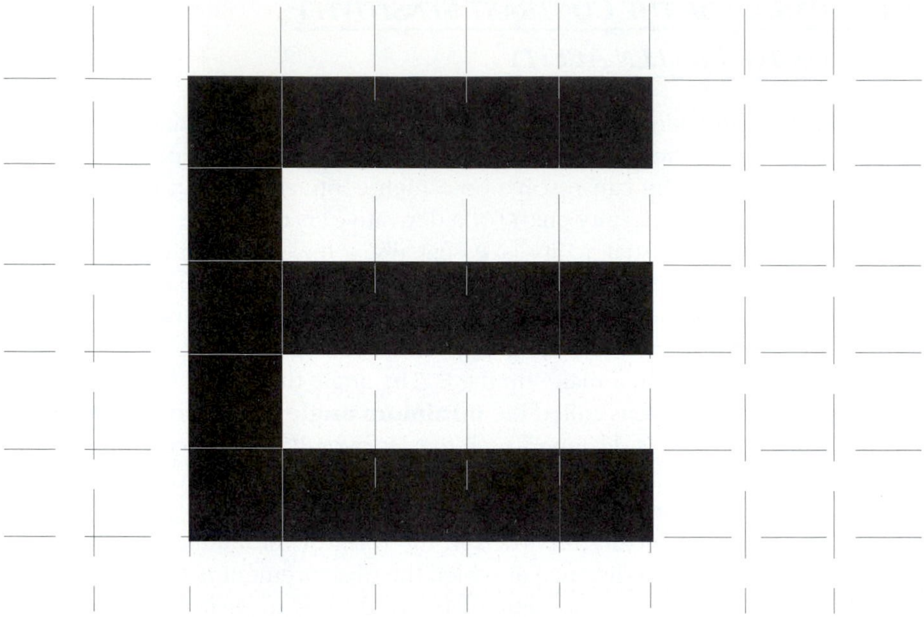

**FIGURE 7–19.** Construction of the optotype **E.** The detail (a bar or a gap) is one fifth of the overall size of the optotype.

of 20 ft); and the patient's MAR is 1′ arc. Let us now relate this 20/20 Snellen fraction more directly to the patient's CSF. What is the expected high-frequency cutoff of a patient with 20/20 acuity?

The first step is to realize that a Snellen fraction of 20/20 corresponds to a MAR of 1′ arc (i.e., each bar, or gap, of the threshold optotype **E** subtends 1′ arc at the patient's eye). Referring back to Figure 7–18, we can see that the combination of a bar and a gap corresponds to a cycle of a spatial grating. A patient with 20/20 acuity can just barely resolve a grating with bars (or gaps) that subtend 1′ arc; therefore, the just resolvable grating subtends 2′ arc. As spatial frequency is typically given in cycles per degree, we must make the following conversion:

$$\left(\frac{1\text{ cycle}}{2'\text{ arc}}\right)\left(\frac{60'\text{ arc}}{1\text{ degree}}\right) = 30\text{ cycles/degree}$$

This tells us that a Snellen acuity of 20/20 is equivalent to a high-frequency CSF cutoff of 30 cycles/degree.

## CLINICAL IMPLICATIONS OF THE CONTRAST SENSITIVITY FUNCTION

We have spent a considerable amount of time developing the concepts associated with the human CSF. What is the clinical value of this knowledge? Of primary interest is that the optical correction of refractive errors improves only a limited aspect of a patient's spatial vision. An optical correction improves high-frequency acuity; it has little effect on low frequencies.

In a highly visual society such as ours, high-frequency resolution is critical. Reading road signs, blackboards, computer screens, and books and watching movies and television are all dependent on a high level of visual resolution. Consequently, the demand for the correction of refractive errors is great. It is, however, important to realize that a reduction in acuity, secondary to a refractive error, is often well-tolerated by patients whose acuity demands are not high. All eye care practitioners are occasionally frustrated by the patient whose acuity we have substantially improved, yet who prefers his or her old correction that produces worse visual acuity. These patients illustrate the critical fact that there is more to spatial vision than high-frequency resolution.

Consider the world about you. Certainly many objects are highly detailed and require good acuity to resolve. Yet most objects can be recognized by their moderate frequency content. Consider the tree across the street, the dog in the driveway, or the outline of your spouse's body. All of these objects could be recognized without high-frequency acuity.

Often the novice clinician is surprised by how well a patient with severe central (macular) vision loss performs. This patient may have difficulty reading or driving, but is most often capable of taking care of himself or herself and performing many of the essential tasks of life. The patient's high-frequency spatial resolution is severely impaired, but he or she retains vision at moderate and low frequencies.

Just as a reduction in high-frequency resolution acuity produces a noticeable visual defect, a reduction in contrast sensitivity for moderate and low frequencies also results in a noticeable defect in vision. This situation can pose a problem for diagnosis by the clinician. Suppose we examine a patient who has a deficit at moderate frequencies with only minimal reduction in sensitivity at high frequencies. This patient may present with symptoms of substantially reduced vision. Yet when we perform a standard acuity test, we find normal or near-normal visual acuity.

Fortunately, the preceding situation rarely presents in such a pure form. That is, typically the reduction in sensitivity to moderate frequencies is accompanied by a reduction in acuity or other signs that aid in verifying the complaint. A good example is that of cataracts. (See Fig. 7–20 for an illustration of a cataract and the resultant CSF.) Patients with early cataract formation often complain of a profound reduction in their ability to see; however, a visual acuity task often shows only a moderate reduction in acuity (Hess and Woo, 1978). The discrepancy between the severe complaint and the moderate reduction in acuity lies in the fact that the cataract acts as a diffuser. This diffuser results in a

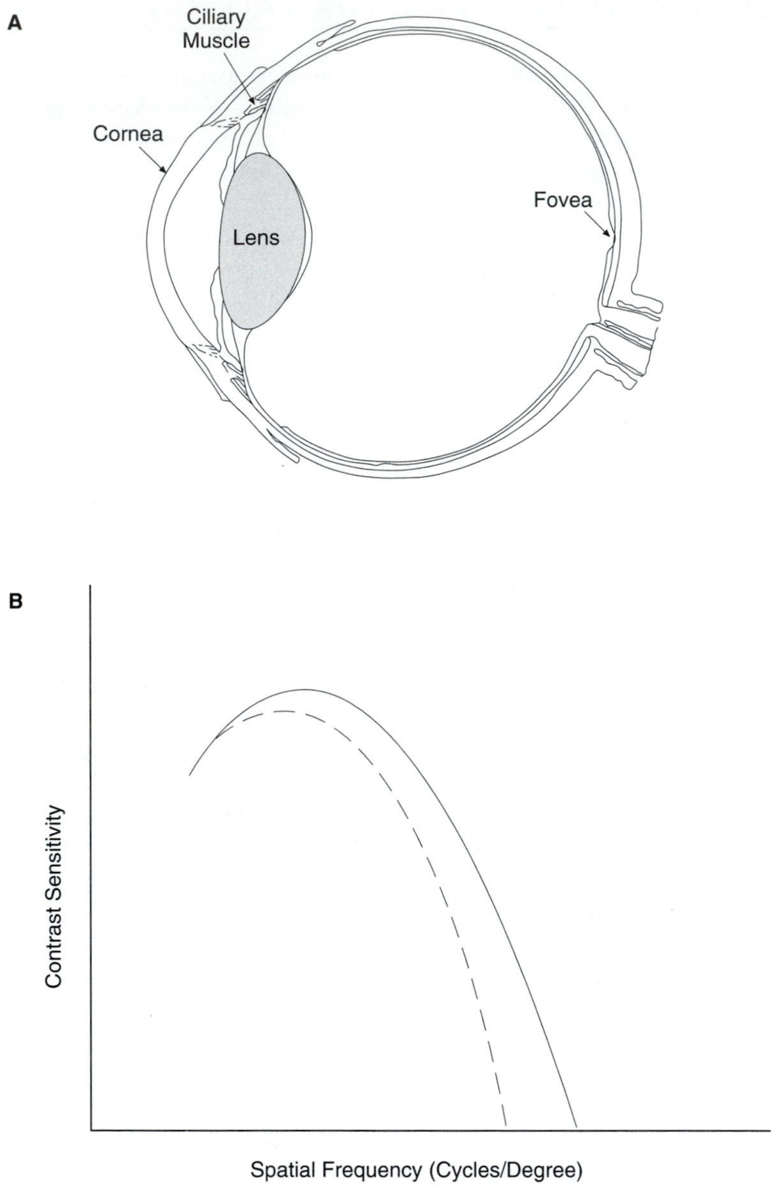


**FIGURE 7–20. A.** A cataract is an opacity of the crystalline lens as illustrated. **B.** This opacity reduces the overall retinal contrast such that the resultant CSF has the form of the dashed curve.

reduction in image contrast across all frequencies. (One can think of the cataract as producing a **"veiling glare."**) This is similar to the example discussed earlier where an optical lens is coated with clear nail polish (see "Spatial Modulation Transfer Function of a Lens" earlier in the chapter.) The patient is handicapped not only at high frequencies, but at moderate and low frequencies as well. Consequently, the patient's complaints are disproportionate to the moderate reduction in acuity.

Patients wearing contact lenses frequently manifest similar symptoms (Hess and Carney, 1979; Woo and Hess, 1979). Contact lenses often produce edema of the cornea. The swelling of the corneal stromal layers (or epithelial cells) results in an increased scatter of light similar to that produced by a cataract. This results in a reduction in contrast sensitivity across all frequencies. Not surprisingly, these patients often have normal or near-normal acuity, but complain of poor vision. (For example, the patient may have 20/20 vision yet complain of blur.)

Scarring of the stromal layers secondary to trauma or refractive surgery (i.e., incisions from refractive keratometry or haze following photorefractive procedures) can cause clinically significant light scatter, with a resultant reduction in contrast sensitivity at moderate frequencies. Swelling of the stroma, as occurs in Fuchs endothelial dystrophy, can also lead to loss in sensitivity at moderate frequencies. It is important to keep in mind that patients with reductions in contrast sensitivity at moderate frequencies may have only a slight reduction in acuity (e.g., 20/25) yet complain of severe visual impairment.

In summary, we must be aware that Snellen acuity samples only a small portion of the patient's spatial vision. Cataracts, corneal edema, and other conditions commonly produce reductions in contrast sensitivity at spatial frequencies other than those measured in an acuity task (Bodis-Wollner and Camisa, 1980). Consequently, complaints of reduced vision, not proportionate to the reduction in Snellen acuity, warrant careful investigation. On the other hand, when dealing with healthy eyes with defects that are only optical in nature, we must not overestimate the benefits of optical correction on the performance of many daily activities.

## CLINICAL DETERMINATION OF THE CONTRAST SENSITIVITY FUNCTION

Determination of a CSF is not a common clinical procedure. It is time consuming and costly, and often provides information that could be determined otherwise.

The most accurate clinical methods display gratings on a video monitor that is driven by a microprocessor. Such instruments are costly and typically available only in large eye clinics. Less costly methods employ gratings displayed on a chart (VISTECH) or a series of cards (Arden plates). The reliability and validity of the latter tests have been called into question (Reeves et al, 1991).

A promising clinical approach is the determination of visual acuity with low-contrast optotypes rather than the high-contrast optotypes typically used to measure visual acuity. This may be done with the Bailey–Lovie low-contrast acuity chart (Bailey and Lovie, 1976). The concepts associated with this test are illustrated in Figure 7–11. A variation on this theme is the Pelli–Robson approach, which measures the threshold contrast using optotypes rather than gratings (Pelli et al, 1988). The concepts associated with this task are also illustrated in Figure 7–11. Either the Bailey–Lovie low-contrast chart or the Pelli–Robson test would be appropriate for the typical eye-care office. They are efficient and alert the clinician to a reduction in contrast sensitivity at moderate frequencies.

## *OTHER FORMS OF VISUAL ACUITY*

Our discussion of visual acuity has centered on resolution acuity and recognition acuity. **Resolution acuity** involves distinguishing a pattern (e.g., a grating) from a uniform patch of light of equal luminance (see Fig. 17–9). The determination of the high-frequency cutoff of the CSF, using spatial gratings, is an example of resolution acuity. For a young, healthy adult, the high-frequency cutoff is from 40 to 60 cycles/degree, which is equivalent to a MAR of 0.75 to 0.50 minutes of arc. (When gratings are used to determine resolution acuity, the task is sometimes referred to as **grating acuity.**)

**Recognition acuity** is a form of resolution that requires the subject to be familiar with the object that must be resolved. Snellen acuity is an example of recognition acuity because the patient must be familiar with the alphabet to read the optotypes on the chart. Young adults typically manifest Snellen acuities of 20/15 to 20/10.

Resolution and recognition acuity are by far the most commonly utilized clinical measures of acuity. This is primarily because of the utility of these acuity tasks in the diagnosis and amelioration of refractive errors.

Other forms of visual acuity also provide useful information regarding the limitations of spatial vision. **Minimum detectable acuity** refers to the smallest object that can be seen. Imagine a thin wire against a blue sky. How thin could this wire be and still be visible? (In this task, the subject does not need to recognize the object, only to detect it.) Figure 7–21 illustrates how we can approach this question. Minimum detectable acuity can be considered to be equivalent to an increment threshold task (see Chaps. 3 and 11). Due to optical imperfections of the eye, the wire will not be in perfect focus on the retina; its image will form what is referred to as a **line spread function.** In order for the line to be detected, the height of the line spread function, which represents the brightest part of the image, must be of a critical value. It turns out that this critical value is the same as the $\Delta I$ in an increment threshold experiment.

Minimum detectable acuity is limited by how thin a line (or small a dot) can be made and still emit sufficient light so that the increment threshold is reached. This has been determined to be 1 second of arc (Westheimer, 1979). Note that this value is considerably smaller than the value for resolution acuity.

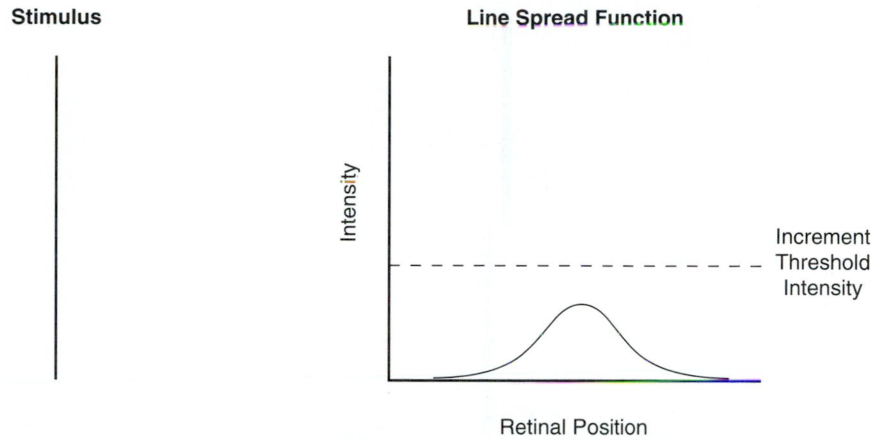


**FIGURE 7–21.** Minimum detectable acuity is determined by making a line progressively thinner until it is no longer visible. The line produces a line spread function with a maximum height that diminishes as the line becomes thinner. Viewed in this manner, minimum detectable acuity can be considered to be an increment threshold task. In the example illustrated, the line would not be detectable because its peak retinal intensity falls below the increment threshold.

Optical defocus, such as caused by an uncorrected refractive error, will result in a reduction in the height of the line spread function, with a resultant reduction in minimum detectable acuity. This reduction, however, is not as marked as with resolution acuity. Minimum detectable acuity is comparatively unaffected by refractive errors.

The final type of acuity that we will discuss is **hyperacuity,** so named because of the exquisite sensitivity manifested by this form of acuity. Several different hyperacuity tasks are given in Figure 7–22. It can be very difficult to align a picture on a wall so that it does not appear tilted because of our excellent abilities at detecting tilt, a form of hyperacuity. Hyperacuity apparently depends on the visual system's ability to sense direction. Consider the **vernier acuity** task in Figure 7–22A. Each bar represents a different direction. When these two bars represent sufficiently different directions, a threshold for this hyperacuity task is reached.

Thresholds for hyperacuity are very low, on the order of 3 seconds of arc (Westheimer, 1979). These low thresholds are presumably related to the visual system's ability to average luminance information across space to arrive at a sense of direction. This process occurs at postreceptoral levels, perhaps in the visual cortex (Levi et al, 1985).

Hyperacuity is very resilient to optical defocus. Whereas refractive errors greatly reduce resolution acuity, they have minimal effects on hyperacuity. Figure 7–23 provides an explanation for this observation. For the resolution task, optical defocus causes the blur circles to overlap, thereby interfering with the

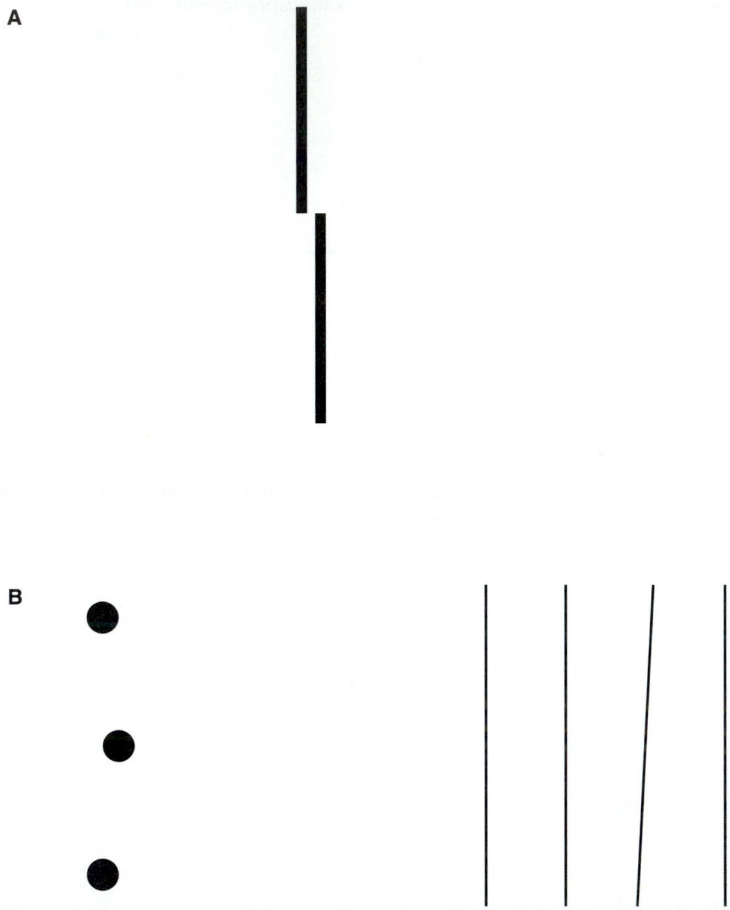


**FIGURE 7–22. A.** Target used to measure vernier acuity, a form of hyperacuity. **B.** Other targets that measure hyperacuity. For the target on the left, the task is to determine if the three circles are in alignment with each other. For the target on the right, the task is to determine which line is tilted.

resolution of the two lines. In comparison, optical defocus does not interfere with the integration of information across the retina that enables the positions of the two lines to be determined. The peaks of the luminance profiles of the two lines are in different positions and this leads to the perception of a different location for each line.

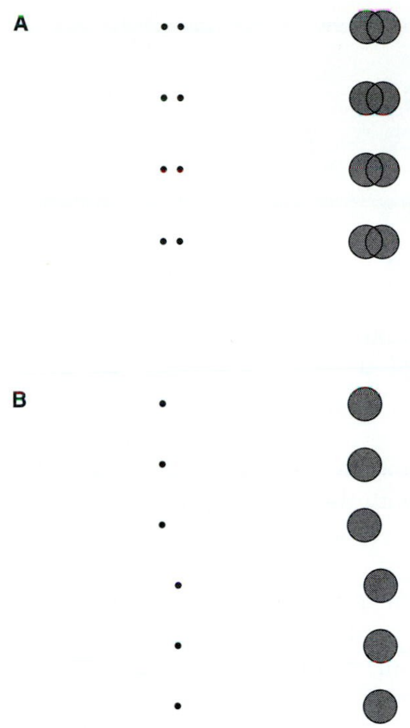

**FIGURE 7–23. A.** Each line in a resolution task can be considered to be constituted of points. Defocus leads to overlapping blur circles, thereby reducing resolution acuity. **B.** In spite of optical blur, the luminance profiles of the blurred lines of a vernier target provide sufficient information to distinguish their positions.

## *SUMMARY*

Contrast sensitivity functions provide a powerful tool for characterizing spatial vision capabilities. The common clinical measurement of visual acuity (resolution acuity) assesses only a small portion of the patient's spatial vision; however, this is the aspect of spatial vision that prompts most visual complaints and is amenable to optical correction. Nonetheless, we should keep in mind that reductions at frequencies other than the highest frequencies do occur and are of clinical importance.

# Self-Assessment Questions

1. Determine the predicted high-frequency contrast sensitivity function cutoff, in cycles/degree, for the following visual acuities: **A.** 20/15. **B.** 20/80. **C.** 20/150.

2. A visual acuity task is to be performed with a Snellen chart at 20 ft. Calculate the expected Snellen fractions for patients with the following high spatial frequency cutoffs: **A.** 5 cycles/degree. **B.** 20 cycles/degree. **C.** 60 cycles/degree.

3. A patient's visual acuity is 20/100. **A.** What is the overall physical size, in mm, of the smallest letter the patient can read on a Snellen chart at a distance of 20 ft? **B.** What is the size of the detail, in mm, of this letter?

4. A patient has a Snellen fraction of 20/80. What would you predict the Snellen fraction to be when acuity is measured at 10 ft?

5. A patient shows a high-frequency contrast sensitivity function (CSF) cutoff of 30 cycles/degree when tested at 20 ft. **A.** What is the expected high-frequency CSF cutoff, in cycles/degree, when the procedure is repeated at 10 ft? **B.** What is the width of a single bar of the threshold grating, in mm, when the test is performed at 20 ft? **C.** What is the width of a single bar of the threshold grating when the test is performed at 10 ft?

6. You measure a patient's visual acuity with a projected Snellen chart. In a dark room, the acuity is 20/20. **A.** What happens to the measured visual acuity when you turn on the overhead room lights? **B.** Why?

# 8

# Temporal Aspects of Vision

Whereas spatial vision involves the analysis of changes in luminance across space, temporal vision—time-related vision—concerns the analysis of changes in luminance over time. Examples of spatial vision tasks include reading a letter on an eye chart and recognizing a face. In comparison, a temporal vision task could involve the detection of the flicker produced by a flashing light. Temporal vision is closely related to the ability to perceive motion.

Temporal vision and motion analysis have been the subject of much recent scientific inquiry. These studies suggest that temporal and motion vision are analyzed by specialized visual pathways that feed into motion analysis areas within the cerebral cortex. This knowledge has been applied clinically to devise tests to aid in the diagnosis of certain diseases of the visual system.

## STIMULUS CONSIDERATIONS

Temporal vision is frequently studied with stimuli with luminance that varies sinusoidally over time (Fig. 8–1). Such a stimulus is the temporal equivalent of a spatial sine wave grating. Whereas a spatial grating manifests a sinusoidal change in luminance across space, a temporal sinusoid manifests a sinusoidal change in luminance over time.

A temporally modulated stimulus is produced by a light source (e.g., a computer monitor) that turns on and off. To produce a temporal sinusoid, the light source must turn on and off with a sinusoidal time course.

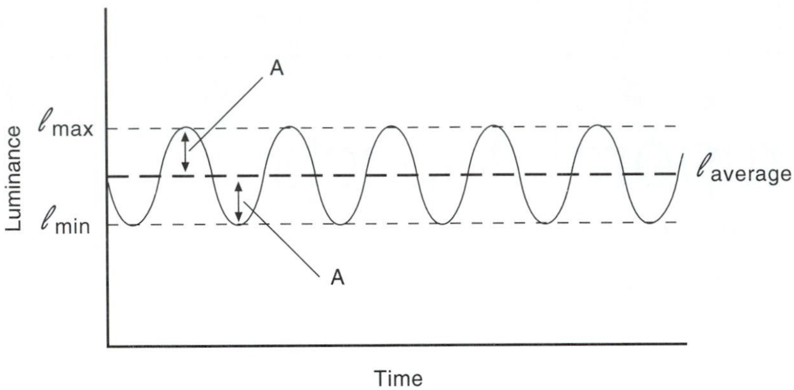


**FIGURE 8–1.** Luminance profile for a stimulus with luminance that is temporally modulated in a sinusoidal manner over time. A computer screen that turns on and off with a sinusoidal time course would produce a luminance profile similar to that given in this figure. "A" refers to amplitude of modulation.

## *Depth of Modulation*

The visibility of a temporally modulated stimulus is related to its depth of modulation. The stimulus in Figure 8–2A has a relatively low depth of modulation. A light source that is modulated at this low depth appears steady; no perception of flicker is noted. In comparison, the stimulus in Figure 8–2B manifests a relatively large depth of modulation. A light source modulated at this greater modulation depth is not perceived as steady; it appears to flicker.

The preceding example is analogous to the detection of spatial gratings. A spatial grating of very low contrast appears as a uniform gray surface. Only when the contrast is sufficiently high is the grating resolved. Likewise, a temporally modulated stimulus of low modulation depth is not resolved; it appears steady. As the modulation depth is increased, however, it is resolved and seen as flickering.

The **percentage depth of modulation** of a temporally modulated stimulus is given by the relationship

$$\text{percentage modulation} = \frac{A}{l_{ave}}(100)$$

where

$$A = \text{amplitude of modulation}$$
$$l_{ave} = \text{time-averaged luminance}$$

Note that this formula is essentially the same as that for spatial contrast, except that the stimulus is temporally modulated rather than spatially modulated.

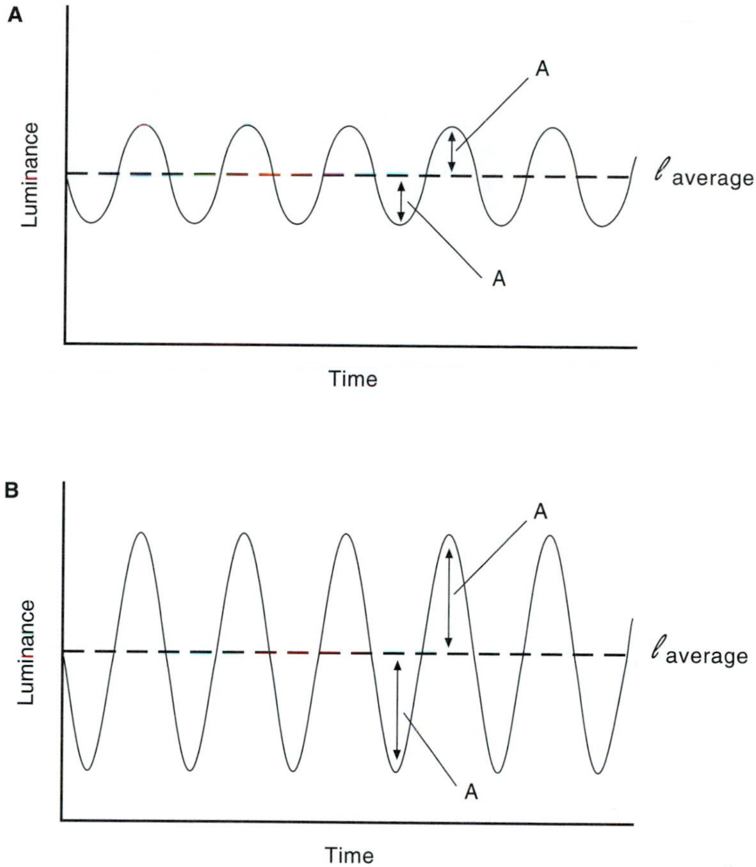


**FIGURE 8–2. A.** Temporal sinusoid with a low modulation depth. **B.** Temporal sinusoid with a high modulation depth.

## *Temporal Frequency*

Just as it is possible to vary the frequency of a spatial grating, it is also possible to vary the frequency of a temporal sinusoid (Fig. 8–3). A low temporal frequency stimulus appears to flicker at a slow rate, whereas a higher temporal frequency stimulus is seen as flickering at a faster rate.

As the temporal frequency is increased, a frequency is reached at which flicker can no longer be resolved. This temporal frequency is referred to as the **critical flicker fusion frequency (CFF).** The CFF is analogous to spatial resolution acuity. As the frequency of a spatial grating is increased, it appears to consist of increasingly thin bars. At the high spatial frequency cutoff, the bars are not resolvable; the stimulus appears as a uniform gray surface. Likewise, as

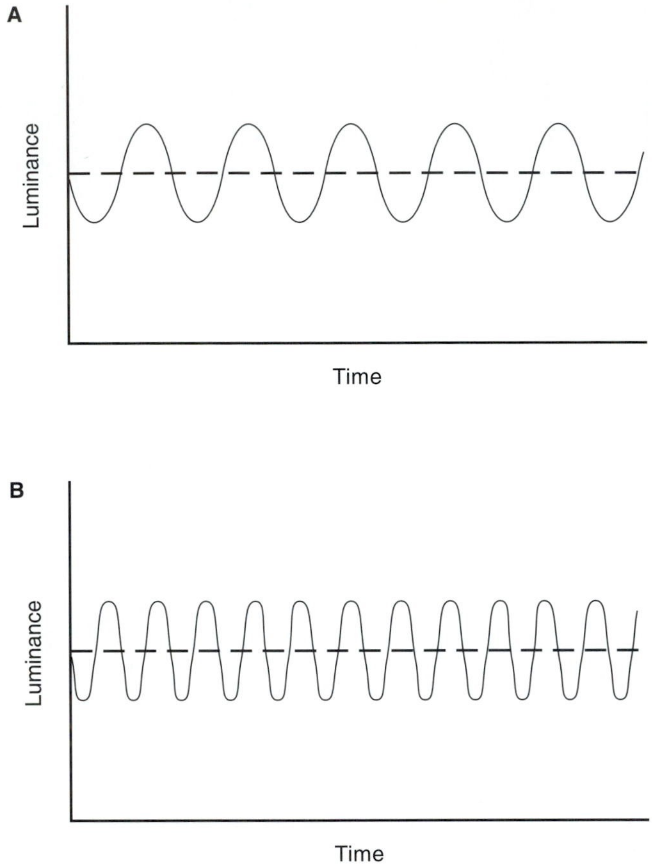


**FIGURE 8–3. A.** Temporal sinusoid modulated at a low temporal frequency. **B.** Temporal sinusoid modulated at a high temporal frequency.

the frequency of a temporally modulated stimulus is increased, the flicker appears more rapid. A frequency is eventually reached that cannot be resolved; the stimulus appears steady. This temporal frequency, the CFF, represents the high temporal resolution limit of the visual system for a given depth of modulation. Temporal frequency is typically given in hertz (Hz). One hertz is equal to one cycle per second.

## *TEMPORAL MODULATION TRANSFER FUNCTIONS*

The advantage of sinusoidal stimuli is that they allow the application of linear system analysis (Fourier analysis) (de Lange, 1958). In Chapter 7, we learned that any spatial stimulus can be constructed by the proper combination of spatial sine wave gratings. Similarly, a temporal stimulus can be constructed by the appropriate combination of temporal sinusoids.

Spatial vision is characterized by the contrast sensitivity function (CSF). Likewise, temporal vision is characterized by the temporal modulation transfer function (TMTF). To determine a TMTF, an individual views a light source (e.g., a computer screen) that is modulated at a given temporal rate. Initially, the modulation depth is very low and the screen appears steady. The depth of modulation is slowly increased until the subject reports that the screen is flickering. The percentage modulation at which the person first sees flicker is the threshold. The reciprocal of this threshold percentage modulation represents the relative sensitivity (relative to the background illumination) for flicker resolution. This procedure is repeated for a large number of temporal frequencies to obtain a TMTF.

A typical human TMTF is given in Figure 8–4. This graph shows relative sensitivity (the reciprocal of threshold percentage modulation) as a function of temporal frequency. Stimuli that fall outside of the TMTF are seen as fused or

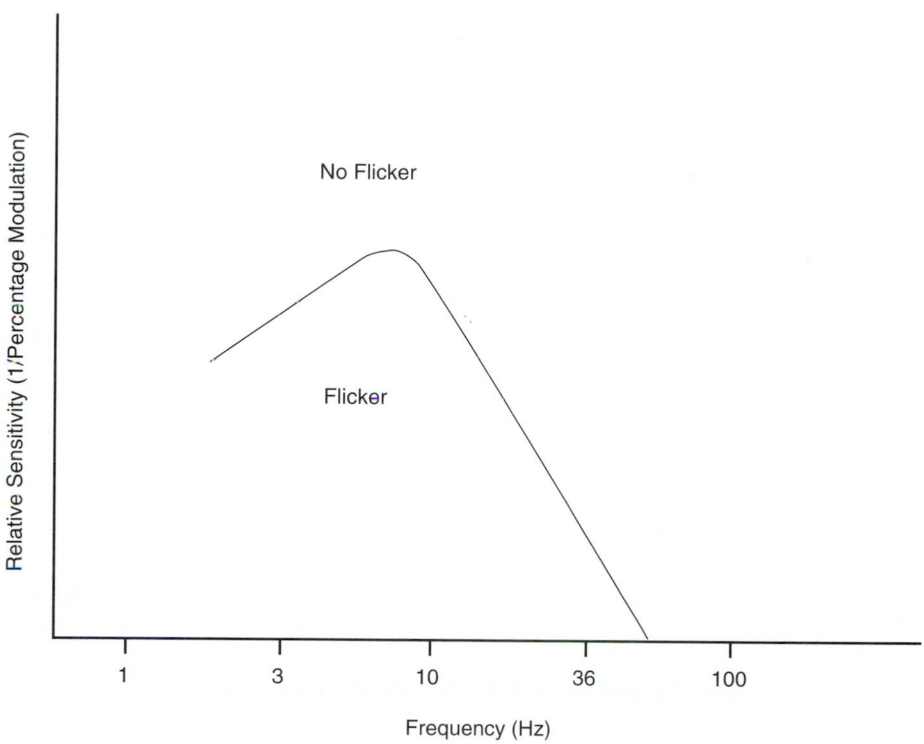


**FIGURE 8–4.** Typical temporal modulation transfer function. Graph is plotted on log coordinates.

steady; they are not temporally resolved. Those stimuli that fall under the graph are temporally resolved and perceived as flickering.

The TMTF presented in Figure 8–4 has a band-pass shape; sensitivity for the detection of flicker falls off at both low and high temporal frequencies. Stimuli modulated at moderate frequencies are detected at a lower percentage modulation than are other stimuli.

### *Reduction in Sensitivity for Low Temporal Frequencies*

The band-pass shape of the TMTF makes intuitive sense. Consider the low-frequency reduction in sensitivity. Very gradual or slow changes in illumination are not seen. An example is the change in illumination that occurs as the sun sets. Although we are aware of the changing illumination, we do not actually perceive the change itself. Another example is the minute hand on a watch. Although we know that the minute hand moves, we do not actually see it move.

The inability to perceive **stabilized retinal images** is a manifestation of the visual system's reduced sensitivity to low temporal frequencies (Riggs et al, 1953). Consider the retinal blood vessels that lie on top of the photoreceptors. Relative to the retina, these vessels are stabilized; they move as the eye moves and manifest a temporal frequency of zero. Only when a moving light is shined into the eye, which casts moving shadows on the photoreceptors, is it possible for us to visualize our own retinal vessels. (To observe your retinal vasculature, place a penlight against your closed eyelid and jiggle the penlight.) The retinal vasculature, when visualized in this manner, is referred to as the **Purkinje tree.**

Another example of the reduced sensitivity to low temporal frequencies is provided in Figure 8–5. Steady fixation of the top fixation point causes the blurred border to disappear; however, fixation of the bottom fixation point does not cause the sharply focused border to disappear. This phenomenon is due to the interaction of eye movements with the stimulus border.

The eyes continuously move, even when fixating a target (Ratliff and Riggs, 1950). These eye movements are involuntary. If these eye movements occur across a blurred border (Fig. 8–5A), the changes in retinal illumination produced by this border are of a very low temporal frequency, approaching 0 Hz. Because we are not sensitive to low temporal frequencies, the border disappears. The disappearance of low temporal frequency stimuli is referred to as the **Troxler phenomenon** (Troxler, 1804). Eye movements across the sharply focused border in Figure 8–5B result in the introduction of moderate temporal frequencies. Because we are very sensitive to these frequencies, the border does not disappear.

### *Reduction in Sensitivity for High Temporal Frequencies*

The high-frequency drop-off of the TMTF is demonstrated by the inability to perceive the temporal modulation displayed by household incandescent light

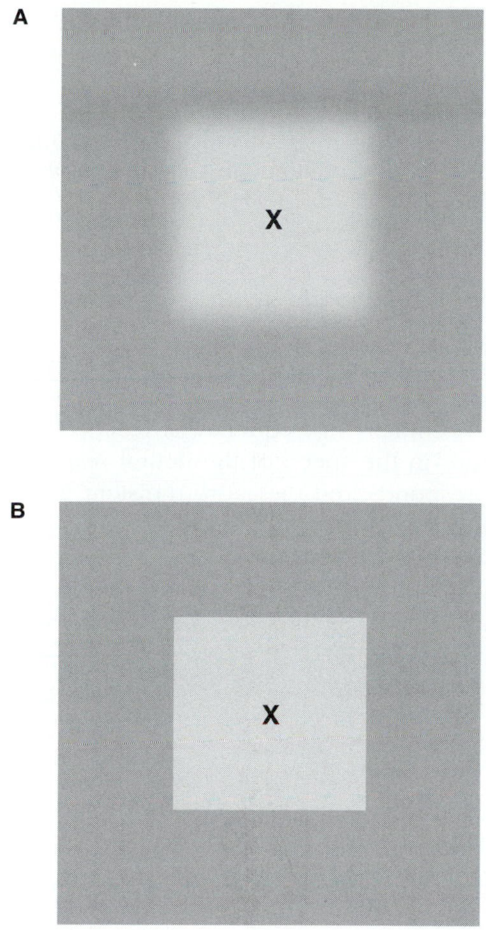


**FIGURE 8–5. A.** Steadily fixate the "X." Note that the blurred border disappears. **B.** The sharply focused border usually does not disappear when the "X" is fixated. (*Adapted from Cornsweet T.* Visual Perception. *New York: Academic Press; 1970.*)

bulbs. These bulbs are modulated at 60 Hz, yet they appear steady. Because we are relatively insensitive to this high-frequency temporal modulation, these bulbs are perceived as steady, rather than flickering.

Interpretation of the TMTF is very similar to interpretation of the contrast sensitivity function (CSF). In both cases, sensitivity is plotted as a function of frequency. In the case of a CSF, sensitivity, expressed in terms of spatial contrast, is plotted as a function of spatial frequency. For a TMTF, sensitivity, expressed in terms of percentage modulation, is plotted as a function of temporal frequency.

Both the CSF and TMTF show a band-pass shape, indicating maximal sensitivity to moderate frequencies. For spatial vision, this means that a sinusoidal spatial grating of about 4 cycles/degree is seen at a lower spatial contrast than are gratings of lower or higher spatial frequencies. Likewise, a stimulus temporally modulated at moderate rates is seen as flickering at lower percentage modulations than are stimuli of lower or higher temporal frequencies.

A high-frequency cutoff is manifested by both the CSF and the TMTF. For the CSF, this high-frequency cutoff represents the highest spatial frequency that can be resolved at 100 percent spatial contrast. For the TMTF, this high-frequency cutoff represents the highest temporal frequency that can be resolved at 100 percent modulation.

### *Origins of the Low and High-frequency Temporal Modulation Transfer Function Drop-offs*

The high-frequency cutoff of the TMTF is due to neural limitations in coding high temporal frequency information. Eventually, a frequency is reached that cannot be resolved because of limitations in the speed of the neural response (Fig. 8–6). The faster a neural system responds and the more transient its response, the greater is its temporal resolution.

The reduction in sensitivity to low frequencies is due to time lags inherent in lateral inhibitory interactions (lateral inhibition) within the retina (see Chap. 12). Low temporal frequency stimuli maximize these inhibitory interactions with a resultant reduction in sensitivity (Ratliff et al, 1963).

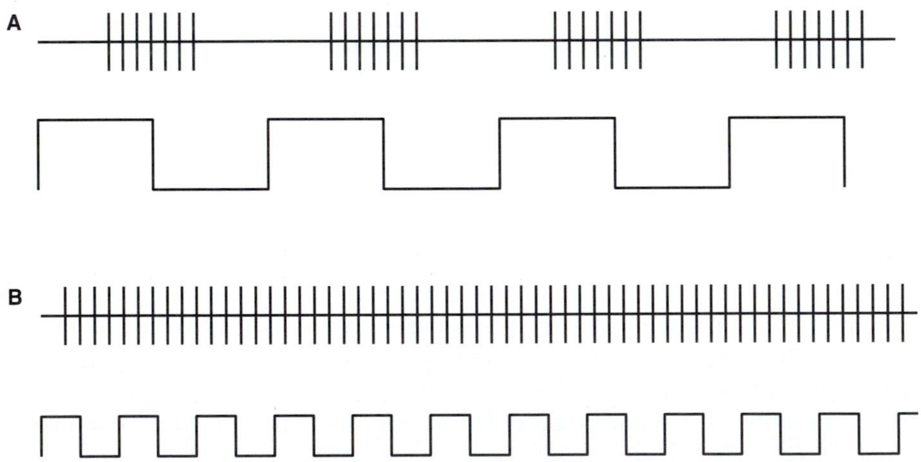


**FIGURE 8–6. A.** A moderate temporal frequency stimulus produces a nicely modulated neural response. The neuron is capable of resolving this moderate-frequency stimulus. **B.** The neuron's response is neither sufficiently fast nor sufficiently transient to allow temporal resolution of this high-frequency stimulus.

## CRITICAL FLICKER FUSION FREQUENCY

The critical flicker fusion frequency is the highest or lowest temporal frequency that can be resolved at a given percentage modulation. The example in Figure 8–7 shows the CFF for 4.0 percent modulation. This corresponds to a relative sensitivity of 1/4.0, or 0.25. A line extended from this point intersects the TMTF at two points: 4 and 10 Hz. These frequencies represent the low and high-frequency CFFs for 4.0 percent modulation. At this percentage modulation, stimuli of less than 4 Hz or greater than 10 Hz are seen as fused. Other frequencies are resolved and perceived as flickering. (Note that when not specified, the CFF typically refers to the high-frequency CFF.)

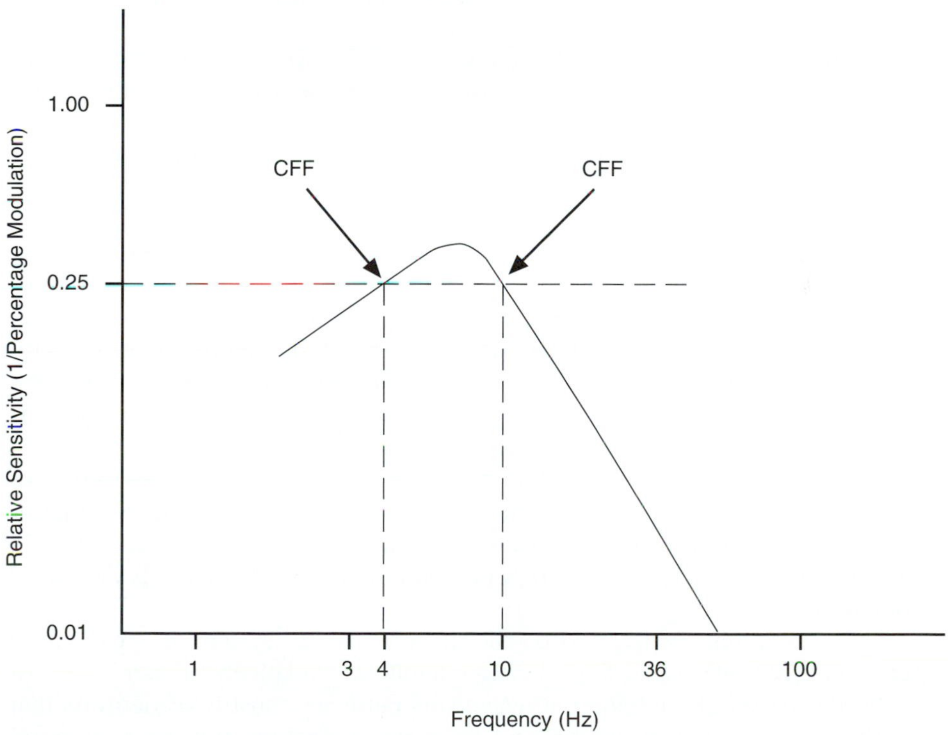


**FIGURE 8–7.** The low-frequency critical flicker fusion frequency (CFF) for 4 percent modulation is 4 Hz; the high-frequency CFF is 10 Hz. Stimuli of 4 percent modulation that are below 4 Hz or above 10 Hz are not resolved; they appear steady.

### *Effect of Illumination on the Critical Flicker Fusion Frequency*

Figure 8–8A displays TMTFs obtained under various levels of retinal illumination. Note that increasing the background illumination has different effects on relative sensitivity for low and high temporal frequencies (Kelly, 1961). For low temporal frequencies, increasing the illumination has no effect on relative sensitivity. This is demonstrated by the overlap of the low-frequency aspects of the TMTFs.

In comparison, high-frequency relative sensitivity increases as the background illumination increases. Related to this is an increase in the high-frequency CFF with increasing levels of illumination.

The high-frequency CFF increases approximately linearly with the log of the retinal illumination. This is referred to as the **Ferry–Porter law** (Fig. 8–8B) (Ferry, 1892; Porter, 1902). The physiologic basis for this increase in the CFF is most likely related to a general speeding up of retinal processes that occurs at increasing levels of light adaptation.

### *Effect of Stimulus Size on the Critical Flicker Fusion Frequency*

The **Granit–Harper law** states that the CFF increases with the log of the stimulus area (Granit and Harper, 1930). Consequently, for a given percentage modulation, flicker is more likely to be perceived if the stimulus is large.

The Granit–Harper law is consistent with the observation that the peripheral retina is better at detecting movement and flicker than is the central retina. (A large stimulus falls on more of the peripheral retina than a small stimulus.) The peripheral retina is considered to be a portion of an alerting **"where" system,** which signals the presence of those visual stimuli that require our attention (Livingstone and Hubel, 1987, 1988). To perform this task, the peripheral retina is adapted to detect high-frequency temporal alterations, such as those produced by rapidly moving stimuli. This system does not, however, manifest highly developed spatial resolution; the visual acuity of the peripheral retina is poor, approximately 20/200.

The physiologic pathway that accounts for the high temporal resolution of the peripheral retina is most likely the magno pathway. This retinocortical pathway consists of neurons that respond in a transient manner to visual stimuli; consequently, it manifests high temporal resolution. (This pathway is discussed in detail in Chap. 13.)

Once a stimulus is detected by the magno "where" system, it is examined with foveal (central) vision. Foveal vision manifests a relatively greater contribution by the parvo physiologic pathway. This pathway consists of neurons that show excellent spatial resolution and color discrimination, but poor temporal resolution. The parvo pathway forms a **"what" system,** which enables the observer to examine a visual stimulus in detail such that the stimulus can be identified (Livingstone and Hubel, 1987, 1988).

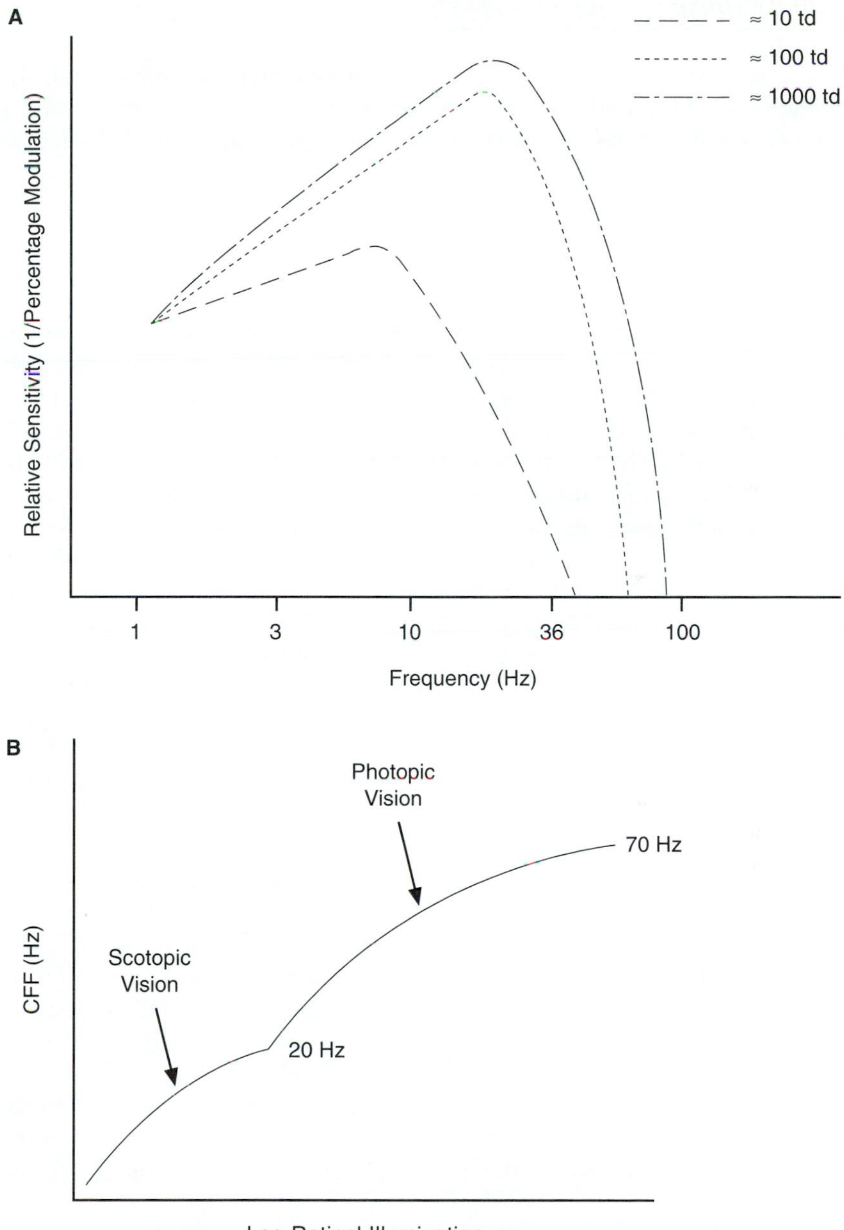


**FIGURE 8–8. A.** Temporal modulation transfer functions for background retinal illuminations of 10, 100, and 1000 td. Note that increasing illumination has no effect on low-frequency sensitivity and enhances high-frequency sensitivity. (*Adapted from Kelly DH. Visual responses to time-dependent stimuli. 1. Amplitude sensitivity measures.* J Opt Soc Am. *1961;51:422-429.*) **B.** Graphic representation of the Ferry–Porter law showing that the critical flicker fusion frequency (CFF) increases with the log of the retinal illumination. The CFF for scotopic vision is about 20 Hz, while for photopic vision it is 70 Hz.

## OTHER TEMPORAL VISUAL EFFECTS

In this section, several assorted temporal phenomena are introduced. These phenomena are frequently referred to in the vision science literature and provide important information regarding the basic operating characteristics of the visual system.

### *Broca–Sulzer Effect*

The Broca–Sulzer effect is that suprathreshold flashes of light with a duration on the order of 50 to 100 milliseconds appear brighter than stimuli of either shorter or longer durations (Broca and Sulzer, 1902, 1904). This effect is demonstrated by having an observer compare the brightness of two flashes of light, a test flash and a control flash. The test flash is of variable duration and constant intensity. The control flash is of constant duration and variable intensity. The observer's task is to adjust the intensity of the control flash such that it matches the brightness of the test flash. Over the course of an experiment, the test flash is presented at a large number of durations, and for each duration the observer adjusts the intensity of the control flash so that it matches the brightness of the test flash. The result is a plot of brightness as a function of pulse duration that reveals durations of about 50 to 100 milliseconds to be the brightest (Figure 8–9A).

Can the Broca–Sulzer effect be explained by the temporal response profiles of ganglion cells? Figure 8–9B shows the temporal response profile of a ganglion cell when exposed to a flash of light. These data are replotted in Figure 8–9C as the frequency of action potentials as a function of time that the stimulus is on. This function reveals a maximum sometime after the onset of the stimulus and then falls off. It has a form very similar to the Broca–Sulzer effect.

This similarity has led some to conclude that the Broca–Sulzer effect is due to the frequency of action potentials generated in visual neurons when exposed to a flash of light (LeGrand, 1968). This correlation is, however, an illusory or false correlation (Wasserman and Kong, 1974; Schwartz, 1992). The false nature of this correlation is made evident by observing that the independent variable for the two experiments is not the same. For the psychophysical Broca–Sulzer effect, the independent variable is duration, whereas for the neural discharge, the independent variable is time. As the independent variables are different, the apparent correlation between the psychophysical and physiologic results is false.

To determine if the frequency of action potentials accounts for the Broca–Sulzer effect, it would be necessary to repeat the physiologic experiment using duration as the independent variable. If this were done, one would find that there is no aspect of the neural response that increases to a peak and then decreases, as the duration is increased. Consequently, the action potential profile of a ganglion cell does not provide a straightforward explanation for the Broca–Sulzer effect.

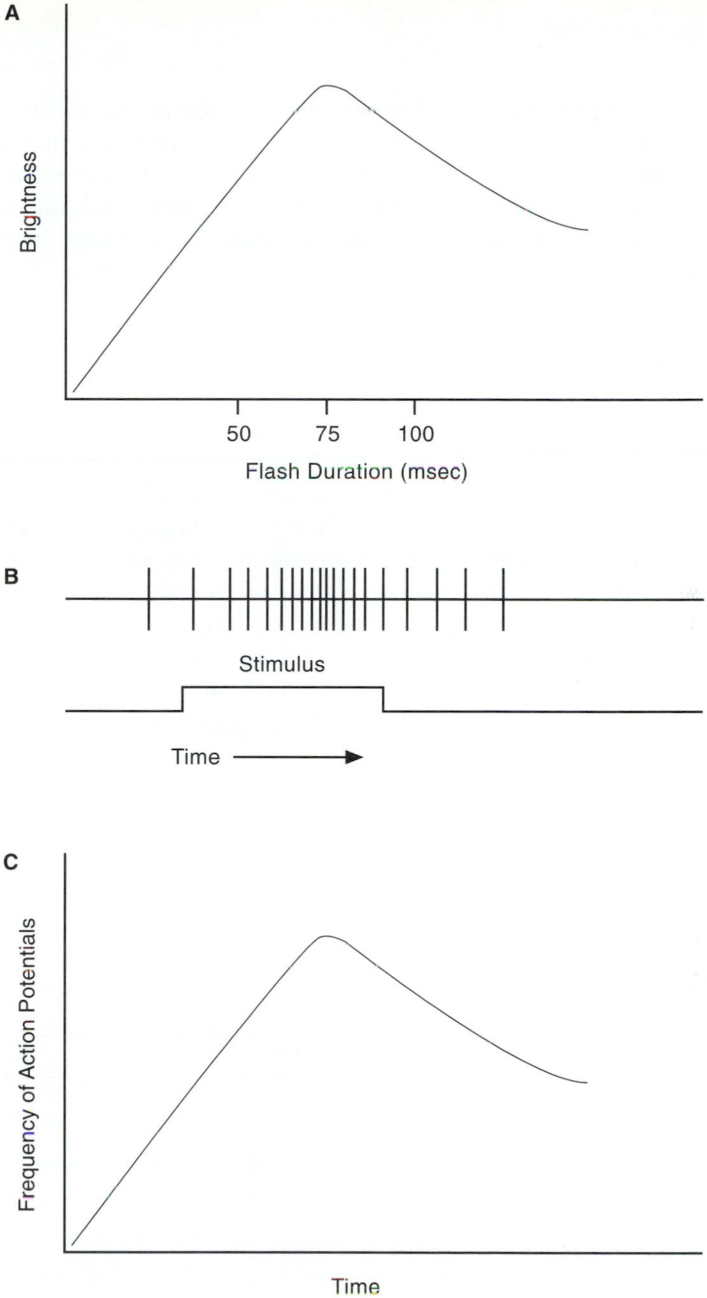


**FIGURE 8–9. A.** Graphic representation of the Broca–Sulzer effect. Stimuli with a duration of 50 to 100 milliseconds are perceived as brighter than stimuli with a duration of less than or greater than this value. **B.** A flash elicits action potentials in a ganglion cell. The frequency of these action potentials gradually increases and then decreases. **C.** The neural response in B is replotted as frequency of action potentials as a function of time. Note the similarity of this function to the form of the Broca–Sulzer effect; however, also note that the independent variables for these two phenomena are different. For the Broca–Sulzer effect, the independent variable is duration; for the neural response, it is time.

We have spent a considerable amount of time discussing the illusory correlation between the Broca–Sulzer effect and the form of the neural discharge. The purpose of this discussion is to illustrate the challenging nature of establishing reliable linkage between psychophysical phenomena and the underlying physiology. Models of visual function that propose such linkage must be critically examined.

### *Brücke–Bartley Effect*

The Brücke–Bartley effect, which is also referred to as brightness enhancement, is a manifestation of the Broca–Sulzer effect (Bartley, 1938). The Brücke–Bartley effect is that a light presented at approximately 10 Hz, which is seen as flickering, appears brighter than a steady light of the same average luminance.

The relationship between the Broca–Sulzer and Brücke–Bartley effects is illustrated by Figure 8–10A, which shows a temporal square wave stimulus with a frequency of 10 Hz. Each cycle is one tenth of a second or 100 milliseconds. Therefore, the duration of each increment of light is 50 milliseconds. This is approximately the same duration associated with the Broca–Sulzer effect. For both effects, stimuli of about 50-millisecond duration appear brighter than stimuli of other durations.

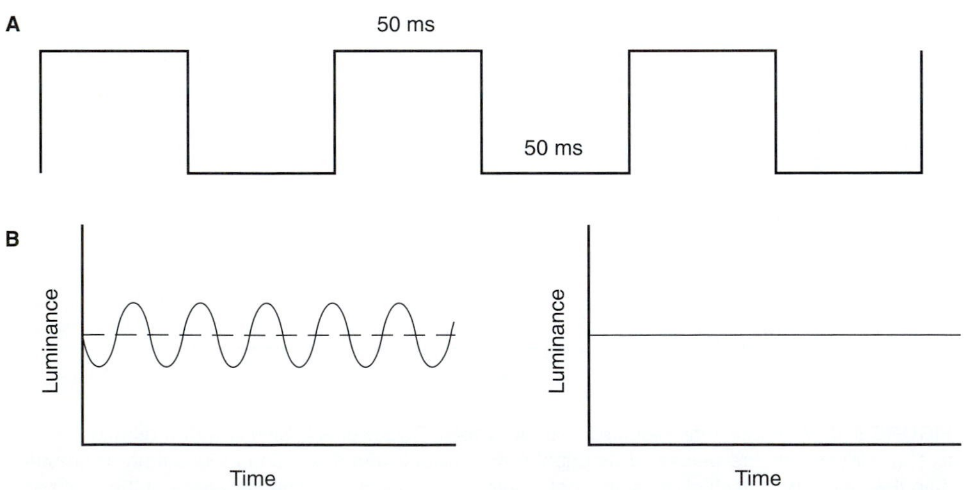


**FIGURE 8–10. A.** A square wave stimulus of 10 Hz can be thought of as consisting of half-cycles of 50-millisecond duration. **B.** The Talbot–Plateau law states that the brightness of a temporally modulated stimulus that is fused is equal to the brightness of a steady light of the same average luminance.

### *Talbot–Plateau Law*

The Talbot–Plateau law states that the brightness of a temporally modulated stimulus, when fused, is equal to the brightness of a steady light with the same time-averaged luminance (Fig. 8–10B). For this law to apply, the temporally modulated light must be presented at a rate beyond the CFF.

## *MASKING*

Masking involves the use of one stimulus, the **mask,** to reduce the visibility of another stimulus, the **target** (Breitmeyer, 1984). Masking phenomena provide information regarding both spatial and temporal processing of visual information. Although physiologic models have been proposed to account for these phenomena, these models are beyond the scope of this textbook. The various types of masking are briefly summarized here.

### *Simultaneous Masking*

In simultaneous masking, both the mask and the target are present at the same time. An example is the use of spatial gratings of a given frequency (the mask) to interfere with the detection of spatial gratings of a similar frequency (the target). As both frequencies share the same spatial frequency channels, there is a reduction in the visibility of the target gratings.

Simultaneous masking is more pronounced in patients with amblyopia (see Chap. 17) than in patients whose vision developed normally. Consequently, the acuity in an amblyopic eye is better when viewing isolated letters than when viewing a row of letters, such as in a typical eye chart. This reduction is acuity caused by surrounding spatial patterns is referred to as the **crowding phenomenon** (Flom et al, 1963).

### *Backward Masking*

In backward masking, the target precedes the mask. Even though the mask occurs after the target, it reduces the visibility of the target. This typically occurs when the mask is substantially brighter than the target. Because it is brighter, the mask is transmitted along the neural pathways at a relatively rapid rate. This enables it to surpass the preceding target and interfere with its detection.

### *Forward Masking*

In the case of forward masking, the mask precedes the target. The mask reduces the visibility of the subsequently presented target.

### *Metacontrast*

Metacontrast is a form of backward masking where the mask and target are spatially adjacent. The visibility of a briefly presented target is reduced by the subsequent presentation of a spatially adjacent mask (Fig. 8–11). Lateral processing (inhibition) within the retina is thought to account for metacontrast. In addition, stimulation of the faster magno pathway appears to be critical for producing metacontrast (Breitmeyer, 1992).

### *Paracontrast*

Paracontrast is a form of forward masking where the target and mask are spatially adjacent. A mask reduces the visibility of a subsequently presented, spatially adjacent target.

## CLINICAL CONSIDERATIONS

The diagnosis of primary open angle glaucoma (POAG) is often problematic. In POAG, the intraocular pressure (IOP) is typically, but not always, elevated. The IOP presumably damages the retinal ganglion cells. This ganglion cell damage manifests as visual field defects (scotomas).

Although increased IOP is correlated with visual field loss, it is not a reliable predictor of whether an individual will develop field loss. A minority of pa-

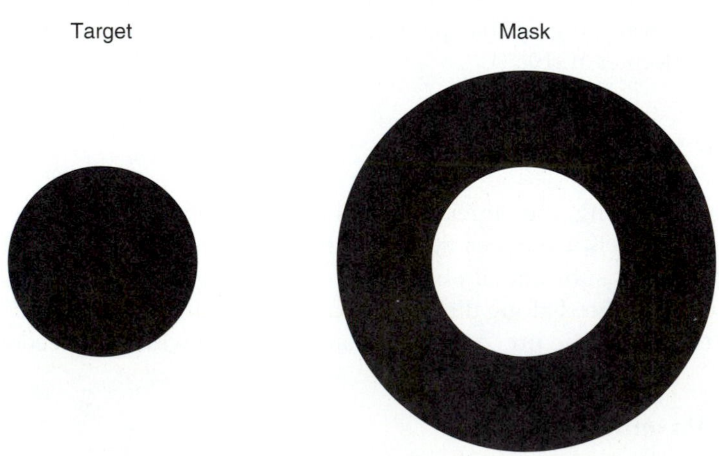


**FIGURE 8–11.** In metacontrast, the visibility of the target is reduced by the subsequent presentation of a spatially adjacent mask.

tients with elevated IOPs develop visual field defects. As a consequence, practitioners often do not initiate treatment until visual loss is demonstrable on visual field testing. Unfortunately, visual field testing is not as sensitive an indicator of loss of ganglion cell function as once was believed. A substantial proportion of the ganglion cells are damaged by the time early visual field defects manifest (Quigley et al, 1982). Consequently, there is interest in developing more sensitive psychophysical measures of ganglion cell loss.

Temporal modulation transfer functions and related temporal psychophysical tasks offer promise for assisting in the early diagnosis of glaucoma (Tyler, 1981; Johnson, 1995). Data obtained on patients with ocular hypertension (elevated IOPs with normal visual fields) suggest that TMTFs may be a more sensitive indicator of ganglion cell loss than are standard visual fields.

Figure 8–12 shows TMTFs typical of a healthy person and certain patients with ocular hypertension. The patient with ocular hypertension manifests no vi-

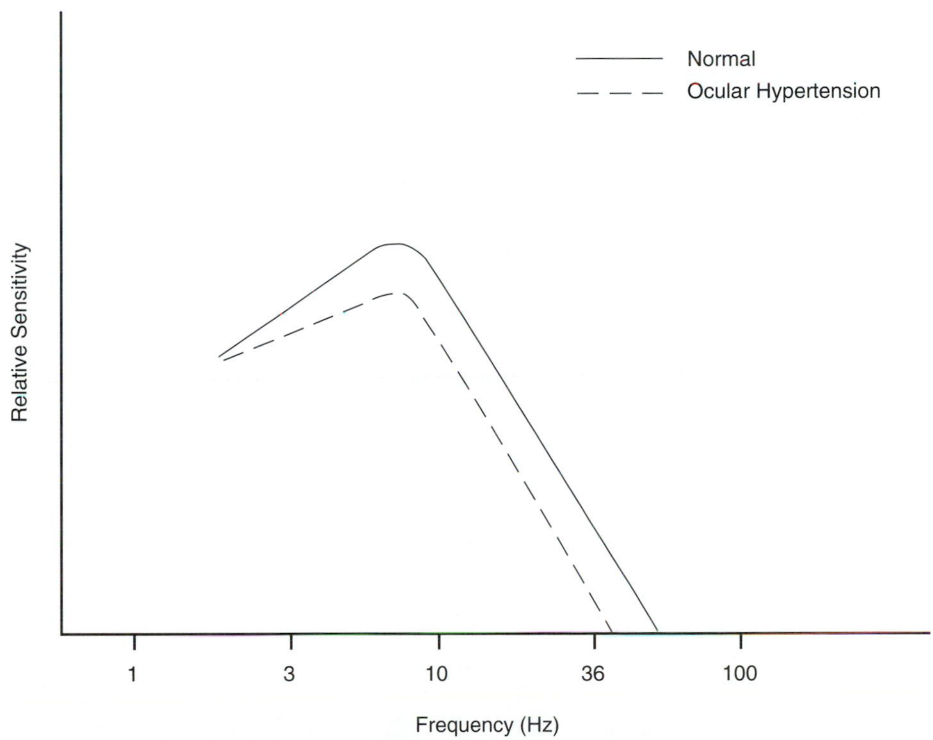


**FIGURE 8–12.** Expected temporal modulation transfer functions for a healthy patient and a patient with glaucoma, but normal visual fields (ocular hypertension). (*Adapted from Tyler CW. Specific defects of flicker sensitivity in glaucoma and ocular hypertension.* Invest Ophthalmol Vis Sci. *1981;20:204–212.)*

sual field defects; therefore, he or she may not be diagnosed as having glaucoma. Yet this patient manifests substantial losses in sensitivity to temporally modulated stimuli. Note that the most obvious loss of temporal sensitivity is at moderate and high temporal frequencies. This is typical of glaucomatous patients.

The high temporal frequency loss manifested in glaucoma may provide insight into the basic mechanisms of this disease. Both psychophysical and physiologic data support the notion that the magno pathway codes high temporal frequencies (see Chap. 13). Consequently, the high-frequency loss suffered in glaucoma suggests that the magno pathway is particularly vulnerable to glaucomatous damage. This is consistent with anatomic data that show a disproportionate loss of presumed magno fibers in glaucomatous eyes (Quigley et al, 1987).

Temporal modulation transfer functions also provide useful clinical information regarding retinitis pigmentosa and age-related macular degeneration (Tyler et al, 1984; Mayer et al, 1992). Although the testing of temporal aspects of vision is foreign to most eye care practitioners, there is increasing evidence suggesting that deficits in temporal processing may prove to be as useful in the diagnosis of certain eye diseases as are defects in spatial processing.

## SUMMARY

The same principles that apply to understanding spatial vision also apply to temporal vision. Temporal capabilities are assessed by determining transfer functions. Similar to spatial transfer functions, temporal transfer functions assess sensitivity as a function of frequency. The low and high-frequency drop-offs of these functions reflect basic limitations of neural processing.

Although not yet commonly used for clinical purposes, analysis of temporal vision holds promise. Further clinical applications await the development of practical clinical instrumentation.

# Self-Assessment Questions

1. A square wave stimulus has a frequency of 20 Hz. Calculate, in milliseconds, the duration of the on phase of each cycle. (*Hint:* Draw a diagram of the stimulus and label the duration of a cycle.)

2. A stimulus is on for 20 milliseconds and off for 20 milliseconds. This stimulus is presented continuously. Calculate its temporal frequency in Hz. (*Hint:* Draw a diagram of the stimulus and label it.)

3. Figure 8–8 shows that relative sensitivity, at low temporal frequencies, remains constant as the background illumination increases. Is this a manifestation of Weber's law? Explain. (*Hint:* See Chapter 11.)

# 9

# Motion Perception

Changes in the spatial distribution of light, over time, can lead to the perception of motion. Think of a person jogging across your field of vision. The spatial distribution of light that falls on your retina changes from moment to moment as you watch the person jog. This change in the spatiotemporal distribution of light leads to the perception of motion.

Consider the jogger in more detail. His or her arms are moving in opposite directions; they are swinging back and forth. As one leg extends forward, the other leg moves relatively little. The torso is moving slower than the leg that is stepping forward. A careful analysis of the jogger reveals that several different components of his or her body are moving at different rates and in different directions, but are perceived as a single unified object moving forward.

A growing body of knowledge provides insight regarding the complex mechanisms of motion perception. It is becoming evident that motion is processed along a specialized visual pathway, the parietal processing stream. This localization of function provides the basis for tests of motion perception that can be useful in the diagnoses of certain neurologic disorders. This chapter concentrates on certain psychophysical aspects of motion perception. The physiologic basis of motion perception is discussed in Chapter 15.

## MOTION PERCEPTION CAN BE STUDIED WITH SIMPLE STIMULI

When we observe a jogger, we are perceiving real motion; the image slides across the retina. Much of the motion that we experience, however, can be classified as **apparent** or **illusory motion.** For instance, when spatially separated lights are sequentially flashed, with a proper interval between the flashes, a sense of motion is elicited (Fig. 9–1) (Korte, 1915; Bartley, 1963). Referred to as **stroboscopic motion,** or the **phi phenomenon,** this effect is commonly used by businesses to create lighted signs that have the illusion of motion. An example is a bowling alley that advertises itself with a sign consisting of a lighted bowling ball that appears to move down an alley toward the awaiting pins. This illusion is created by the sequential flashing of the various lights constituting the sign at the proper rate.

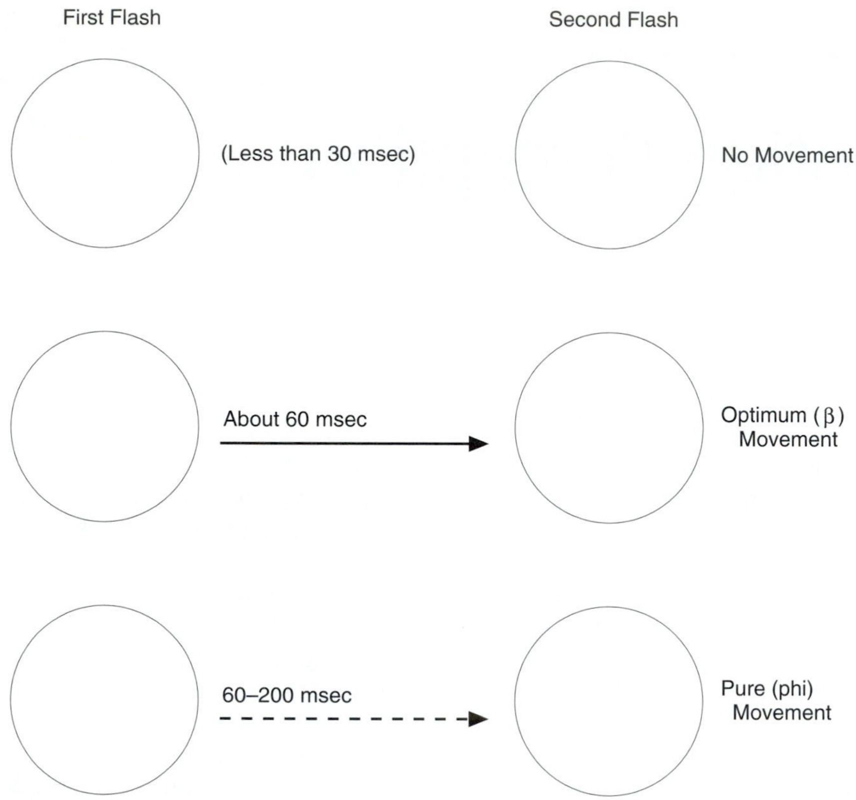


**FIGURE 9–1.** Stroboscopic movement. Various sensations of movement are produced by different intervals between the two flashes of light. An interval of 60 milliseconds produces a realistic sensation of the spot moving from position A to position B **(optimum** or **beta movement).** An interval of less than 30 milliseconds produces no sensation of movement, whereas durations of 60 to 200 milliseconds produce a partial illusion of movement **(pure** or **phi movement).**

Movies, television, and computer monitors all create a sense of motion by the use of stroboscopic stimuli. Each frame in a movie, television picture, or computer display has a spatial configuration slightly different from that of the preceding frame. These frames are presented at a temporal rate that creates the illusion of smooth motion.

While earlier studies of apparent motion used pairs of stroboscopic stimuli flashed in sequence, recent investigations frequently use sine wave gratings that are presented on a computer screen. The luminance profile of the spatial sine wave grating is sinusoidally modulated over time (Fig. 9–2). The resulting stimulus is a sine wave grating that appears to drift in a given direction.

The stroboscopic and sine wave stimuli that we have discussed up to this point are comparatively simple: they consist of a linear exchange of light for

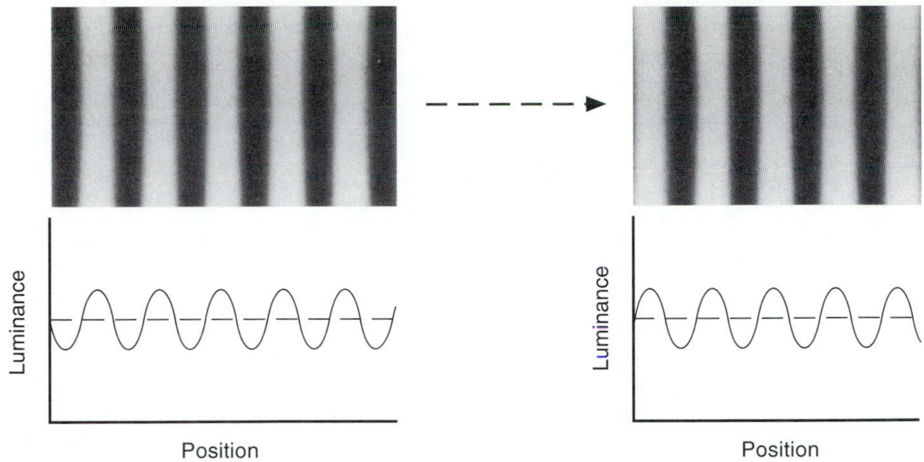


**FIGURE 9–2.** A sinusoidal grating is phase shifted sinusoidally over time to produce a grating that appears to drift or move.

dark (or vice versa). Such stimuli are referred to as **first order** stimuli for motion. We can, however, extract motion information from more complex stimuli, sometimes referred to as **second order, or global,** stimuli for motion (Logothetis,1994).

## *RANDOM DOT KINEMATOGRAMS CAN BE USED TO STUDY GLOBAL MOTION PERCEPTION*

Figure 9–3 shows how **random dot kinematograms** are used to study global (second order) motion perception. In panel A, the dots are moving in random directions; by definition, the pattern shows no coherence. As we proceed from panel B to panel C, an increasing percentage of the dots move in a common direction and the percent coherence increases from 50 percent to 100 percent. One measure of a person's ability to detect global motion is the **coherence threshold,** which is defined as the smallest percent coherence that results in the perception of motion in a defined direction (e.g., up, down, left, or right) (Newsome and Paré, 1988; Silverman et al, 1990).

Random dot kinematogram stimuli can also be used to study other aspects of motion perception (Fig. 9–4) (Nakayama, 1985). The minimum distance that the dots must move in a given direction to elicit the perception of motion is referred to as the **minimum displacement threshold ($D_{min}$).** Likewise, the maximum distance the dots can move and still elicit motion perception is called the **maximum displacement threshold ($D_{max}$).**

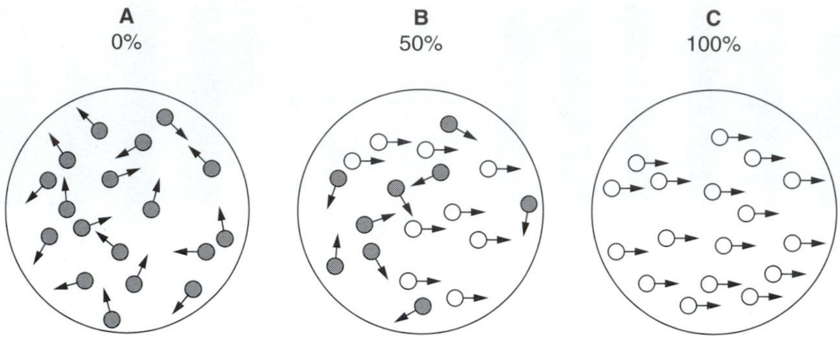


**FIGURE 9–3.** Random dot kinematograms are used to study global motion perception. **A.** When the dots are moving in random directions, there is no coherence. **B.** At 50 percent coherence, the direction of movement of 50 percent of the dots is correlated. **C.** All the dots are moving in the same direction when the coherence is 100 percent.

The detection of motion elicted by random dot kinematograms is more complex than is the case with stroboscopic stimuli (Nakayama and Tyler, 1981). Whereas stroboscopic motion (first order motion perception) can be explained by local luminance changes on the retina, such an explanation will not suffice for random dot kinematograms (second order motion perception). In order for random dot stimuli to elicit the perception of motion, the visual system must integrate information from many dots over a broad expanse of the retina. This requires sophisticated neural processing that apparently occurs in *higher level* motion centers in the cortex (Newsome and Paré, 1988).

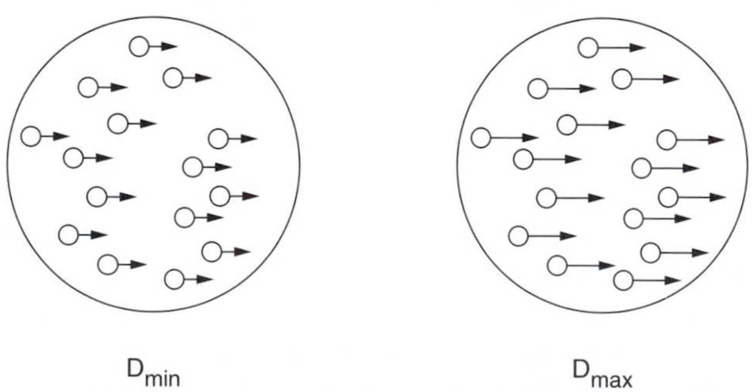


**FIGURE 9–4.** The minimum movement that elicits the perception of motion is referred to as the minimum displacement threshold ($D_{min}$), while the maximum movement that elicits movement is the maximum displacement threshold ($D_{max}$). (*Adapted from Bullimore MA, Wood JM, Swenson K. Motion perception in glaucoma.* Invest Ophthalmol Vis Sci. *1993;34:3526–3533.*)

## *Motion Is Processed Along a Specialized Pathway*

From the retina to the striate cortex, motion information is processed primarily along the magno pathway (see Chaps. 2 and 13). While the parvo pathway is not blind to motion cues, it apparently plays less of a role in motion perception than does the magno pathway (Newsome and Wurtz, 1988; Maunsell et al, 1990). Interestingly, amblyopes (see Chap. 17) show reduced senstivity to slow velocities, apparently due to an impairment of the parvo pathway (Steinman et al, 1988).

Motion information is disseminated from the striate cortex to adjoining cortical areas, with a convergence of motion information apparently occurring at visual area 5, which is also known as the **middle temporal area, MT, or V5** (see Figs. 14–3 and 15–1). This cortical pathway, which originates at the striate cortex and continues through visual area 5 to the prefrontal cortex, is variously referred to as the **parietal** pathway, the **dorsal** processing stream, or the **where** system (Mishkin et al, 1983).

Cells in V5 have features that make them well-suited to play a major role in motion perception (Maunsell and Van Essen, 1983). As discussed in Chapter 15, neurons in V5 respond to global stimuli, including random dot kinematograms. Electrical stimulation of cells in V5 of a monkey alters the animal's motion perception (Salzman and Newsome, 1994). Underscoring the centrality of this area to motion perception, damage to V5 can impair the perception of motion (akinetopsia) (Zihl et al, 1983; Barton et al, 1996). The functional physiology of V5 is discussed in more detail in Chapter 15.

## *Luminance Is a Stronger Stimulus for Motion Than Color*

Ample evidence suggests that the magno pathway plays an important role in the perception of motion. An interesting question is whether the perception of motion can be elicited by stimuli defined solely by color, such as isoluminant gratings, that are thought to be poor stimuli for the magno pathway (Livingstone and Hubel, 1987, 1988). Isoluminant gratings consist of bars of various hues, with each bar having the same luminance (see Chaps. 5 and 13). The grating is visible only because the bars that constitute it have different hues.

Consider the isoluminant grating that is schematically represented in Figure 9–5. The bars are moving to the right. Would an individual perceive the movement of the bars of this isoluminant grating as motion? The answer is complicated (Cavanagh, 1996). Under certain isoluminant conditions, the perception of motion is impaired. The perception may be weak or not as fast as the actual movement of the bars. Adding luminance contrast (i.e., making one bar brighter than the other) improves the perception of motion. This psychophysical finding is consistent with a predominant role for the magno pathway in processing motion information. Under certain other isoluminant conditions, however, the per-

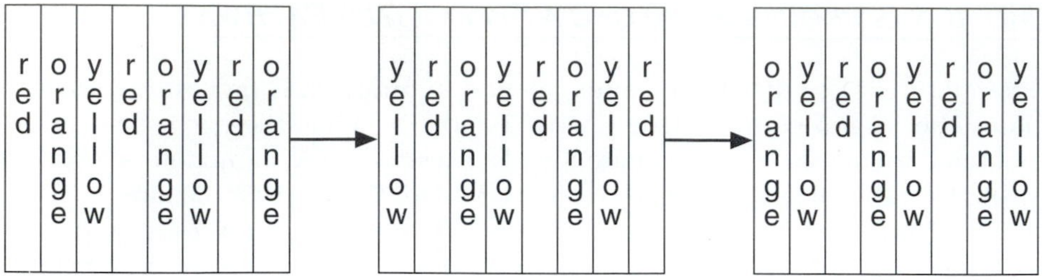


**FIGURE 9–5.** The bars that constitute an isoluminant grating all have the same luminance. The perception of movement as the bars drift to the right is impaired by the absence of luminance contrast.

ception of motion is robust, pointing to a role for the parvo pathway in coding motion (Cropper and Derrington, 1996).

## *SPATIAL RESOLUTION IS AFFECTED BY STIMULUS MOVEMENT*

Many of the visual stimuli that we encounter are not stable, but are moving. What effect does the velocity of a moving stimulus have on visual acuity? As stimulus velocity increases, resolution acuity remains relatively constant until the stimulus velocity reaches about 60 to 80 degree/second (Miller and Ludvigh, 1962). Beyond this velocity, the ability to resolve a moving stimulus, commonly referred to as **dynamic visual acuity,** deteriorates (Fig. 9–6). The reduction in dynamic visual acuity at increasing target velocities is apparently due to our inability to accurately follow the stimulus with tracking (or following) eye movements, referred to as **smooth pursuit eye movements** (Barmack, 1970).

## *THE WORLD IS NOT SMEARED DURING SACCADIC EYE MOVEMENTS*

Place your two index fingers at arms length, separated by about one foot. Now, look back and forth between your two fingers. This ballistic eye movement between two fixation points is referred to as a **saccadic eye movement.** Note that as you move your eyes from finger to finger, or from any one object to a another object, the visual world remains still and clear. This is in spite of the movement of the image of the world across your retinae as you move your eyes.

Vision is suppressed shortly before, during, and shortly after saccadic eye movements. These phenomena, variously referred to as **saccadic suppression** and **saccadic omission,** enable us to look from one object to another without

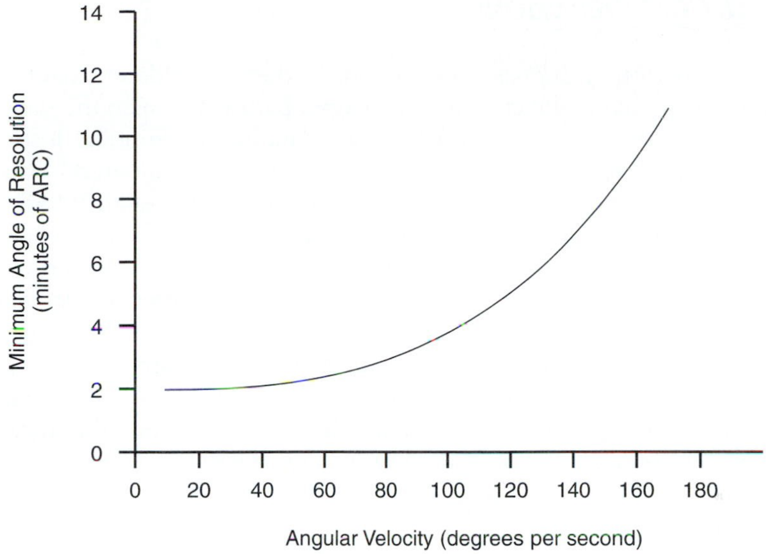


**FIGURE 9–6.** The minimum angle of resolution remains relatively constant as the velocity of an acuity target increases up to about 60 to 80 degrees per second. Beyond this velocity, there is a degradation in resolution acuity. (*Adapted from Miller JW, Ludvigh E. The effect of relative motion on visual acuity.* Survey Ophthal. *1962;7:83–116.*)

a smearing of our vision that would otherwise be caused by the rapid movement of the image across the retina (Matin, 1974; Ciuffreda and Tannen, 1995).

Saccadic suppression is apparently due to a selective suppression of the magno pathway. This makes sense when you consider that the image movement across the retina during saccades is very fast and consists of high temporal frequencies. Since the magno pathway (not the parvo pathway) is most sensitive to high temporal frequencies (see Chaps. 2 and 13), it needs to be suppressed to avoid a smearing of our vision.

The mechanism whereby the magno pathway is suppressed during saccades is not known for certain. Some hypothesize a centrally initiated suppression whereby the signal to move the eyes is also the signal to suppress the magno pathway (Burr et al, 1994). This makes sense because the suppression begins prior to the actual eye movement. The suppression, however, is very similar to reductions in sensitivity due to masking. This observation has led to the suggestion that the movement of the image across the retina acts as a mask that is selective for the magno pathway (Matin et al, 1972; Schwartz and Godwin, 1996).

## CLINICAL CONSIDERATIONS

As we have previously discussed (see Chap. 8), there is evidence that the neural damage in glaucoma is selective for the magno pathway. Given the data in support of a critical role for the magno pathway in motion perception, it should not be surprising that tests of motion perception have been evaluated to determine if they are useful for the early diagnosis of glaucoma (Trick et al, 1995).

Recent studies of motion perception in glaucoma have used random dot kinematograms. *Minimum displacement thresholds* have been found to be elevated in glaucoma suspects (Bullimore et al, 1993). In patients with glaucomatous field defects, *motion coherence thresholds* are higher in those regions of the visual field showing glaucomatous damage than in comparatively unaffected regions of the visual fields (Bosworth et al, 1997). These results suggest that motion deficits occur relatively early in the disease process and that measures of motion perception may be valuable in early diagnosis.

## SUMMARY

The perception of motion requires the analysis of spatial displacements over time. Basic (first order) motion perception that is elicited with simple stroboscopic stimuli can be explained by processing that occurs early in the visual system (V1 or earlier). The perception of motion that is elicited by global cues (such as random dot kinematograms), however, apparently depends on an analysis in higher visual centers—in particular, V5. (Additional evidence in support of this view is discussed in Chap. 15.)

V5 is part of the parietal processing stream. This pathway originates in the striate cortex, passes through V5, and continues on to the prefrontal cortex. The major precortical input to the parietal processing stream is the magno pathway.

It has been proposed that diseases resulting in selective damage to the magno pathway may lead to deficits in motion perception. This hypothesis has led to studies of motion perception in glaucoma that demonstrate impaired motion perception in the early stages of the disease. The practicality of tests of motion perception for routine clinical practice awaits further study.

# Q Self-Assessment Questions

1. Describe an experiment that would allow you to locate the areas of the human cortex that are most responsible for analyzing motion information. (*Hint:* See Chap. 1.)

# 10

# Depth Perception

Human observers are very adept at judging the relative distances of objects. As you look around the room in which you are sitting or look out the window, it is a straightforward task to judge which objects are close and which are located further away.

A common misconception regarding depth perception is that it depends on the use of both eyes—that it is solely a binocular phenomenon. If one eye is covered, however, a strong sense of depth persists. This tells us that monocular cues (monocular information) play a large role in depth perception. Binocular vision does, nonetheless, play a significant role in depth perception. Although depth is noted monocularly, it is generally enhanced when viewing binocularly.

In this chapter, we discuss both monocular and binocular cues to depth. To discuss binocular cues, we touch on some of the processes involved in binocular vision. Our discussion of binocular vision is limited to the presentation of background material sufficient to gain a basic understanding of stereopsis. More detailed discussions of binocular vision are found in texts dealing exclusively with this broad topic.

## MONOCULAR DEPTH CUES

Monocular depth cues are perceived just as strongly when viewed with one eye as when viewed with both eyes. The major classes of monocular depth cues are pictorial depth cues, motion parallax, and accommodation.

### *Pictorial Depth Cues*

Pictorial depth cues are those cues that can be presented in a two-dimensional representation, such as a photograph or a painting. The sense of depth that can be created by the cues is substantial. Artists are masterful at manipulating pictorial cues to create a strong sense of depth.

Pictorial depth cues (size, linear perspective, texture, interposition, clarity, and lighting and shadow) are of critical importance in our day-to-day judgements of depth. Monocular individuals manifest surprisingly sophisticated depth perception largely due to the ever-present pictorial cues in our visual world.

***Size.*** Consider the following experiment. You observe two illuminated balloons in a pitch black room. The only objects illuminated are the balloons. Such a scene may appear similar to that illustrated in Figure 10–1 (Ittleson and Kilpatrick, 1951). When asked to judge the relative distances of the two balloons, most observers assume that the larger balloon is closer and the smaller balloon is farther away. They do so although the balloons are the same distance from the observer, with the larger one being more inflated than the smaller one.

The aforementioned experiment shows that the perceived distances of objects are often determined by the relative sizes of the retinal images they produce. If two objects are thought to be the same size, the object that produces the smaller retinal image size is perceived as being farther away. **Relative size** is an important depth cue when viewing a scene, such as in Figure 10–1, that includes several objects with sizes that can be compared.

**Familiar size** is a cue to depth that is used when we view objects of known size. For instance, imagine a barn surrounded by nothing but snow. Relative size is not a useful cue to depth because there are no other objects to which the barn can be compared. To judge the distance of the barn, we would probably assume it is the size of a typical barn. If the barn produces a small retinal image, it would be seen as far away.

***Linear Perspective.*** Linear perspective is related to relative size. Figure 10–2 provides an example of linear perspective. A strong sense of depth is experienced because it is assumed that the horizontal lines on the bottom of the picture and those at the top of the picture are identical objects having the same actual size. Because the lines at the top of the picture produce a smaller retinal image sizes, they are perceived as further away.

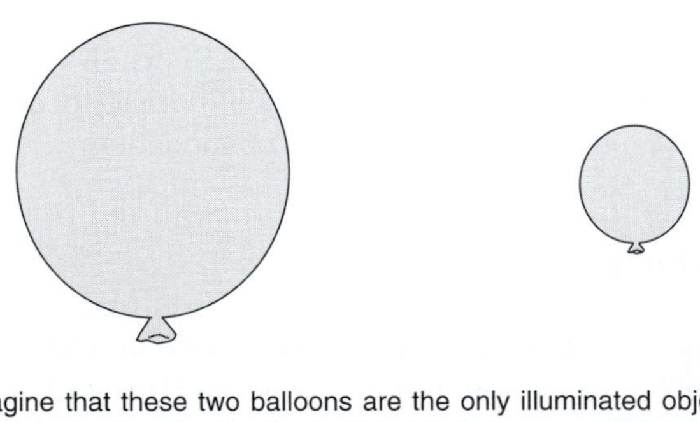

**FIGURE 10–1.** Imagine that these two balloons are the only illuminated objects in an otherwise dark room. In these circumstances, the less inflated balloon may appear to be located farther away than the more inflated balloon.

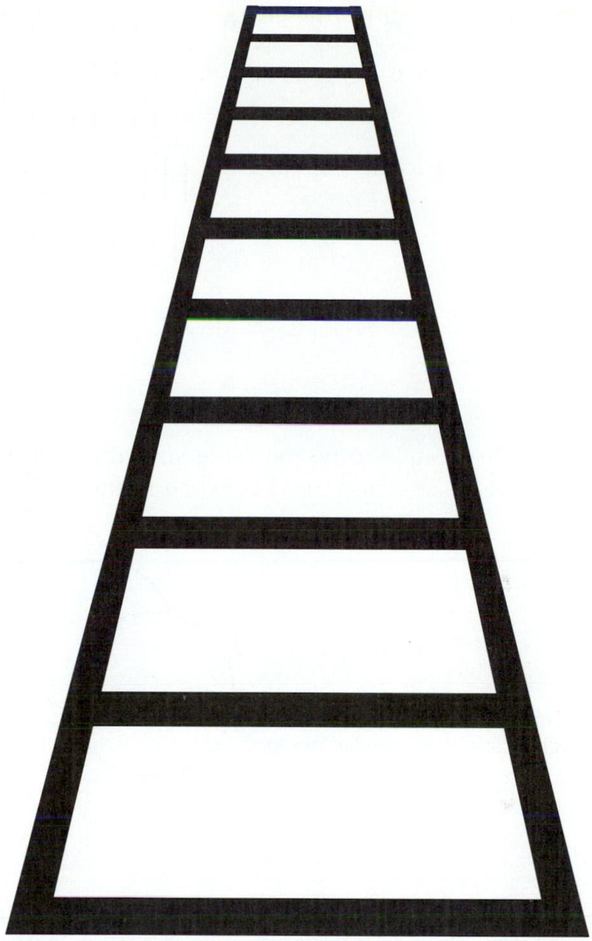

**FIGURE 10–2.** Linear perspective is a monocular cue to depth. The top of the diagram is perceived to be at a greater distance than the bottom.

***Texture.*** Texture is also related to relative size. Figure 10–3A shows that the smaller, more densely packed objects appear farther away than the larger, less densely packed objects. The observer assumes that all the objects are the same size; those that produce the smaller retinal image size are perceived as more distant.

***Interposition.*** Interposition occurs when one object blocks the view of another object (Fig. 10–3B). The result of this interposition is that the blocked object appears farther away from the observer than the object that does the blocking.

A

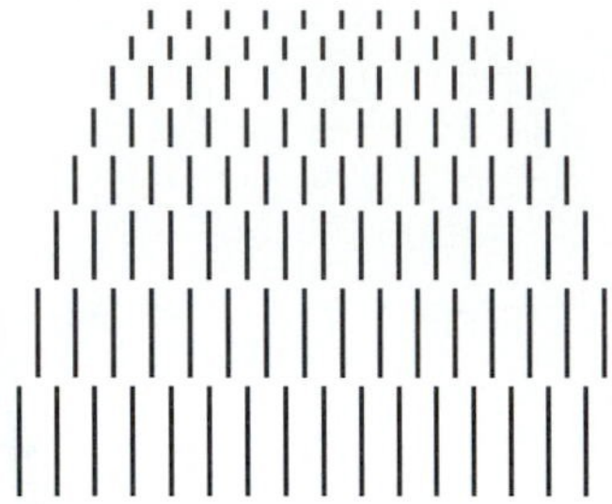

B

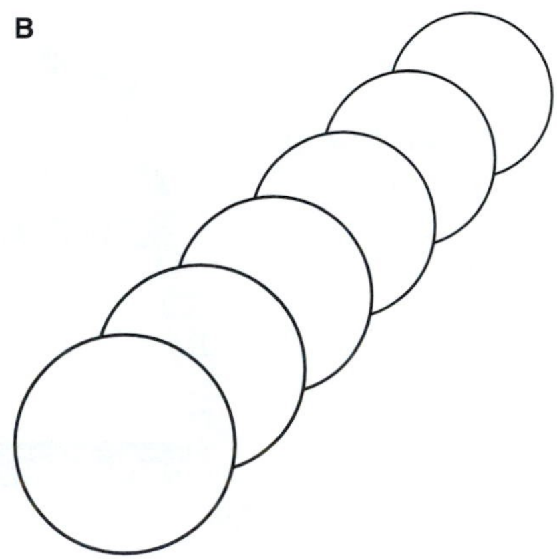

**FIGURE 10–3. A.** Texture is a monocular cue to depth. **B.** Interposition is also a monocular cue to depth.

***Clarity.*** Clarity is essentially a form of interposition. Objects in a photograph, picture, or actual scene that appear clear are interpreted as being nearer than those objects that appear hazy. Fog, smoke, rain, and smog act as interposing elements that contribute to making the obscured objects appear farther away.

***Lighting and Shadow.*** When light falls on an object, the object casts a shadow. The shadow is interpreted as falling behind the object; consequently, a sense of depth is created.

### *Motion Parallax*

Motion parallax is a **kinetic monocular depth** produced by the relative motion of two or more objects. It is nicely demonstrated by making the following observation. Place your two index fingers directly in line with each other, with one located 15 cm from your right eye and the other located 30 cm from your right eye. Close your left eye. Fixate on the distant finger while moving your head sideways. Without changing your fixation, notice that the near finger appears to move in the opposite direction of your head (against-motion). Now fixate the near finger and again move your head sideways. This time, notice that the far finger appears to move in the same direction as your head (with-motion). The preceding demonstration shows that the relative motion of objects provides information regarding their relative distances.

Motion parallax has useful clinical applications when viewing ocular structures with a monocular instrument, such as a monocular ophthalmoscope. Consider the example of a small, dot-like opacity that is observed during monocular ophthalmoscopy. If the clinician fixates on the pupil and moves his or her head sideways, the opacity shows against-movement if located anterior to the iris. Likewise, with-motion is noted if the opacity is located posterior to the plane of the iris.

### *Accommodation*

During accommodation, the dioptric power of the lens increases. This allows near objects to be clearly focused on the retina. The signal to accommodation contains information regarding the distance of viewed objects, but the extent to which this information is used for the determination of depth is not known.

## *BINOCULAR DEPTH CUES*

### *Stereopsis*

Consider the situation illustrated in Figure 10–4. A square is fixated by the subject. Distant to this square is a triangle and proximal to this square is a circle. An observer, while fixating the square, is able to judge the distances of the triangle and circle relative to this square. It is obvious to the individual that the triangle is farther away than the square, and the circle is closer. This is because the retinal locations on which the images of the objects fall signal the distances of these objects. The observer would perceive depth even in the absence of any other cues to depth (e.g., relative size, interposition). Because the observer is instructed to fixate on the square, images of the square fall on the two foveas. The two foveas correspond to the same direction in space and are referred to as **corresponding points** (Ogle, 1950).

Consider the retinal images produced by the triangle. The light rays from the triangle pass through the nodal points of the eyes and strike the retinas nasal to the foveas. The distance between the corresponding points (in this case, the foveas) and the image locations is referred to as **retinal disparity,** and provides information that allows the visual system to judge the triangle as being distant to the fixated object. In this case, where the retinal images fall nasal to the corresponding points, we have **uncrossed retinal disparity.**

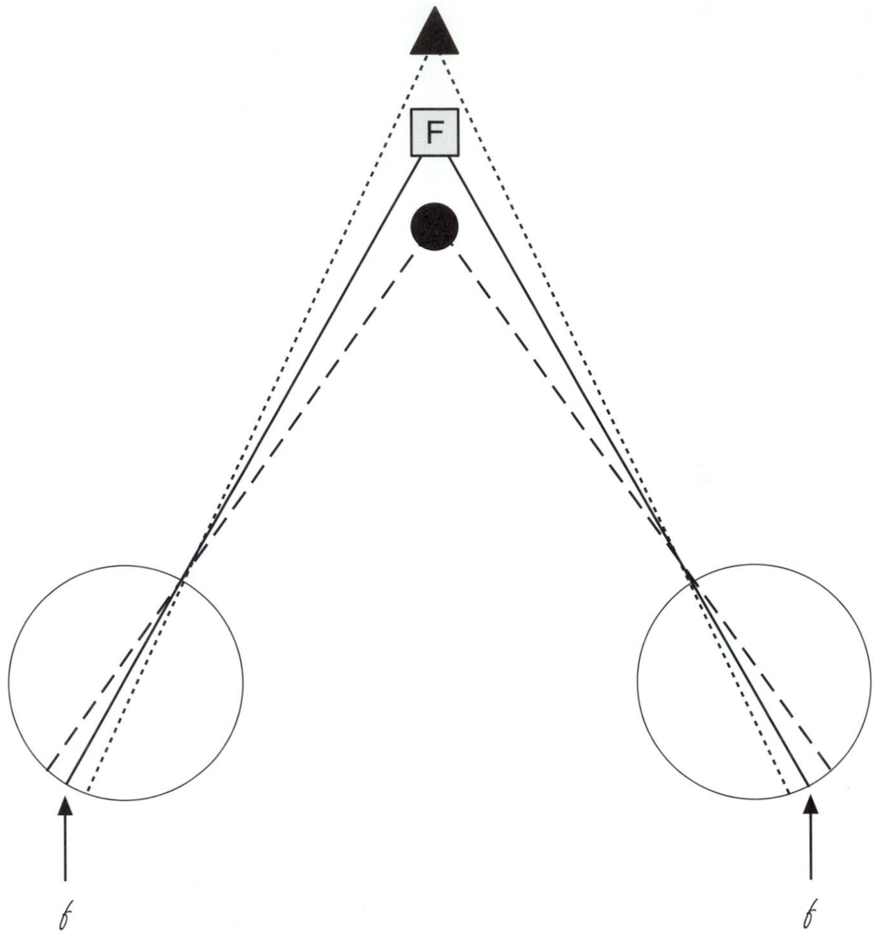


**FIGURE 10–4.** The square is fixated and its image falls on each fovea. The triangle produces uncrossed retinal disparity, which causes it to be perceived as farther away than the square. The circle produces crossed retinal disparity, causing it to be perceived as closer than the square. A sense of depth—stereopsis—is obtained because the retinal disparities fall within Panum's fusional area on the retina.

Now take the case of the circle. The rays emitted by the circle strike the retinas temporal to the foveas. This is referred to as **crossed retinal disparity** and signals that the circle is located closer than the object of regard (the square).

The perception of the depth that is produced by binocular retinal disparity is referred to as **stereopsis.** Stereopsis is important for providing finely tuned depth perception at near distances (particularly within arm's length), especially when other depth cues are absent. Stereopsis is less important when viewing objects at far distances because the threshold for retinal disparity, which is specified as an angle at the eye, requires such objects to be separated by great distances.

Binocular disparity produces stereopsis only if the retinal disparity is not too great. If the retinal disparity is not too great, the retinal images are fused with a resultant sensation of depth—stereopsis. The area on the retina that corresponds to this area of binocular fusion is referred to as **Panum's fusional area.** If the retinal disparity is too great, binocular fusion does not occur. The images fall on retinal positions that signal grossly different directions, resulting in **physiological diplopia** (double vision).

Demonstration of stereopsis and physiologic diplopia is straightforward. Hold one index finger about 15 cm from your nose, and hold your other index finger directly behind it at arm's length. Fixate on the near finger. Notice that the distant finger is doubled. Now slowly move the distant finger toward your nose while maintaining fixation on the near finger. Note that before you reach the near finger, the physiologic diplopia disappears and only the sense of depth is noted. At this point, the retinal images of the two fingers fall within Panum's fusional area.

Figure 10–5 illustrates a slightly different way of understanding stereopsis. It has been mentioned that images falling on the two foveas signal the same direction (i.e., they are corresponding points). In fact, each retinal point has a corresponding point in the other eye, and each of these pairs of corresponding points signals the same distance. Plotting these corresponding points (for a given fixation distance) results in a curved plane referred to as a **horopter** (Ogle, 1950). All points on the horopter stimulate corresponding retinal points and are perceived as being at the same distance. (The horopter is curved, rather than flat, because of the curvature of the retina.)

Figure 10–5 shows that those objects that fall relatively close to the horopter are fused. For these stimuli, the retinal disparity falls within Panum's fusional area and the result is stereopsis. For those objects located at greater distances from the horopter, the disparity is too great for the objects to be fused, and the result is physiologic diplopia.

There is convincing evidence that stereopsis is coded by cortical neurons (Barlow et al, 1967). As discussed in Chapter 14, binocular cortical neurons are maximally responsive to a stimulus at a specific distance from the eyes. The same stimulus, when positioned at other distances, elicits a less vigorous neural response. These neurons act as **disparity detectors.**

### *Convergence*

As we view objects at various distances, the eyes converge and diverge. The degree of convergence potentially provides information regarding the distance of objects; however, the manner in which this information is incorporated into the conscious perception of depth, if at all, is unresolved (Brenner and Van Damme, 1998).

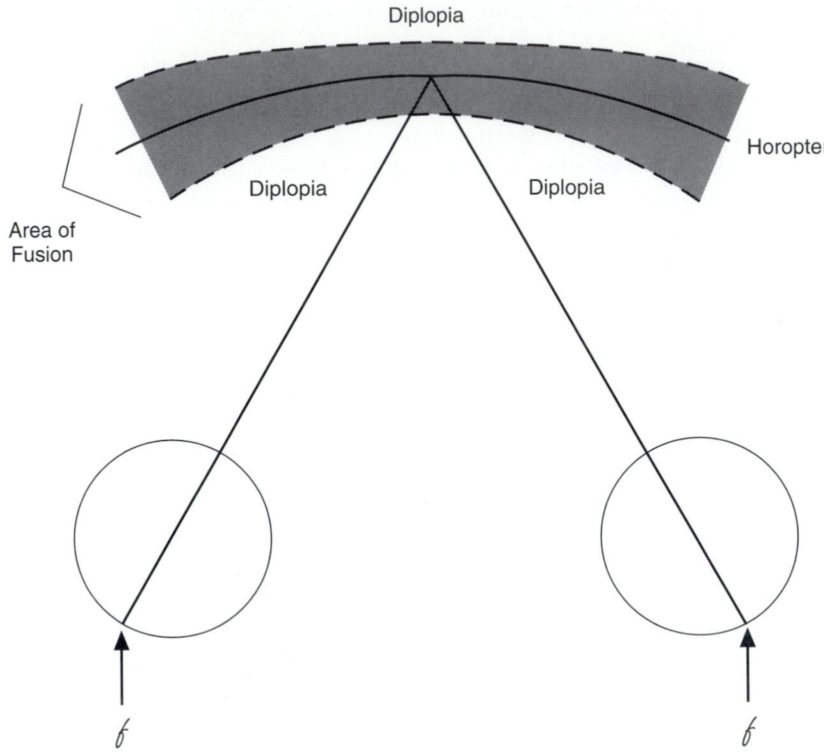


**Figure 10–5.** Objects located on the horopter all appear at the same depth. Objects located within the shaded area produce retinal disparities that fall within Panum's fusional area. Consequently, objects located within the shaded area are fused and produce stereopsis. Objects falling outside of Panum's fusional area are not fused and produce physiological diplopia.

## *VISUAL ILLUSIONS*

Visual illusions are erroneous perceptions. Certain of the most commonly encountered visual illusions result when pictorial depth cues are used to judge the size of unfamiliar objects.

The apparent size of an object does not normally change with viewing distance. Despite the difference in retinal image size, an automobile that is nearby is not seen as larger than an automobile that is farther away. Our visual system compensates for differences in retinal image size by taking into account the relative distance of an object, a phenomenon referred to as **size constancy.** When judgments of distance are erroneous, such as occurs when viewing a flat picture, size constancy may fail. The result is a type of visual illusion that is called a **size illusion.**

In the **corridor illusion** (Fig. 10–6), size constancy fails because monocular depth cues provide incorrect information regarding the relative distances of the circles. Although the two circles are at the same distance from you, the top circle is perceived as further away. This leads to the illusion that the top circle is larger. In fact, the two circles are the same size.

The well-known **moon illusion** is considered by many to be a size illusion (Kaufman and Rock, 1962). The moon, when viewed on the horizon, appears larger than when viewed directly overhead in the cloudless sky. The angular subtense of the moon, however, is the same under both conditions. The illusion occurs because the moon does not appear to be at the same distances when on the horizon and directly overhead (Fig. 10–7). Because of the background presented by the horizon (trees, houses, fields, etc.), the moon appears farther away than when viewed directly overhead; consequently, it appears larger on the horizon.

One of the most famous illusions is the **Müller–Lyer illusion** (Fig. 10–8). This size illusion is thought to result from the lines mimicking the corner of a

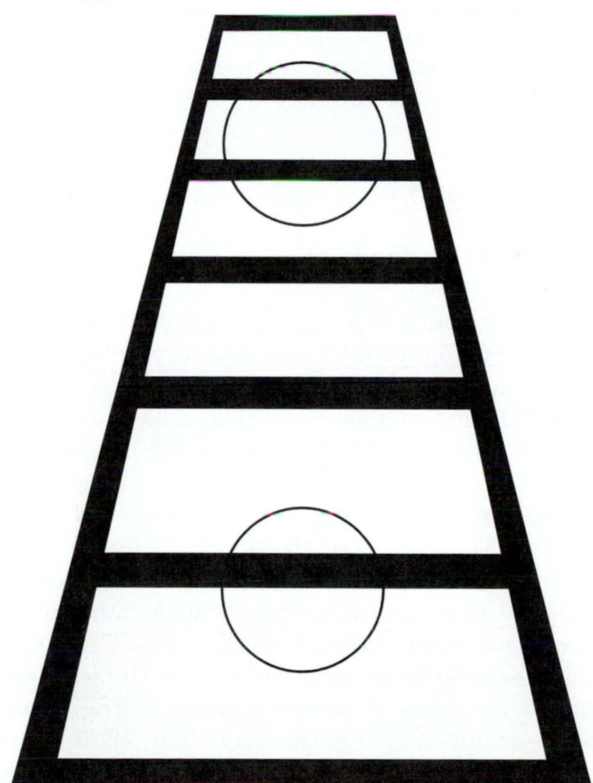

**FIGURE 10–6.** Corridor illusion. Both circles are the same size, but the top circle appears larger than the bottom circle.

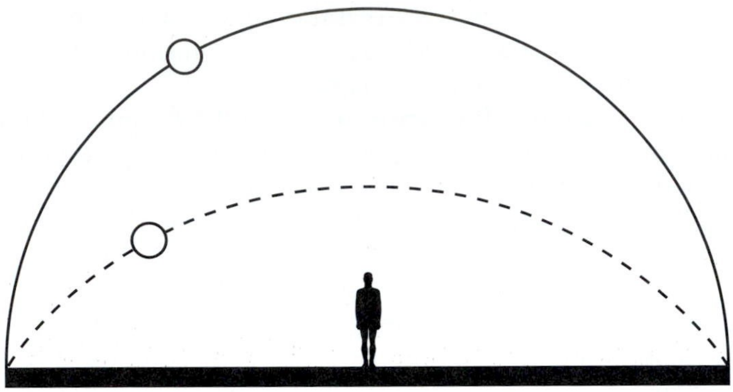

**FIGURE 10–7.** The actual trajectory of the moon is given by the solid line and the perceived trajectory by the dashed line. When viewed on the horizon, the moon is judged as farther away than when viewed overhead. Since the angular subtense of the moon is the same under both conditions, the moon looks larger on the horizon.

room (Gregory, 1978). The line that appears as an outgoing corner is judged as farther away than the line that appears as an ingoing corner. Because the lines are equal in length, the more "distant" line is perceived as longer.

## *CLINICAL CONSIDERATIONS*

### *Stereopsis and Visual Development*

The measurement of a patient's degree of stereopsis provides important information regarding the status of his or her visual system. Stereopsis is measured clinically by asking a patient to view a flat surface that has two identical figures separated by a very small distance. Using Polaroid or red and green glasses, only one object is presented to each eye. The separation of the images is designed to produce retinal disparity, and this disparity results in stereopsis. In a typical stereopsis test, the minimum amount of disparity that allows the patient to perceive depth is determined. This threshold disparity is referred to as the patient's **stereoacuity** (a form of hyperactivity) and can be as small as 3 seconds of arc.

Highly developed stereoacuity is dependent on a normal complement of binocular neurons in the visual cortex. For these cortical neurons to be present, the visual system must have been exposed to a normal visual environment during its development. Disorders of binocular vision, such as anisometropia and strabismus, alter the infant's visual environment and retard the development of binocular cortical neurons (see Chap. 17). The result is a reduction in stereoacuity (Birch and Stager, 1985). Consequently, the clinical measurement of stereoacuity provides important information regarding a patient's visual development and current binocular status.

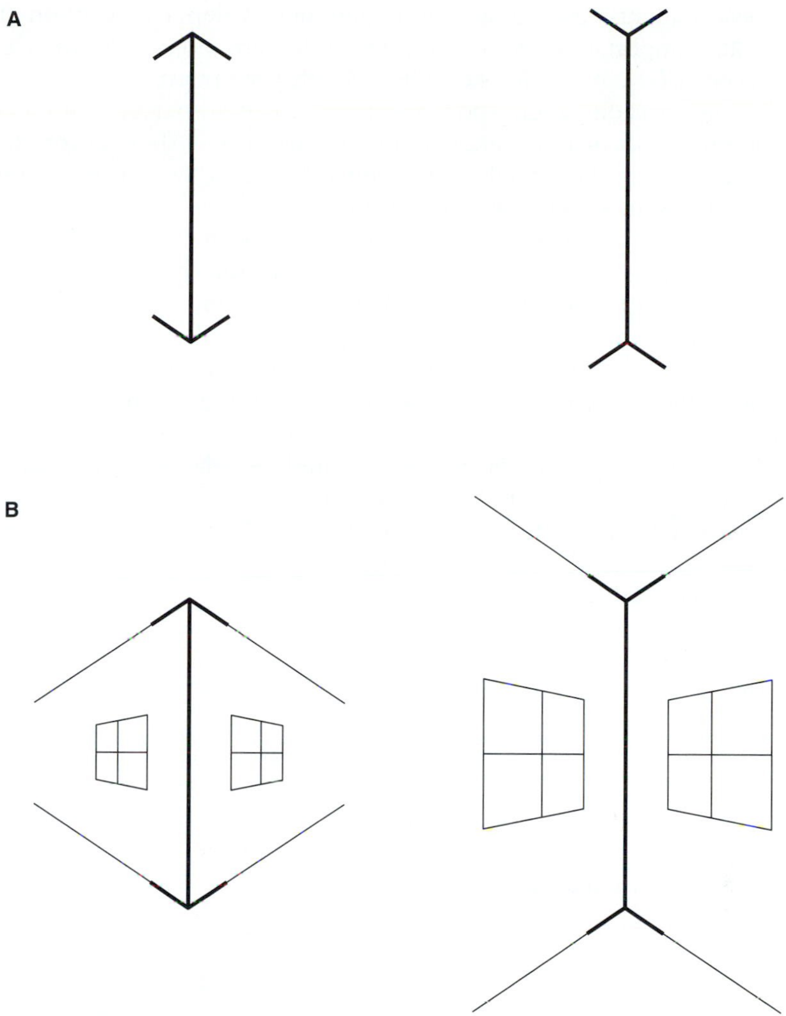


**FIGURE 10–8. A.** The Müller–Lyer illusion. The two lines are the same length. **B.** One explanation for the illusion is that the arrows may be likened to outgoing and ingoing corners of a room.

### *Monovision Contact Lenses*

It is common clinical practice to correct one eye of a presbyope for distance vision and the other eye for near vision. This enables the presbyope to alternate between the two eyes to see both distant and near objects clearly. (Diplopia typically does not occur because the blurred foveal image from the unused eye is suppressed.) This arrangement may reduce stereopsis because the patient is essentially monocular at all distances. However, contrary to what is often believed, these patients retain a substantial amount of depth perception. This is because many important cues to depth perception are monocular. In fact, a patient with only one eye manifests excellent depth perception.

Will a monovision patient show a reduced ability to perceive distances relative to normal binocular viewing conditions? The answer depends on the task. Stereopsis is an important depth cue for near distances, especially within arms length, but is less important at greater distances.

A question that often arises is whether monovision contact lenses cause a reduction in stereopsis that interferes with driving safety. This is not an easy question to answer because each individual adapts to monovision at a different rate and to a different extent. Some patients perform well with monovision; others do not. While many of the judgments of distance required in driving are for far distances, where stereopsis is less important, other judgements are for near distances.

At a minimum, monovision patients should be advised of a reduction in depth perception that could potentially interfere with their driving. Spectacles that compensate for the reduced distance vision in the near eye may be recommended for wear over the contact lenses. Alternatively, distance contact lenses may be worn on both eyes when driving.

## SUMMARY

Depth perception is a major feature of our visual world. The cues for depth perception are both monocular and binocular in nature. Stereopsis, a form of binocular depth perception, is dependent on normal visual development. For this reason, the clinical measurement of stereoacuity provides important information regarding visual development.

# Self-Assessment Questions

1. Could monovision contact lenses interfere with a pilot's ability to safely fly an airplane? Explain.

# 11

# Psychophysical Methodology

Much of the basic and clinical research that provides insights regarding visual processing is psychophysical in nature. Moreover, psychophysical procedures are frequently used in routine eye care. Visual acuity testing, refraction, visual fields, phoria testing, and color vision testing are all examples of clinical psychophysical tests. An understanding of psychophysical theory and methodology better enables the clinician to perform these tests and interpret their results in a meaningful manner.

The past several decades have seen substantial progress in the understanding of basic visual processes. This information is now being applied to the diagnosis and treatment of clinical entities. Clinical applications largely take the form of non-invasive psychophysical tests that enable the clinician to diagnose disease at an early stage and to monitor the effectiveness of treatment.

## THRESHOLD

Psychophysical experiments and psychophysically based clinical procedures frequently involve the determination of a threshold. A threshold is the minimum quantity of a stimulus that can be detected. For example, in a visual acuity test, the threshold is the minimum angle of resolution (MAR). For a visual field test, the threshold is the minimum light intensity that can be detected. Likewise, for an increment threshold experiment, such as illustrated in Figure 11–1A, the threshold is the minimum light intensity that can be detected. The determination of a threshold is complicated by the fact that humans (and other animals) are not perfect observers. A perfect observer would give the same threshold each time the experiment is performed. In reality, the threshold varies on repetition of the measurement.

Figure 11–1 shows the results of a psychophysical experiment conducted with a hypothetical ideal observer (Fig. 11–1B) and a real observer (Fig. 11–1C). The experiment itself is an increment threshold procedure: the participant is asked to detect a light (stimulus) that is flashed on a surrounding background. The task is performed for a range of intensities, from a very dim stimulus to an intense stimulus. The percentage of stimuli detected is then plotted as a function of stimulus intensity to produce a **psychometric function.**

The hypothetical ideal observer manifests a perfect threshold (Fig. 11–1B). Below the threshold intensity, *T,* the perfect observer never sees the stimulus. Above the threshold intensity, the perfect observer always sees the stimulus. In comparison, a real observer produces results similar to those in Figure 11–1C. As the intensity of the stimulus is increased, the probability of seeing the stimulus also increases. There is no clearly defined intensity, however, below which the stimulus is never seen and above which it is always seen.

As there are no perfect observers, scientists define threshold on the basis of theoretical considerations. Threshold is usually defined as the intensity that results in detection of the stimulus on one half of the presentations. This value is read off the psychometric function as indicated in Figure 11–1C.

Humans are not perfect observers because they are complex biologic systems rather than simple mechanical systems. A stimulus results in neural activity. If this neural activity is sufficiently strong, the stimulus is seen. Random neural noise is inherent within the visual system, however, and the signal produced by the stimulus must be perceived as different than this neural noise. As will be discussed later in this chapter, this neural noise can be thought of as varying over time. At any given moment, the amount of neural noise against which a signal must be detected is unpredictable. Therefore, the threshold is variable.

Other factors also play a role in the variation in threshold. Attention, motivation, and fatigue are all important factors that affect threshold determination.

## DETERMINATION OF THRESHOLD

Over the years, a number of procedures have been developed to measure threshold. We now introduce several of these methods along with some of their advantages and disadvantages.

### *Method of Ascending Limits*

In the method of ascending limits, the stimulus is at first nonvisible; it is below threshold. During a trial, the stimulus is presented at increasingly intense levels from presentation to presentation until it is visible. For example, in an increment threshold experiment, the intensity of the stimulus is increased in a systematic manner until the observer sees the stimulus. A number of trials are performed and a psychometric function is plotted based on the results.

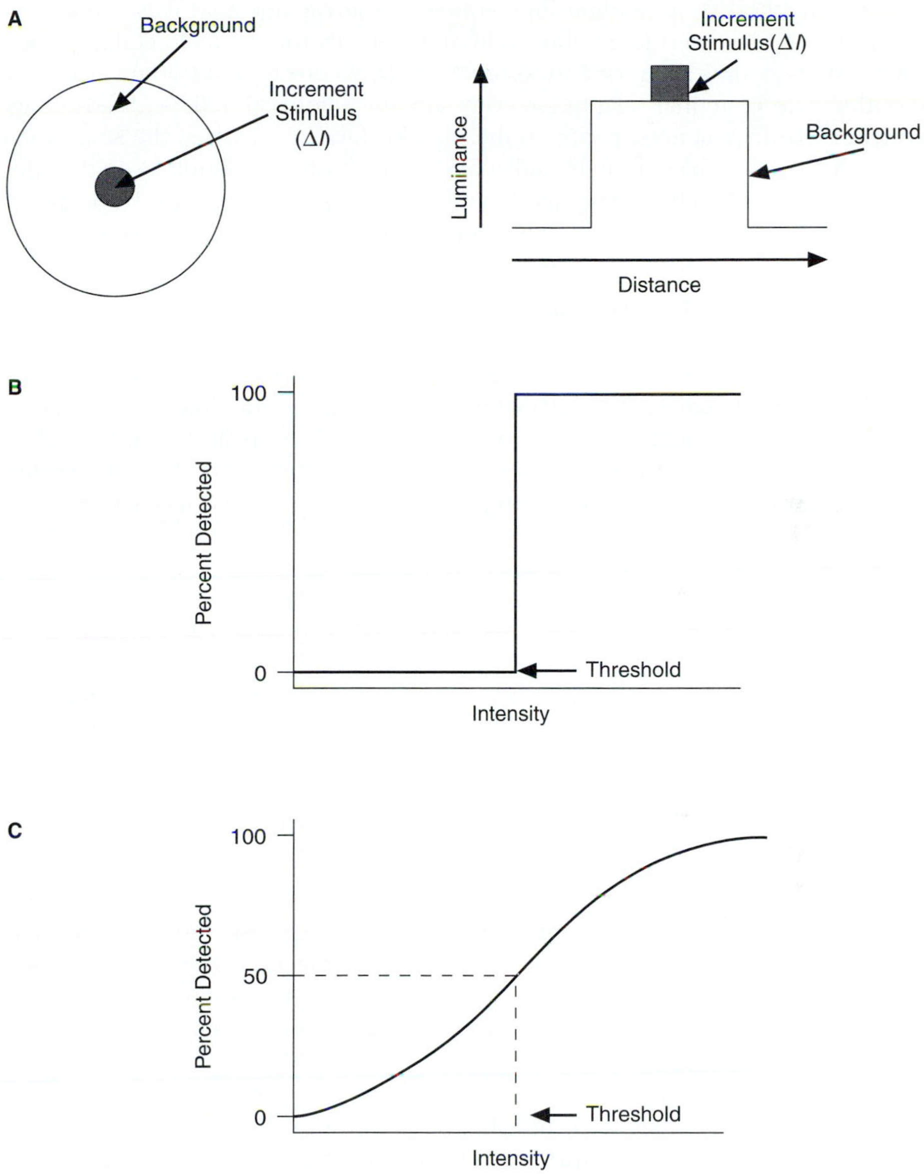


**FIGURE 11–1. A.** The diagram on the left shows an increment stimulus on a background. This is how the stimulus appears to the observer. The diagram on the right is a luminance profile of the stimulus and background. **B.** A psychometric function for a hypothetical ideal observer. Such observers do not actually exist. **C.** A typical psychometric function for a real observer.

The method of ascending limits offers the advantage that it is a relatively quick method to determine a threshold. It is also advantageous in certain procedures, such as dark adaptometry (see Chap. 3), where it is important not to affect the state of retinal adaptation with suprathreshold stimuli. A disadvantage concerns participant anticipation. If the stimulus intensity starts at the same value on each trial, the observer may anticipate when he or she "should" see the stimulus based on when he or she saw it on the previous trial. This disadvantage can be mitigated by beginning each trial with a stimulus of a different intensity.

### *Method of Descending Limits*

The method of descending limits is essentially the reverse of the method of ascending limits. A trial commences with a clearly visible stimulus, the visibility of which is decreased until it can no longer be seen. Whereas in the method of ascending limits we go from nonseeing to seeing, in the method of descending limits we go from seeing to nonseeing.

The determination of visual acuity is a descending limits task. Typically, the patient is asked to read the Snellen eye chart from top to bottom. The letters are readily resolvable at the top (suprathreshold) and become less resolvable as the patient progresses down the chart. Threshold is determined when the letters are too small to be resolved.

Similar to the method of ascending limits, the method of descending limits suffers from observer anticipation. This can be addressed by starting each trial at a different level of visibility.

### *Staircase Method*

The staircase method of determining a threshold is a combination of the methods of ascending and descending limits. A stimulus is presented to an observer in discrete steps of increasing visibility. This is an ascending staircase and is illustrated in Figure 11–2. Eventually, the observer reports seeing the stimulus. At this point the staircase is reversed, and the visibility of the stimulus is reduced until the observer reports that it cannot be detected. The staircase is again reversed, and the stimulus intensity is increased until it is visible. Threshold is frequently defined as having occurred after three or four reversals.

This strategy provides a quick and reliable method of determining a threshold. It is commonly used in psychophysical experimentation and automated visual field testing.

### *Method of Constant Stimuli*

In the method of constant stimuli, the stimulus visibility is varied from presentation to presentation in a random fashion. A large number of stimuli are presented at each level of visibility and from these data, a psychometric function is con-

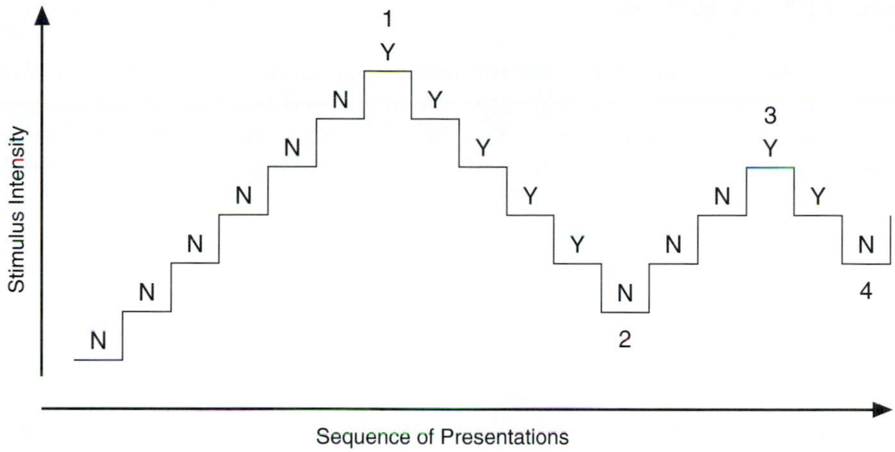


**FIGURE 11–2.** Staircase method for threshold determination. The stimulus intensity is increased from nonseeing (N) to seeing (Y). A reversal occurs at point 1 and, subsequently, the intensity is decreased until another reversal occurs at point 2. Threshold is taken as the intensity at reversal 4.

structed. For example, consider an experiment that involves the determination of an increment threshold. In this case, 20 presentations of 10 different stimuli, each at a different intensity, are randomly presented. The observer is asked on each presentation whether or not she or he sees the stimulus. A psychometric function is plotted and 50 percent visibility is taken as the threshold.

The method of constant stimuli is so named not because the stimulus is kept constant from presentation to presentation, but because the procedure is designed to maintain the observer's expectations at the same level from presentation to presentation. The observer has no legitimate basis on which to anticipate the visibility of an upcoming presentation; consequently, there is little variation in expectations. Because of this, the method of constant stimuli provides valuable information for laboratory experiments. It is, however, time consuming and not typically indicated for clinical applications.

### *Method of Adjustment*

In the method of adjustment, the participants themselves adjust the stimulus intensity until the stimulus is barely visible. This method allows relatively quick determination of a threshold.

A disadvantage of this method is that it suffers, perhaps more than the previous methods, from variations in the participant's threshold criterion. This problem and its remedy are discussed below.

### *Forced Choice Method*

All of the previous methods for determining a threshold share a common flaw: there may be variability in the threshold criteria used by observers. For example, some observers have a strict threshold criterion. These observers do not indicate that they see a stimulus until they are absolutely certain they see it. This strict threshold criterion results in a relatively high threshold (low sensitivity). Other observers have a lax criterion. These observers indicate that they see a stimulus even though they may have a great deal of uncertainty regarding their decision. This lax criterion results in a relatively low threshold (high sensitivity).

Not only may the threshold criterion vary from person to person, it may vary from trial to trial for the same observer. At some times during an experiment, an observer may be more willing to guess that he or she sees a stimulus than at other times. In addition, an observer may apply different criteria for different types of stimuli. For example, an observer may use one criterion when detecting stimuli under photopic conditions and another when detecting stimuli under scotopic conditions. These variations in threshold criteria potentially complicate the interpretation of experimental results.

In a forced choice methodology, the role of the individual's criterion is minimized by forcing him or her to choose between several alternative choices, one of which contains the stimulus. An example is given in Figure 11–3A. In this example, the stimulus is randomly presented in one of the two windows. The other window does not contain a stimulus; it is blank. The observer is forced to choose which window contains the stimulus. The role of the observer's threshold criterion is reduced because the observer must choose a window, even if she or he claims not to be able to see a stimulus.

To construct a psychometric function, a large number of stimuli of various visibilities are presented. If the experiment forces the observer to choose among two alternatives, as in the previous example, it is referred to as a two-alternative forced choice (2AFC) experiment. A psychometric function for a 2AFC experiment is given in Figure 11–3A. Note that the lowest percentage correct is 50 percent. It is not 0 percent, as is the case with previously discussed psychophysical methodologies, because even when the participant cannot see the stimulus, he or she is expected to guess correctly 50 percent of the time. (Because there are two windows and the stimulus must be in one of the two windows, the observer guesses correctly on one half of the presentations.) For a 2AFC experiment, the threshold value is typically taken as the point midway between chance performance (50 percent) and perfect performance. As indicated in Figure 11–3A, this corresponds to 75 percent correct.

Forced choice experiments can present the participant with more than two choices. Consider Figure 11–3B, which shows a four-alternative forced choice (4AFC) stimulus array. In this case, the stimulus is randomly presented in one of the four windows, and the observer is forced to choose the correct window. Note that the psychometric function for this experiment shows a chance level

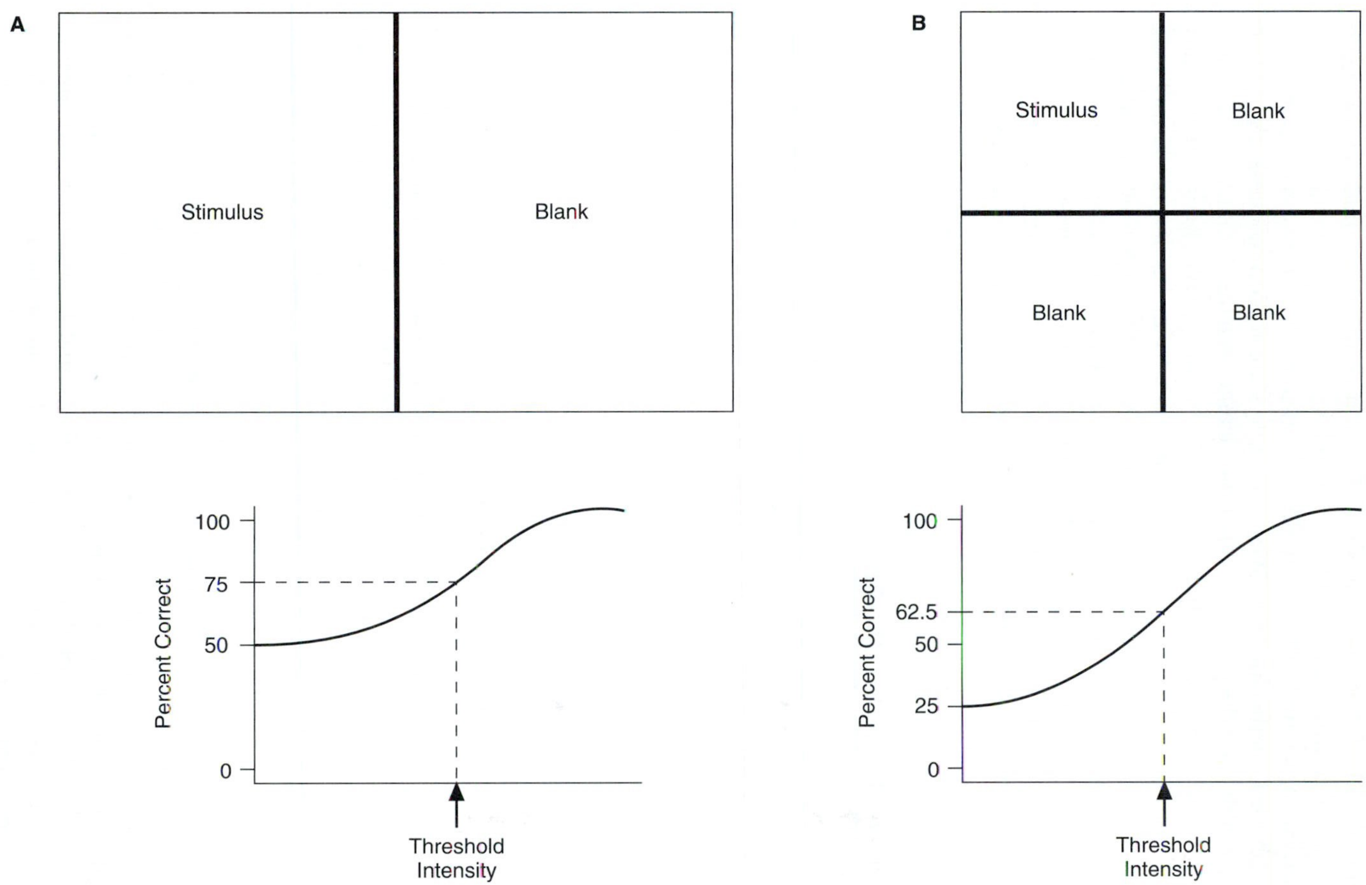


**FIGURE 11–3.** **A.** Two-alternative forced choice (2AFC) methodology. The top diagram shows the stimulus array, and the bottom figure shows a typical psychometric function for a 2AFC experiment. **B.** Stimulus array and psychometric function for a four-alternative forced choice (4AFC) experiment.

performance of 25 percent. Threshold is taken as the point midway between this chance performance and 100 percent, which is 62.5 percent.

Forced choice methodology typically results in lower thresholds than other psychophysical methodologies. When observers are forced to guess, they often do remarkably well despite claims that they cannot see the stimulus.

Forced choice preferential viewing techniques have been successfully used to determine visual acuity and other visual capabilities of infants (see Chap. 17) (Teller et al, 1974). In these procedures, the experimenter observes the infant's gaze as he or she views a 2AFC display (see Fig. 17–9). The experimenter is then forced to choose the location of the stimulus based on observation of the infant's eyes. By using a forced choice methodology, the criterion (i.e., strict or lax) used by the experimenter does not become a confounding factor.

## SIGNAL DETECTION THEORY

From our previous discussion regarding threshold, we know that human observers do not manifest a perfect threshold. Threshold fluctuates depending on a number of variables including decision criteria, attention, and internal neural noise.

Signal detection theory formally addresses the role these factors play in the determination of threshold (Swets et al, 1961). It is important to keep in mind that although signal detection theory presents a useful predictive model, it is, nonetheless, only a model.

Signal detection theory assumes that within the visual system there is a randomly fluctuating level of background neural noise. The stimulus produces a signal that is superimposed on this noise. The observer's task is to differentiate the signal and noise combination from the background noise alone. An analogy would be listening to static (white noise) and attempting to distinguish a discrete increase in the level of noise (signal) from the white noise itself.

A key element of this model is that the neural noise is randomly distributed over time (Fig. 11–4A). This figure shows the probability of a given level of neural activation at any instant in time. At some times there is much noise; at other times there is little noise. Returning to our analogy of static, think of the level of static as randomly fluctuating over time.

The stimulus produces a signal that is superimposed on the randomly distributed noise (Fig. 11–4B). The signal can be thought of as being a constant. This constant signal is added to the noise distribution (N) to produce the noise plus signal distribution (N + S). It is important to keep in mind that the noise is present in the absence of the signal, and the signal is superimposed on this noise. The observer's task is to determine if what he or she is seeing (or hearing) is noise or signal plus noise.

The larger the signal, the easier it is for the participant to distinguish the signal plus noise from noise alone (Fig. 11–5). As the detectability ($d'$) of the

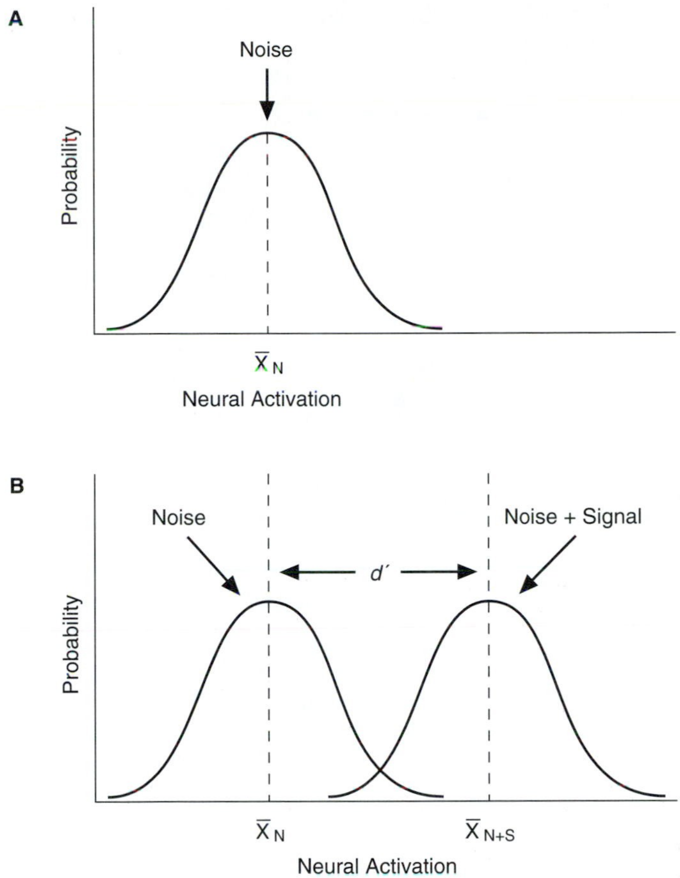


**FIGURE 11–4. A.** In the absence of a stimulus, neural noise is randomly distributed over time. **B.** A stimulus produces a signal that displaces the original distribution of noise to the right. The detectability, $d'$, is a measure of the strength of the stimulus.

stimulus is increased, the distributions of N and N + S become further apart. (Detectability refers to the difference between the means of the N and N + S distributions). With a very large $d'$, there is no overlap of the distributions; therefore, there is no uncertainty regarding whether a stimulus is present.

The situation is not so clear-cut when the stimulus is weak. As indicated in Figure 11–5A, the N and N + S distributions substantially overlap. Consequently, a given level of neural activation may be due to either noise alone or the signal plus noise. For example, the neural activation at point 1 could be produced by noise alone or signal plus noise. There is no way for the observer to be certain whether the stimulus was absent or present. (This level of neural activation re-

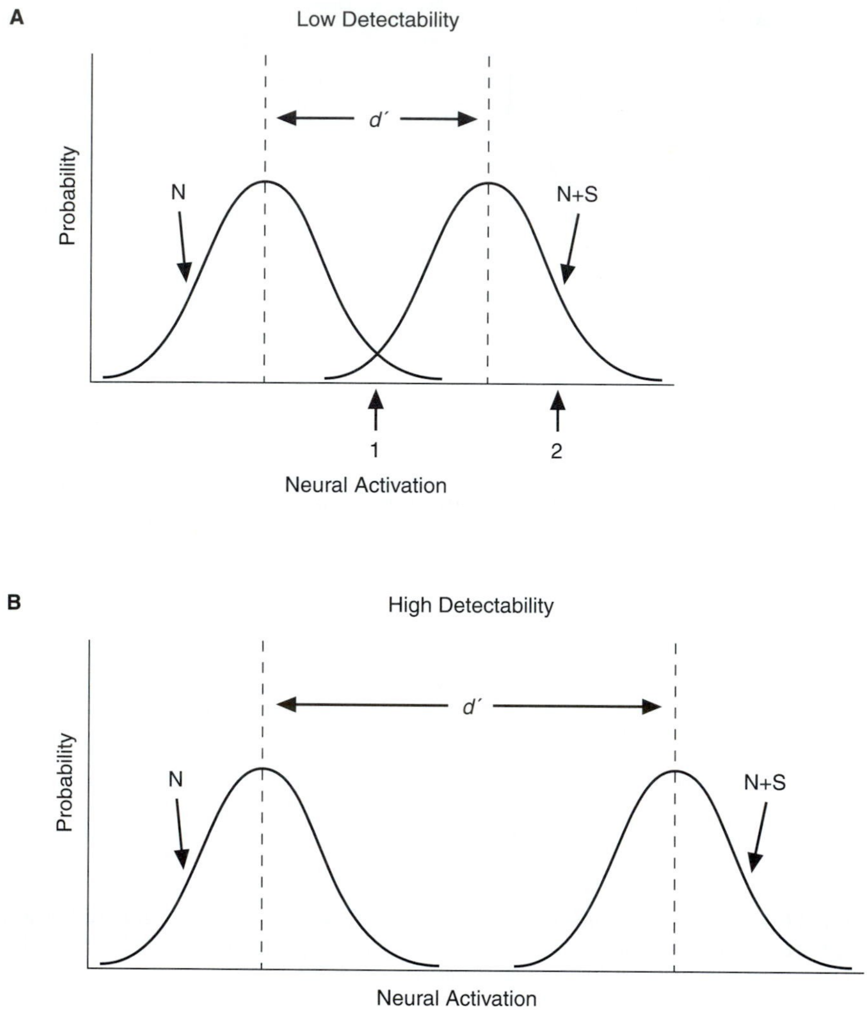


**Figure 11–5.** The larger the detectability of a stimulus, the greater the separation of the noise and noise plus signal distributions. When the detectability is low, a stimulus may not be reliably distinguished from noise alone. This is indicated by point 1 in **A.** When the detectability is high, as in **B,** the signal is easily distinguished from noise.

sults when a stimulus is delivered at a time when the level of neural activation is low.) The same stimulus could also produce a substantial amount of activation, as indicated by point 2. This occurs when the stimulus is delivered at a point in time when the level of noise is very high. As a result, the observer easily sees the stimulus.

### *Effect of Subject Criterion*

Signal detection theory allows us to predict the effect of the observer's criterion on the detection of a stimulus. Consider the situation where the observer has a lax criterion, for example, an intern or resident examining a patient's retina with an ophthalmoscope. The clinician wants to be certain that he or she detects any abnormalities. Therefore, he or she adopts a lax criterion; any deviation from the norm, no matter how small, alerts the doctor.

An example of a lax criterion is given in Figure 11–6A. The dashed line represents the observer's criterion. Any level of neural activation above this lax criterion is interpreted as an event. Levels of activation below this lax criterion do not elicit a response from the observer.

The observer's responses fall into the four categories given in Figure 11–7. When only noise is present, the participant reports seeing a stimulus if the level of activation is greater than the criterion level. This is referred to as a **false positive,** or **false alarm.** If, however, only noise is present, and the level of activation is less than the criterion level, the participant reports that no stimulus is present. This is a **correct reject.**

When the stimulus is present, the observer correctly reports its presence if it produces a level of activation greater than the criterion level. This is a **hit.** Finally, a **miss** occurs when the stimulus is present, but the level of activation is less than the criterion level.

Note that this lax criterion results in many hits and a substantial number of false positives (see Fig. 11–6A); however, there are very few misses. This is the outcome we would expect if a lax criterion is employed by a clinician examining the retina. There may be few misses of retinal disease, yet there may be many false alarms.

Now consider the case of a strict criterion (see Fig. 11–6B). An example is a deer hunter who wants to be absolutely certain that the target in her or his sights is a deer. Note that $d'$ is the same for this strict criterion and the previously discussed lax criterion. The only difference between the two examples is the location of the criterion line.

The strict criterion results in fewer hits than does a lax criterion. A practical implication of this, with respect to our example, is that some deer will not be shot. The payoff, however, is the low number of false positives. By employing a strict criterion, the hunter rarely shoots at targets other than deer.

### *Receiver Operating Characteristic Curve*

The effect of various criteria and levels of detectability ($d'$) can be combined to plot a receiver operating characteristic (ROC) curve. For a ROC curve, probability of a hit is plotted as a function of the probability of a false positive. An example is given in Figure 11–8A, where $d' = 1$ and L represents a lax criterion, S a strict criterion, and M a moderate criterion. This graph expresses what we

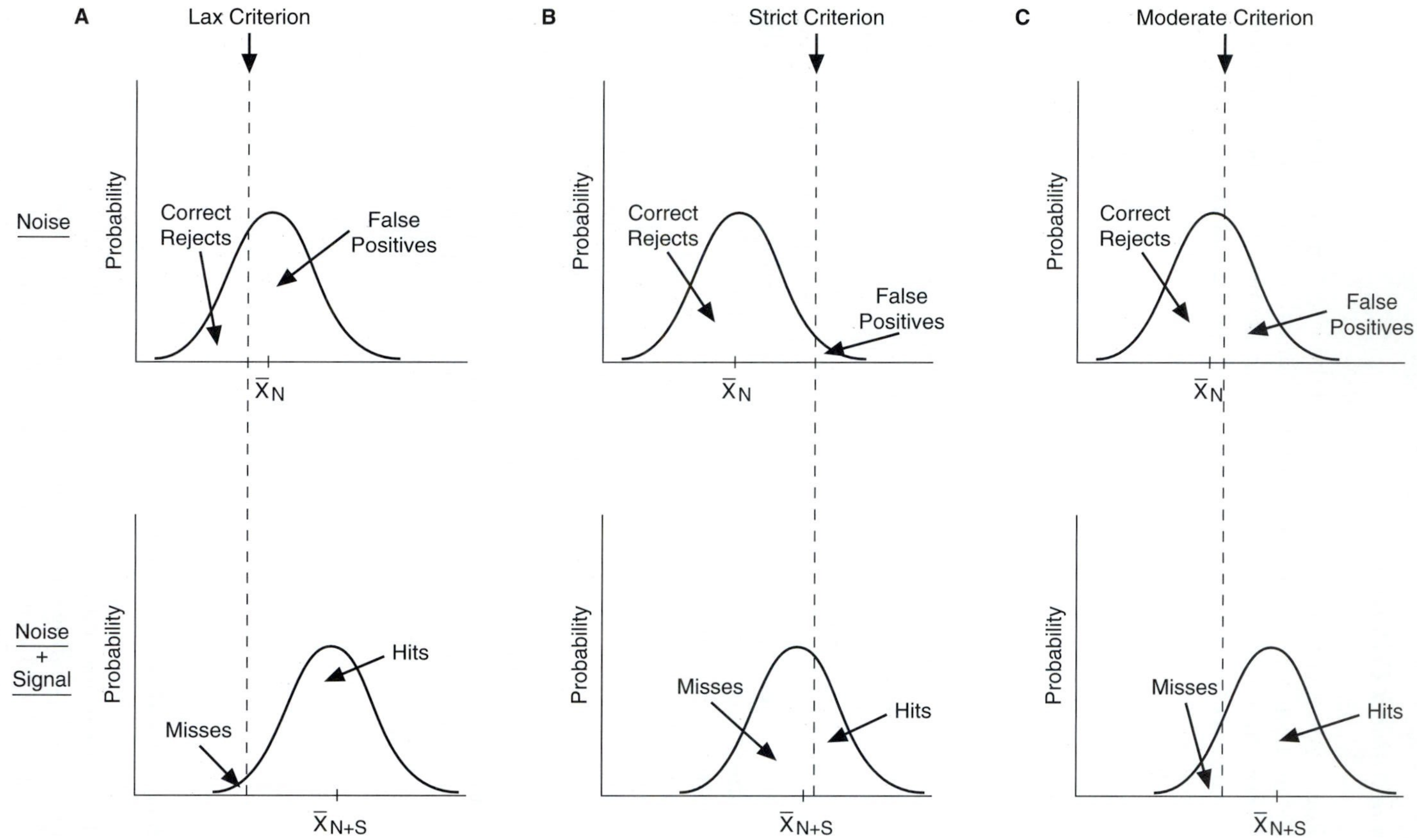


**FIGURE 11–6.** For each of these three examples, the detectability is the same; however, the threshold criterion varies from lax to strict to moderate.

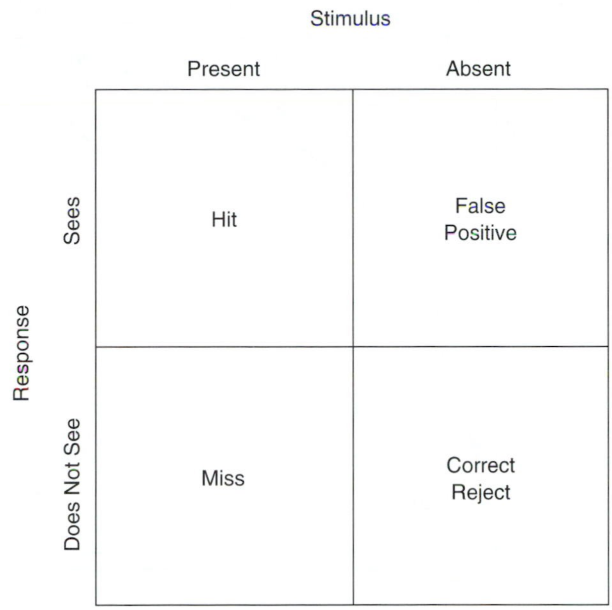


**FIGURE 11–7.** Possible outcomes for a signal detection experiment.

have already learned. For a lax criterion, the probability of a hit is high, but so is the probability of a false positive. For a strict criterion, the probability of a hit is low, but so is the probability of a false positive.

What happens to the form of this ROC curve as the detectability changes? Consider the graph in Figure 11–8B, where $d' = 0$. In this case, the stimulus is so weak that it produces no signal. No matter where the criterion line is drawn, the proportion of hits will exactly match the proportion of false positives. Therefore, when $d' = 0$, the ROC curve is a straight-line function. No matter what the criterion, whether lax or strict, the probability of a hit equals the probability of a false positive.

Now consider the case where $d' = \infty$ (Fig. 11–8B). The stimulus is easily distinguished from noise, regardless of the criterion used by the observer. The observer always sees the stimulus, and there are no false positives.

Figure 11–8B shows that a family of ROC curves exist for different levels of detectability ranging from $d' = 0$ to $d' = \infty$. Experimentally, these curves can be derived by controlling $d'$ and the criterion level. The criterion is controlled by providing rewards for hits and penalties for false positives (a payoff matrix). For example, participants may be told that each time they answer correctly, they will receive \$5; however, an incorrect response will result in a penalty of \$20. This would produce a strict criterion. A lax criterion can be produced by minimizing the penalty for a false positive.

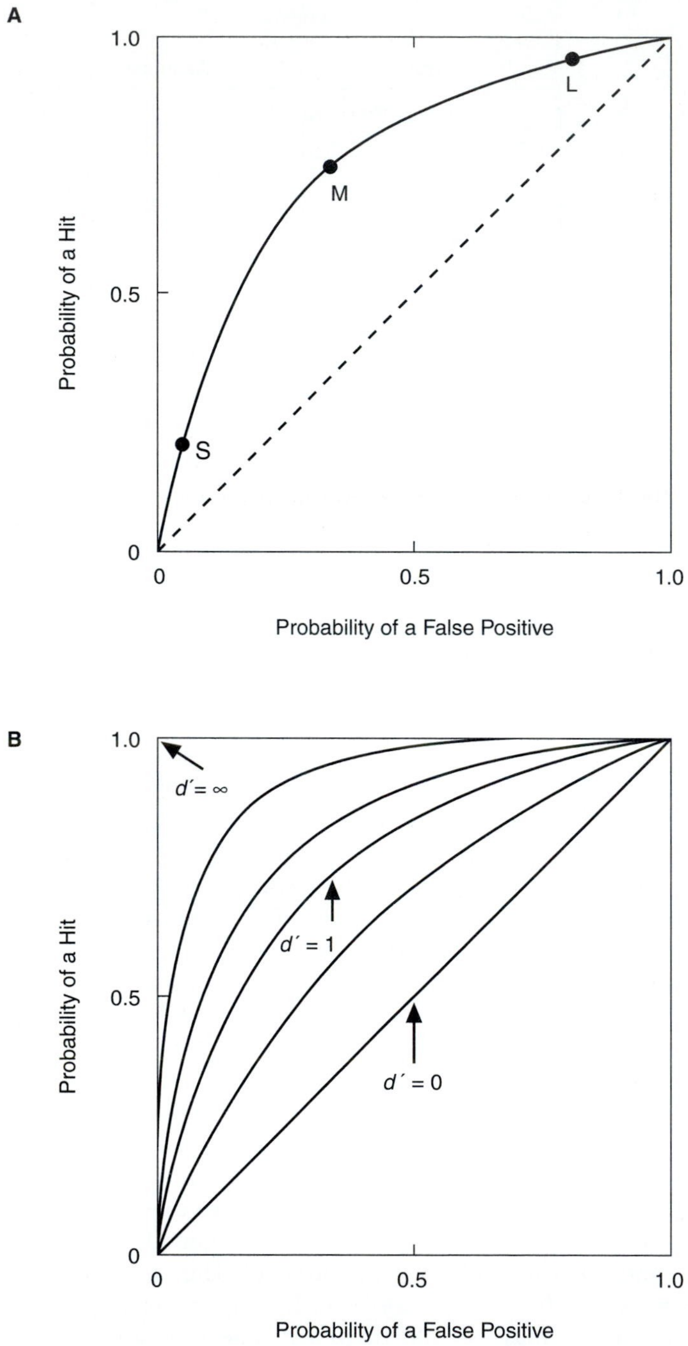


**FIGURE 11–8. A.** Receiver operating characteristic (ROC) curve, where $d' = 1$ (solid curve). S, M, and L represent strict, moderate, and lax criteria. **B.** ROC curves for various levels of detectability.

## *WEBER'S LAW*

Up to now, we have discussed threshold without consideration of the background against which a stimulus is detected. In many psychophysical experiments, however, the task is to discriminate the combination of the stimulus and the background from the background itself.

This can be understood by considering an increment threshold experiment, as illustrated in Figure 11–9A. The observer's task is to detect the increment stimulus. Another way of thinking of this task is that the individual must be able to discriminate the combined stimulus and background from the background itself. For this reason, the threshold stimulus is often referred to as a **just noticeable difference (JND).** (A JND is also referred to as a **difference limen, or DL.)**

The relationship between JNDs and the background on which these JNDs are presented can be quantified by determining increment thresholds as a function of background illumination. An increment, $\Delta I$, is flashed on a background, $I_b$. A JND is the threshold $\Delta I$. It is found that the ratio of the JND to the background intensity remains constant as the intensity of the background increases (Figs. 11–9B and 11–9C). This is referred to as Weber's law and is mathematically expressed as

$$\Delta I = KI_b$$

or

$$K = \frac{\Delta I}{I_b}$$

where

$\Delta I$ = increment threshold (JND)
$I_b$ = background illumination
$K$ = Weber's constant or fraction

Weber's law applies to vision and other sensory modalities. Consider the example of a person who can barely tell the difference between two weights, one of which is 10.0 lb and the other 11.0 lb (the JND is 1 lb). Weber's constant is calculated as (11.0 – 10.0)/10.00 = 0.10. On the basis of this constant, the JND for a 50-lb weight is calculated as follows:

$$\frac{X - 50\text{ lb}}{50\text{ lb}} = 0.10$$

$$X = 55\text{ lb}$$
$$\text{JND} = 55\text{ lb} - 50\text{ lb}$$
$$\text{JND} = 5\text{ lb}$$

The individual will barely be able to tell the difference between weights of 55 and 50 lb. To maintain a constant Weber's fraction of 0.10, the JND is now 5 lb rather than the original 1 lb.

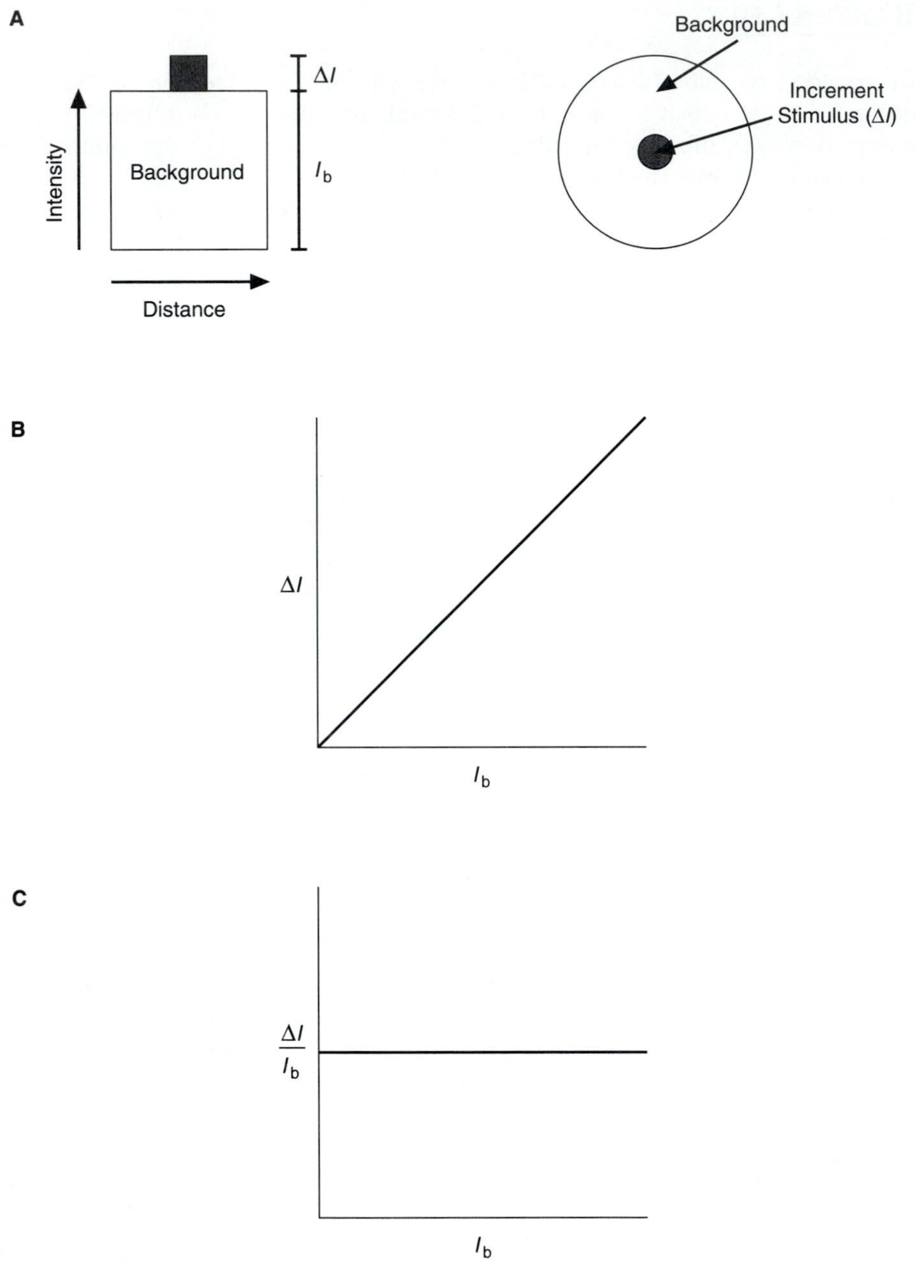


**FIGURE 11–9. A.** Increment threshold arrangement which can be used to demonstrate Weber's law. A luminance profile is on the left, and the observer's view of the stimulus is on the right. **B.** Graphic representation of Weber's law which shows that the ratio of $\Delta I$ to $I_b$ is a constant. **C.** Figure B plotted to show $\Delta I/I_b$ as a function of $I_b$.

Certain implications of Weber's law for vision are illustrated in Figure 11–10, which shows a dark optotype on a gray background under dim illumination (left) and under bright illumination (assume both conditions are photopic). The percentage of light reflected from the dark optotype is 10.00 percent, while that reflected off of the gray background is 10.20 percent. The contrast of the optotype is calculated to be 0.02 under both dim and bright conditions. (The amount of light reflected from the dark and gray surfaces increases at the same rate as we go from dim to brighter lighting conditions, resulting in a constant ratio of optotype to background luminance.) Since Weber's fraction for photopic vision is about 0.02, the optotype is at threshold (barely detectable) under both lighting conditions. The optotype does not become more visible when more light is reflected from it. The visual system is concerned with the difference between the optotype and its background rather than the luminance of the optotype in isolation. A consequence of this characteristic, which is referred to as **lightness constancy,** is that the appearance of objects does not change as the lighting conditions vary. For example, a black and white striped shirt looks the same whether viewed indoors under dim photopic conditions or outdoors under bright photopic conditions.

The preceding example illustrates that the visual system detects stimuli in the context of their background. What is the appearance of a stimulus of constant luminance when viewed against backgrounds of various luminances? Figure 11–11 demonstrates that the brightness of such a stimulus depends on the background, a phenomenon referred to as **simultaneous contrast.** As predicted by

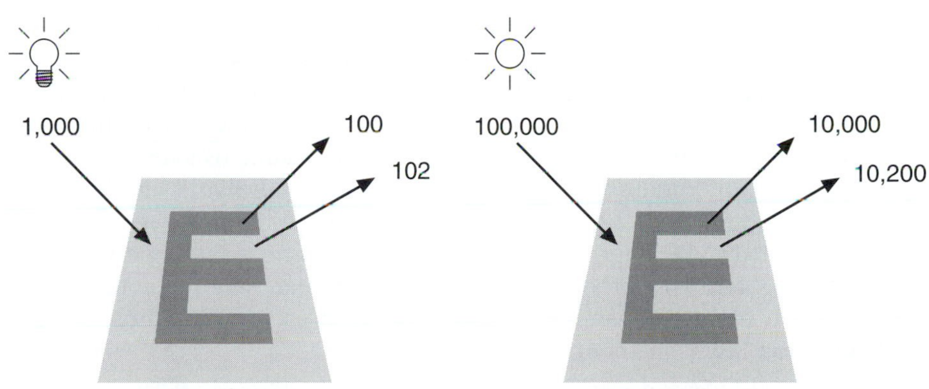


**FIGURE 11–10.** The optotype **E** reflects 10.00 percent of the light incident upon it, while the gray background reflects 10.20 percent. Whether under dim illumination (1000 units of light) or bright illumination (100,000 units of light), the ratio of the optotype to background luminance (contrast) is the same. Since the visual system has evolved to detect contrast, rather than absolute luminance, the appearance of the **E** is the same under both dim and bright lighting conditions. This phenomenon is referred to as lightness constancy.

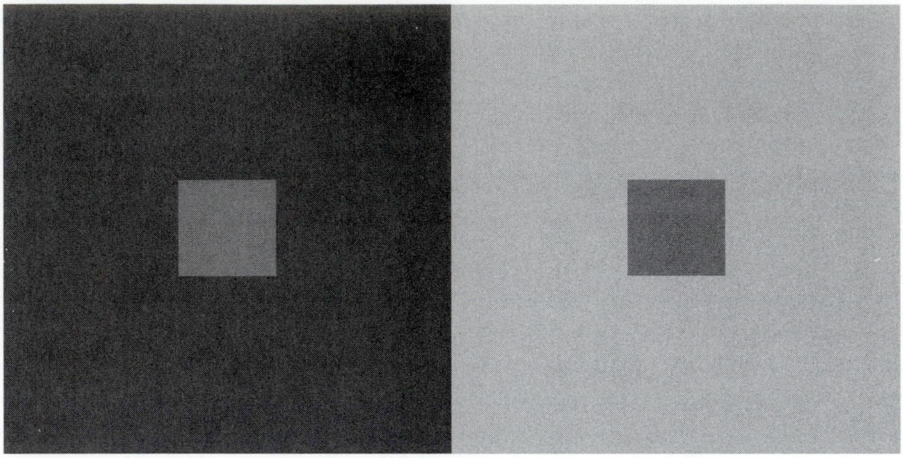

**FIGURE 11–11.** Although the central squares are physically identical (i.e., they each have the same luminance), each has a different brightness. As the background becomes darker, the central square appears brighter. This phenomenon is referred to as simultaneous contrast.

Weber's law, the contrast of the stimulus—not the luminance of the stimulus—is the key factor in predicting its appearance.

## *MAGNITUDE OF SENSATION*

So far we have limited our discussion to the detection of stimuli at threshold. We have not discussed stimuli above threshold: suprathreshold stimuli. It is of interest, however, to quantify the growth in the magnitude of sensation as the intensity of a stimulus is increased to suprathreshold levels. For example, if the intensity of a light bulb is doubled, will it appear twice as bright? Specifically, what is the nature of the relationship between magnitude of sensation and stimulus intensity?

Fechner (1860) addressed this problem by assuming that Weber's law applies to suprathreshold stimuli. For example, if the stimulus intensity is increased by 5 JNDs, Fechner assumed that the stimulus, if a light, would appear five units brighter. This predicted relationship between stimulus intensity and sensation is a log relationship and is graphically presented in Figure 11–12A. **Fechner's log law** is mathematically expressed as

$$S = c \log I$$

where

$S$ = magnitude of sensation (e.g., brightness)
$I$ = stimulus intensity
$c$ = constant related to Weber's constant

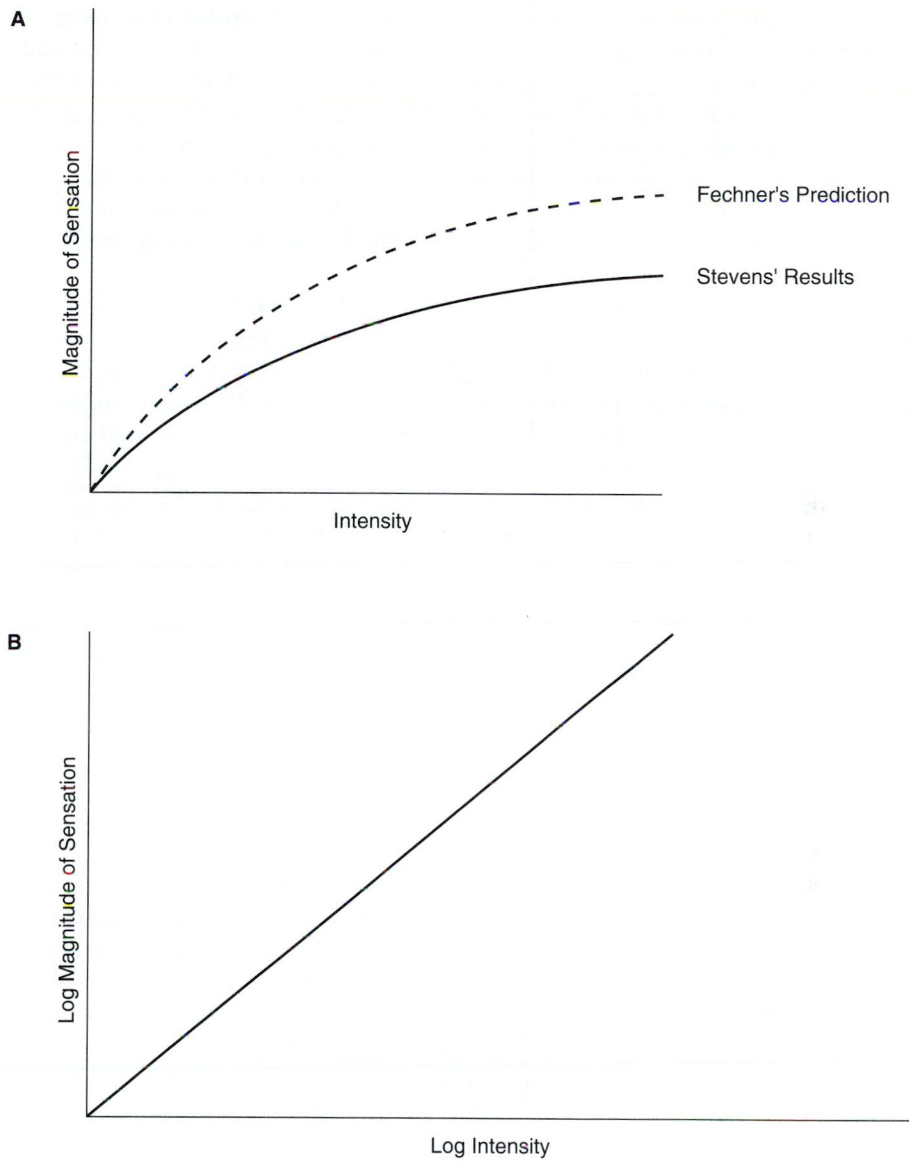


**FIGURE 11–12. A.** Fechner's log law and Stevens' power law plotted on linear coordinates. **B.** Stevens' power law plotted on log–log coordinates.

Fechner provided empirical evidence for this law by **indirect scaling.** Essentially, Fechner determined JNDs and assumed that all JNDs produce equal differences in the magnitude of sensation. For example, Fechner assumed that a JND for a dim background produces the same difference in sensation as does a JND for a bright background. As it turns out, this assumption is incorrect.

In the 1950s, Stevens (1957) applied a remarkably simple paradigm to address this problem. Stevens simply had observers directly assess the intensity of suprathreshold stimuli. This is referred to as **direct scaling,** or **magnitude estimation.**

In an experiment of this nature, an individual is asked to assign a number to the sensation under investigation. When dealing with brightness, he or she is presented with a number of lights of various intensities. The individual is asked to assign a number to the perceived brightness of each of these stimuli. For example, a very dim light is labeled 1, while a very bright light is labeled 10. Sensation, indicated by the numerical values assigned by the observer, is plotted as a function of bulb intensity.

The results of such an experiment, plotted on linear coordinates, are given in Figure 11–12A. When plotted on log–log coordinates, the relationship is seen to represent a power function (Fig. 11–12B). Mathematically, these results are expressed as **Stevens' power law:**

$$S = I^c$$

where

$S$ = magnitude of sensation (e.g., brightness)
$I$ = stimulus intensity
$c$ = constant

By magnitude estimation, Stevens was able to show that the growth in magnitude of sensation follows a power relationship, rather than a log relationship as postulated by Fechner. Although difficult to conceptualize, this means that a constant ratio of sensation is produced by a constant ratio of stimulation.

Stevens' law shows that there is a compression (i.e., saturation) of sensation as stimulus intensity increases. Consider a three-way light bulb that can be set at 0, 50, 100, or 150 watts. The physical difference between each of these settings is the same (50 watts), yet turning the light on (going from 0 to 50 watts) is much more noticeable than adjusting the setting from 100 to 150 watts.

## SUMMARY

The determination of thresholds plays a large role in vision research and clinical eye care. The specific methodology used to determine a threshold may significantly affect the threshold value obtained.

There is frequently a trade-off between ease of measurement and validity of the measurement. For clinical purposes, the repeatability (reliability) of the threshold measurement is often more important than the validity. Consequently, easily applied psychophysical procedures, such as the staircase method or method of limits, provide clinically useful information.

# Self-Assessment Questions

1. **A.** For a three-alternative forced choice experiment, what is the percentage correct used to determine the threshold? **B.** Answer the same question for a five-alternative forced choice experiment.

2. An experiment is conducted where thresholds for the detection of temporally stable gratings are compared to thresholds for gratings that are temporally modulated. What would be the best methodology for determining these thresholds? Explain.

# 12

# Functional Retinal Physiology

This and the following three chapters emphasize data obtained with single-unit electrophysiologic research techniques. In experiments that use these techniques, electrical activity is recorded from single neurons located within the visual system of an anesthetized experimental animal. Two basic methods are used, extracellular and intracellular recording methods.

In **extracellular recording,** a microelectrode placed in close proximity to a neuron records action potentials generated by the neuron. For **intracellular** recording, a microelectrode pierces the membrane of a neuron and records the membrane potential (i.e., the neuron's degree of depolarization or hyperpolarization). This technique, which is technically more challenging than extracellular recording, is necessary when studying neurons that do not generate action potentials. Such neurons, which include several classes of retinal cells, generate **graded** (slow) **potentials.** These potentials cannot be recorded by extracellular procedures.

An advantage of intracellular recording is that the microelectrode (a glass micropipette) can be used to inject a dye into a neuron on completion of the experiment (Fig. 12–1). Subsequently, the experimental animal is sacrificed, and the neuron is located and examined histologically. This allows correlations to be made between the electrophysiologic properties of neurons and their morphology (structure).

## THE RETINA

The retina is a multilayered tissue consisting of many different classes of neurons. These neurons communicate with each other through a multitude of synaptic connections rich in both their diversity and complexity.

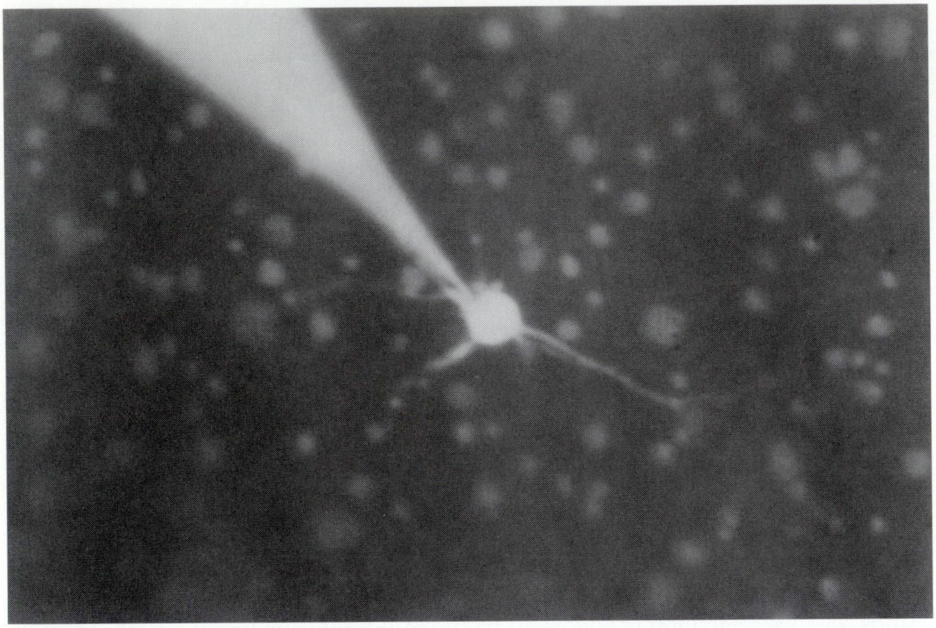

**FIGURE 12–1.** A micropipette (foreground) fills a rabbit ganglion cell with dye following an intracellular recording session. The same micropipette is used to record intracellular potentials from the neuron and to fill the neuron with dye. Note the dendrites that emerge from the neuron's soma. *(Photograph is courtesy of Dr. Ralph Jensen.)*

The retina is not a passive receiver of information. Rather, the optical image that falls on the retina is analyzed and encoded into a complex neural signal that is transmitted to higher visual centers. Because of this complex neural analysis, the retina is considered to be a part of the brain.

In this chapter, basic retinal processing is examined. We begin our discussion by studying the receptive field characteristics of the neurons that represent the final stage of retinal processing, the ganglion cells. We then examine the receptive field characteristics of the major classes of retinal cells that precede the ganglion cells.

## RECEPTIVE FIELDS OF GANGLION CELLS

Consider the electrophysiologic experiment illustrated in Figure 12–2. The fovea of an anesthetized animal, such as a monkey or a cat, is aligned with a point on a screen. A microelectrode is placed in close proximity to a single ganglion cell, such that it records action potentials from this one ganglion cell (extracellular single-unit recording). If a spot of light is directed onto various areas of the screen,

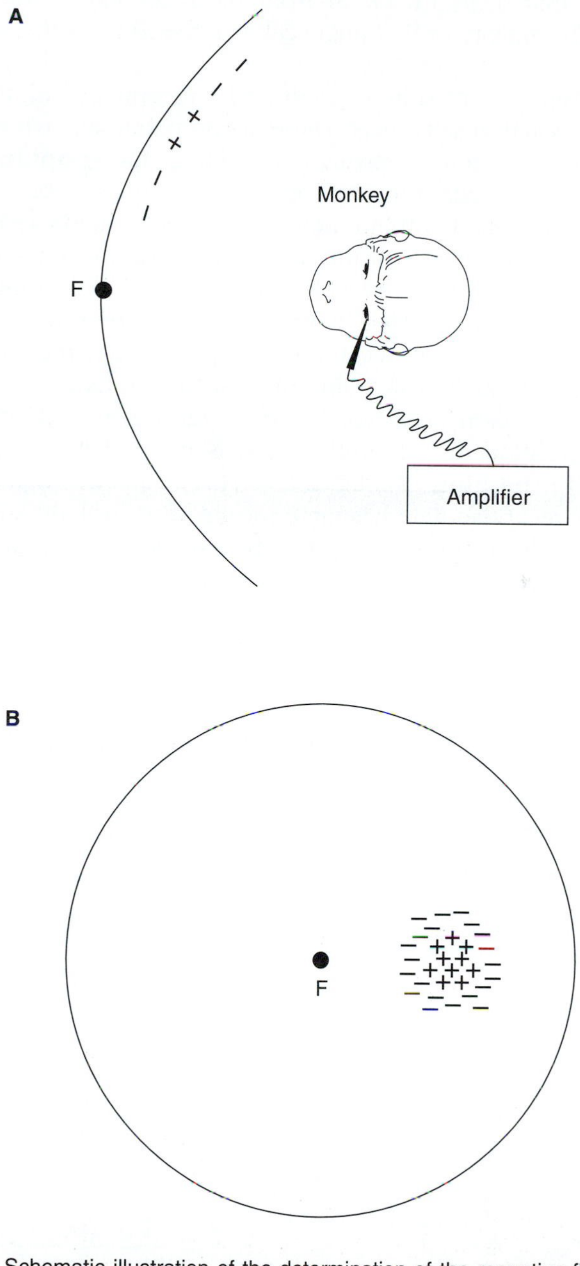


**FIGURE 12–2. A.** Schematic illustration of the determination of the receptive field of an isolated ganglion cell. The animal's eye is aligned with the fixation point, F. Small spots of light are projected onto a screen. Light falling on a certain region of the screen affects the activity of the neuron. This region is the receptive field of the neuron and is indicated by the plus and minus signs. Light falling on the area indicated by plus signs causes the neuron to become excited, whereas light falling on the area indicated by minus signs causes it to be inhibited. **B.** Face-on view of the screen and receptive field.

an area is found that elicits a response from this ganglion cell. The area in space that influences the activity of this single cell is referred to as the **receptive field** of the cell.

Even when light is not shining on the cell's receptive field, the cell spontaneously generates action potentials. These action potentials, which occur in the absence of a stimulus, are collectively referred to as the **spontaneous activity,** or **maintained discharge,** of the neuron.

A stimulus positioned within a neuron's receptive field can either increase or decrease the discharge rate of the neuron (Fig. 12–3). A small light located within the center of this receptive field causes an increase in the frequency of action potentials. This is indicated by the plus signs. The same small light positioned in the surround of the receptive field produces a reduction in the frequency of action potentials. This is indicated by the minus signs.

Mammalian ganglion cells typically have receptive fields with a **center–surround** organization; they manifest what is referred to as **spatial antagonism,** or **lateral inhibition** (Kuffler, 1953). This means that light falling on one part of the cell's receptive field has the opposite effect of light falling elsewhere within the same cell's receptive field. For the ganglion cell in Figure 12–3, light

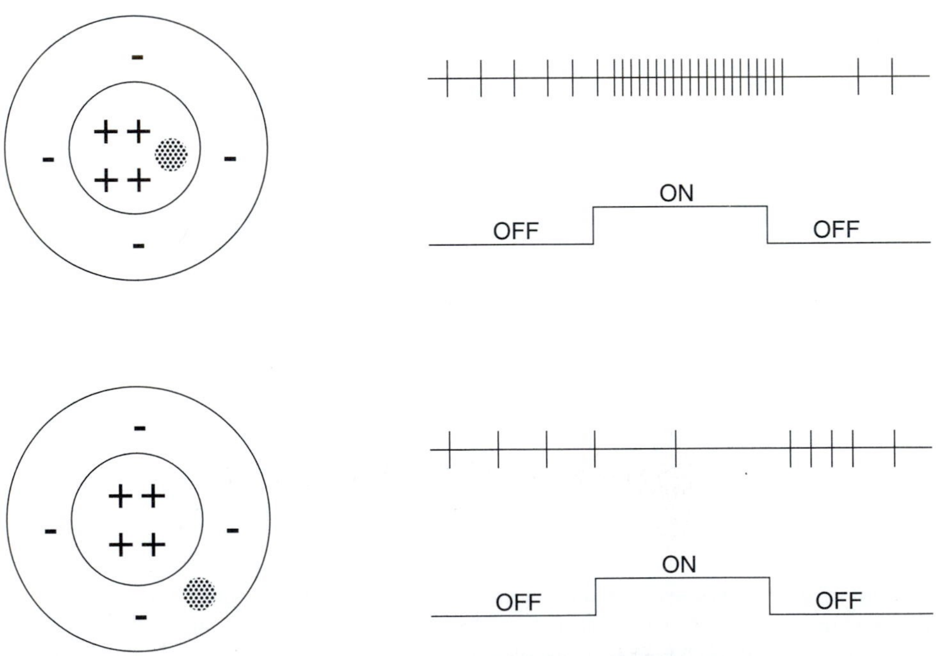


**FIGURE 12–3.** A spot of light falling on the excitatory center of a ganglion cell receptive field causes an increase in the frequency of action potentials. The same spot of light falling on the inhibitory surround causes a reduction in the frequency of action potentials.

falling on the receptive field center excites the cell; it causes an increased frequency of action potentials. In contrast, light falling on the receptive field surround inhibits the cell; it produces a reduction in the frequency of action potentials. (Other ganglion cells have the reverse arrangement. Light falling on the receptive field center produces a decrease in the frequency of action potentials, whereas light falling on the surround produces an increase in frequency.)

The preceding discussion may be confusing if this is your first exposure to this concept. Let us approach it from a slightly different perspective. Consider the following experiment. A single ganglion cell in the retina of a cat is isolated. The cell has a receptive field organization similar to that given in Figure 12–4; it has an excitatory center and an inhibitory surround.

Using a projector, we shine a very small light onto the center of the cell's receptive field. This produces an increase in the frequency of action potentials compared with the maintained discharge. If the experiment is repeated with a slightly larger spot of light, the result is an increase in the frequency of action potentials. This is due to spatial summation that occurs within the receptive field's center.

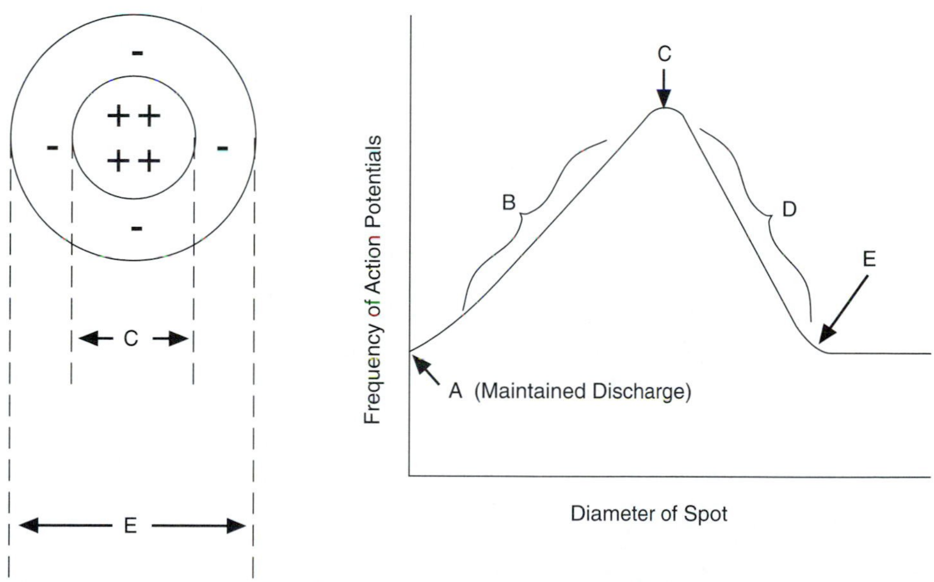


**FIGURE 12–4.** As the diameter of a spot of light is increased, a ganglion cell will manifest spatial summation up to the limits of its receptive field center, point C. This results in an increase in the frequency of action potentials. Beyond this diameter, the light falls on the antagonistic surround; this produces a decrease in the frequency of action potentials. (Point A represents the cell's maintained discharge, area B represents the receptive field center, point C represents the border between the center and surround, area D represents the receptive field surround, and point E represents the termination of the cell's receptive field.)

This result can be represented graphically by plotting the frequency of action potentials as a function of the diameter of the spot of light (Fig. 12–4). As the diameter of the spot increases, the cell's firing rate increases (area B); however, a diameter is eventually reached where the response is maximum (point C), and any further increase in stimulus diameter produces a decrease in the rate of firing (area D). The maximum response is obtained when the stimulus completely fills the receptive field center. The response diminishes as the stimulus becomes larger and falls on the receptive field surround.

The greater the area of the excitatory center that is covered, the more vigorous the response. Once the stimulus is larger than the receptive field's center (point C), however, it encroaches on the antagonistic surround. This inhibitory surround counteracts the excitatory center. The result is a decrease in the cell's response rate (area D).

As the stimulus encroaches on more and more of the inhibitory surround, the response diminishes because of spatial summation within the surround. Eventually, a point is reached where further increases in the stimulus diameter have no effect on the cell's response. This point, indicated by E, represents the termination of the cell's receptive field. Any light falling beyond this point does not influence the activity of the neuron; by definition it falls outside the cell's receptive field.

The firing rate of the neuron, when presented with a very large light (point E), is about the same as when there is no stimulus at all (point A). This demonstrates that ganglion cells are not responsive to diffuse illumination (i.e., the overall level of illumination) (Fig. 12–5).

If diffuse illumination is not an optimal stimulus for a ganglion cell, what is the optimal stimulus? The answer is that retinal ganglion cells are designed to detect one of the most critical features of our visual world: spatial contrast.

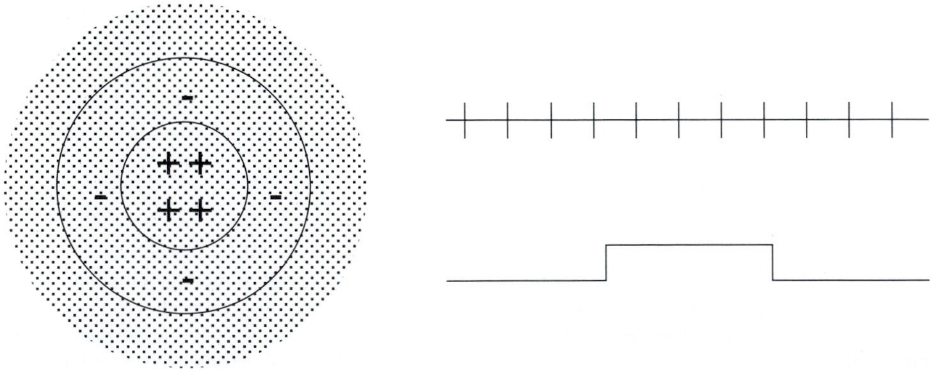

**FIGURE 12–5.** A ganglion cell is not responsive to diffuse illumination. There is no change in the frequency of action potentials from the baseline maintained discharge.

Consider the response of a ganglion cell when presented with a sine wave grating, as illustrated in Figure 12–6. The bright bar falls on the receptive field's center, producing an increase in the frequency of action potentials. The dark bars fall on the receptive field's surround; consequently, any light that could fall on this inhibitory surround, producing a decrease in firing, is blocked. The result is that this spatial grating optimally excites the cell.

This illustrates a critical point. Ganglion cells are selective for spatial contrast, not diffuse illumination. Very early in the visual system, within the retina itself, contrast information is extracted from the visual scene. This should not be surprising. As discussed in Chapter 7, spatial contrast is central to visual perception.

In the remainder of this chapter, we examine how visual information is processed from the photoreceptors through the ganglion cells. The receptive fields of those visual cells that precede the ganglion cells (photoreceptors, horizontal cells, bipolar cells, and amacrine cells) are discussed. We are particularly interested in understanding how the receptive fields of these distal retinal elements contribute to the receptive fields of ganglion cells.

## EXPERIMENT OF WERBLIN AND DOWLING

Before discussing the neurophysiologic properties of retinal cells, let us address a procedural problem. Photoreceptors, along with several classes of retinal neurons, do not generate action potentials. Rather, they generate graded or slow potentials. Extracellular microelectrodes are able to record only action potentials, not graded potentials. Consequently, intracellular recording techniques, in which the microelectrode impales the cell, must be used. This is problematic

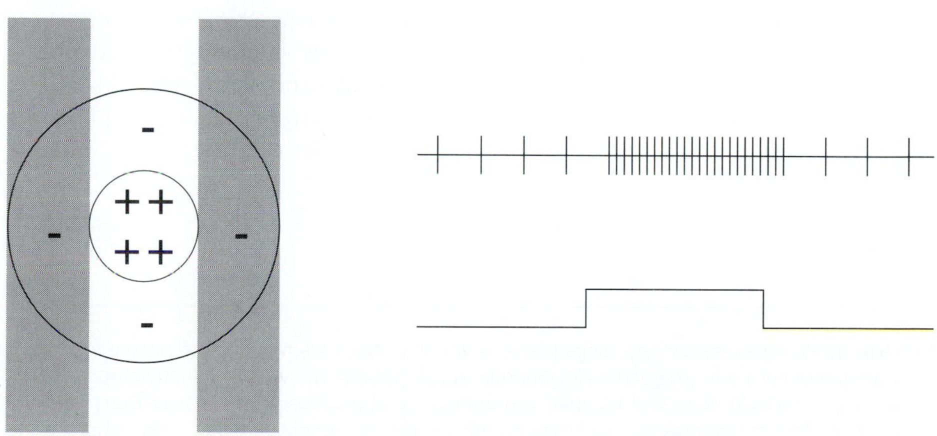

**FIGURE 12–6.** A spatial grating is an optimal stimulus for a ganglion cell. As light falls upon the excitatory center and darkness on the inhibitory surround, the neural response is vigorous.

because photoreceptors and neurons located in the mammalian retina are very small, making it technically difficult to insert an electrode into these cells.

Werblin and Dowling (1969) overcame this obstacle by recording membrane potentials from the unusually large retinal cells of an aquatic salamander, the mudpuppy *(Necturus maculosus)*. The large cells are a result of an aborted metamorphosis in which the cells undergo mitosis without division. By recording from the various classes of retinal cells, Werblin and Dowling (1969) were able to determine the basic outline of information transfer within the retina. Their results are summarized in Figure 12–7. (Modern techniques now allow intracellular recordings from smaller mammalian neurons.)

## PHOTORECEPTORS

Photoreceptors are specialized sensory receptors. They contain a photosensitive pigment that absorbs light quanta and converts this radiant energy into electrical activity. This is the first step in vision.

The manner in which photoreceptors (both rods and cones) respond to light is unexpected. These cells are slightly depolarized relative to a typical neuron. Rather than manifesting a typical resting potential of –70 mV, they have a potential of about –50 mV. When exposed to light, their potential goes from –50 mV to a value closer to –70 mV—they *hyperpolarize* (Tomita, 1970). This is surprising because stimulation is typically thought to cause depolarization rather than hyperpolarization.

The degree of hyperpolarization that a photoreceptor undergoes is related to the intensity of the stimulus. An intense stimulus causes greater hyperpolarization than a less intense stimulus. This is one reason that the potentials produced by photoreceptors are referred to as **graded potentials.**

A summary of the steps that result in the hyperpolarization of a rod are outlined in Figure 12–8 (Lamb, 1986; Pugh and Cobbs, 1986; Stryer, 1986). In the dark, sodium ions ($Na^+$) flow into the rod outer segment through pores, producing a slight depolarization, the so-called **dark current.** The absorption of light by rhodopsin initiates a series of events that result in the blockage of the $Na^+$ pores and the resultant hyperpolarization of the outer segment.

**FIGURE 12–7.** Intracellular recordings from the various neural elements in the mudpuppy retina. Only amacrine cells and ganglion cells generate action potentials; all other retinal neurons generate graded potentials. Note that the spot and annulus elicit responses of opposite signs from the bipolar cell. This is because the spot falls on the bipolar cell receptive field center, whereas the annulus falls on its antagonistic surround. The same effect is also found for the ganglion cell. (*Adapted from Werblin FS, Dowling JE. Organization of the retina of the mudpuppy, Necturus maculosus. II. Intracellular recording.* J Neurophysiol. *1969;32:339–355.*)

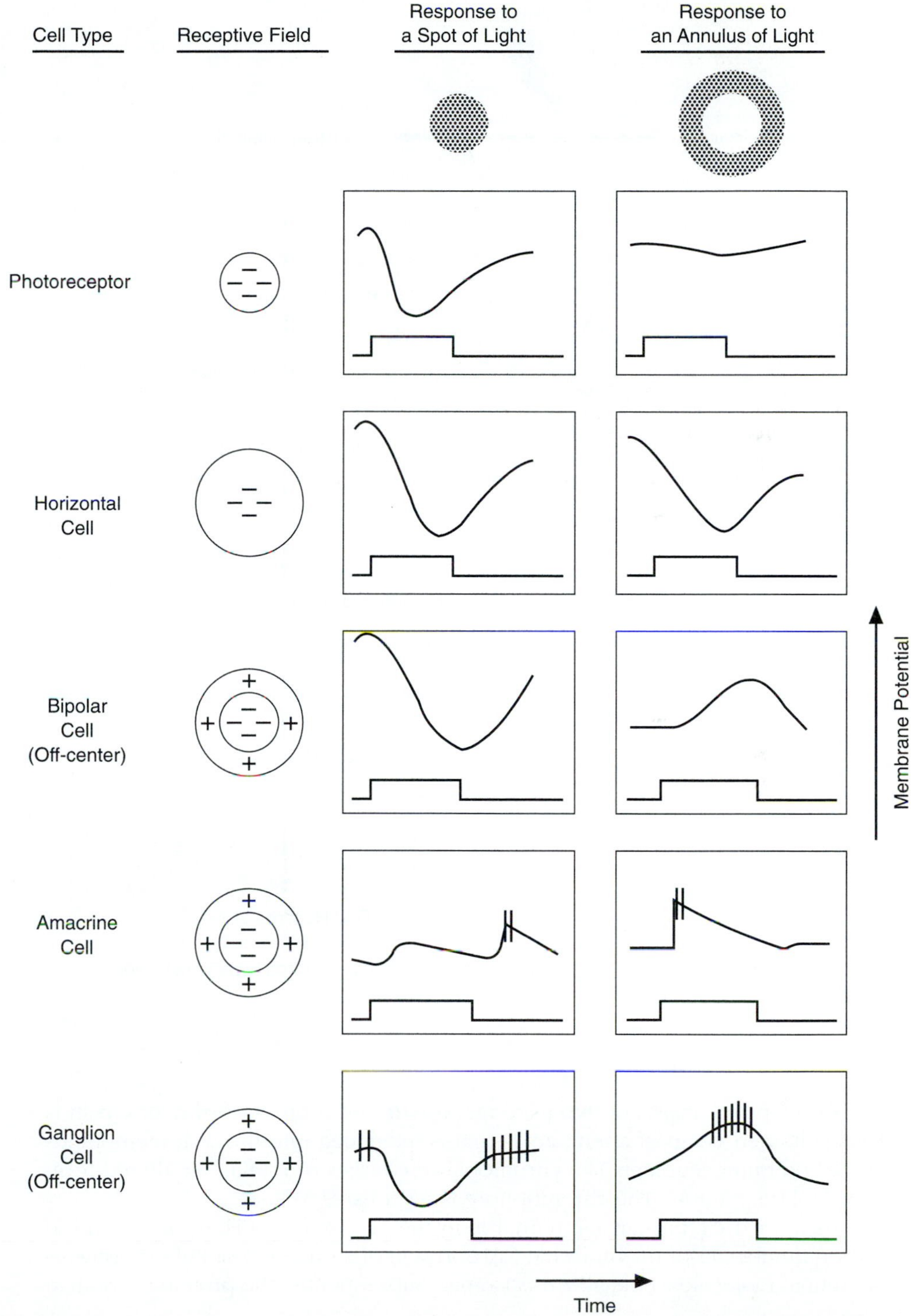
Cell Type
Receptive Field
Response to a Spot of Light
Response to an Annulus of Light
Photoreceptor
Horizontal Cell
Bipolar Cell (Off-center)
Amacrine Cell
Ganglion Cell (Off-center)
Membrane Potential
Time

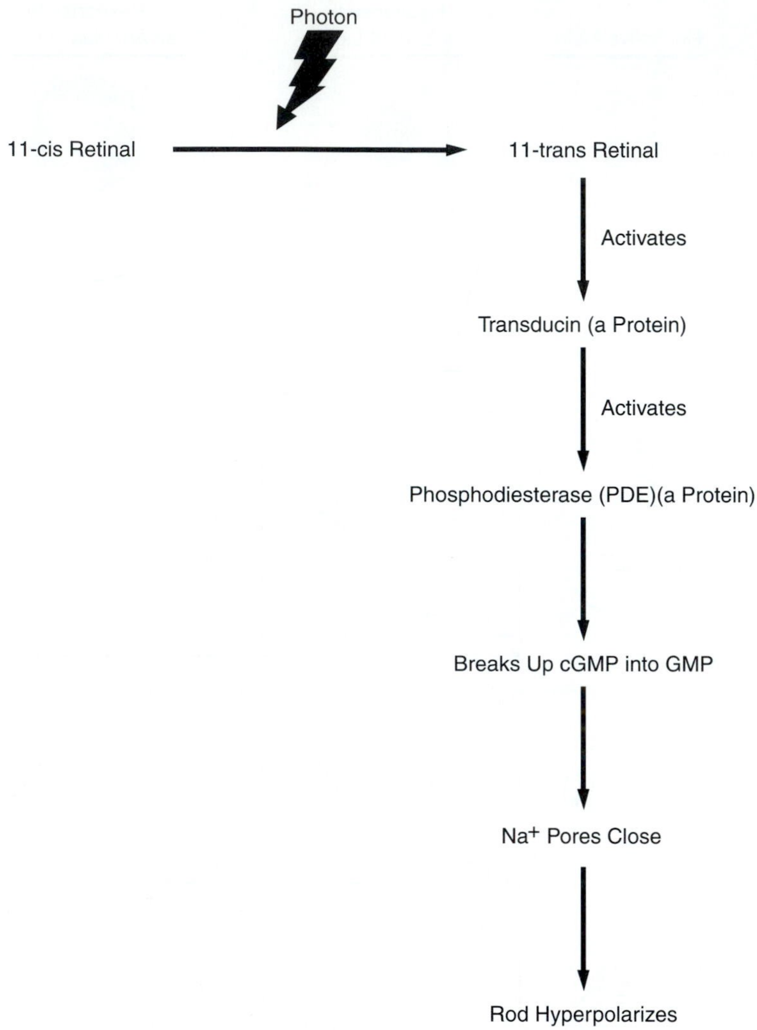


**FIGURE 12–8.** Flow diagram showing the stages that lead to rod hyperpolarization.

Rhodopsin consists of two portions: **opsin** and a **chromophore.** Opsin is a visually inert chain of amino acids that is interlaced into the disk membranes of the rod outer segment. The chromophore consists of retinal, an altered form of retinol (vitamin A). The chromophore is responsive to light.

In normal circumstances, retinal is in the 11-*cis* state. (There is a bend at carbon number 11 of the molecule.) Absorption of a quantum of light transforms the retinal molecule to the all-*trans* isomer. Subsequently, the protein transducin activates the protein phosphodiesterase (PDE). PDE breaks down cyclic GMP (cGMP) into ordinary GMP. A decrease in cGMP levels leads to the closing of the $Na^+$ channels of the rod outer segment. This results in rod hyperpolarization.

The number of sodium channels located in the rod outer segment is limited. This constrains the potential magnitude of rod hyperpolarization (Baylor et al, 1984). When only about 10 percent of a rod's rhodopsin is bleached, a critical number of sodium channels are closed. Consequently, further bleaching of rhodopsin does not result in further hyperpolarization. This helps to explain the psychophysical phenomenon of rod saturation (see Chap. 3). After about 10 percent of rhodopsin is bleached, rods cannot hyperpolarize any further; they are saturated.

## *HORIZONTAL CELLS*

A large number of photoreceptors, distributed over a relatively large area of the retina, synapse with the widely dispersed dendritic tree of a single horizontal cell (Fig. 12–9). Light falling on any of these photoreceptors can affect the neural activity of the horizontal cell. Consequently, horizontal cells manifest substantial spatial summation.

Like the photoreceptors, horizontal cells show a graded hyperpolarization in response to light. Therefore, the synapses between photoreceptors and horizontal cells are referred to as **sign-conserving synapses.**

## *BIPOLAR CELLS*

Bipolar cells are the first (i.e., most distal) retinal cells to display spatial antagonism. The receptive fields of two different types of bipolar cells, along with schematic illustrations of their synaptic connections with photoreceptors and horizontal cells, are given in Figure 12–10. The receptive field on the left is similar to the ganglion cell receptive fields that we have discussed. Light falling on the center of the cell's receptive field cause excitation (depolarization), whereas light falling on the surround causes inhibition (hyperpolarization). These **on-center bipolar cells** tend to form a specialized synapse, referred to as a **triad,** at their synapse with photoreceptors. At this specialized synapse, a bipolar cell and two horizontal cells form an invagination within the photoreceptor (Famiglietti and Kolb, 1976; Stell et al, 1977).

Another class of bipolar cells, also illustrated in Figure 12–10, shows an inhibitory off-center bordered by an excitatory on-surround. The synaptic arrangement associated with this **off-center bipolar cell** is a **conventional flat synapse.**

What occurs within the outer plexiform layer that causes some bipolar cells to have an on-center arrangement and other cells to have an off-center configuration? The answer appears to be that the neurotransmitter **glutamate,** released

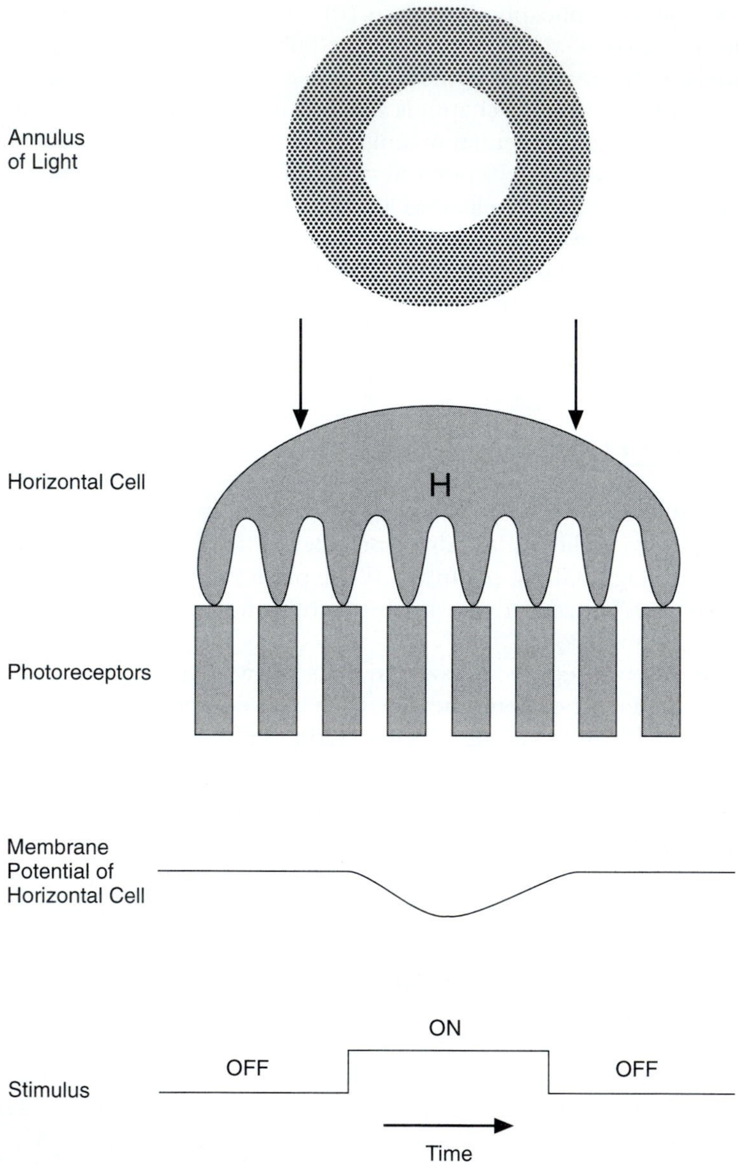


**FIGURE 12–9.** A horizontal cell sums up input from photoreceptors distributed over a large area of the retina. Because of this high degree of spatial summation, an annulus elicits a response from a horizontal cell. The annulus causes the horizontal cell to hyperpolarize. This figure is a schematic.

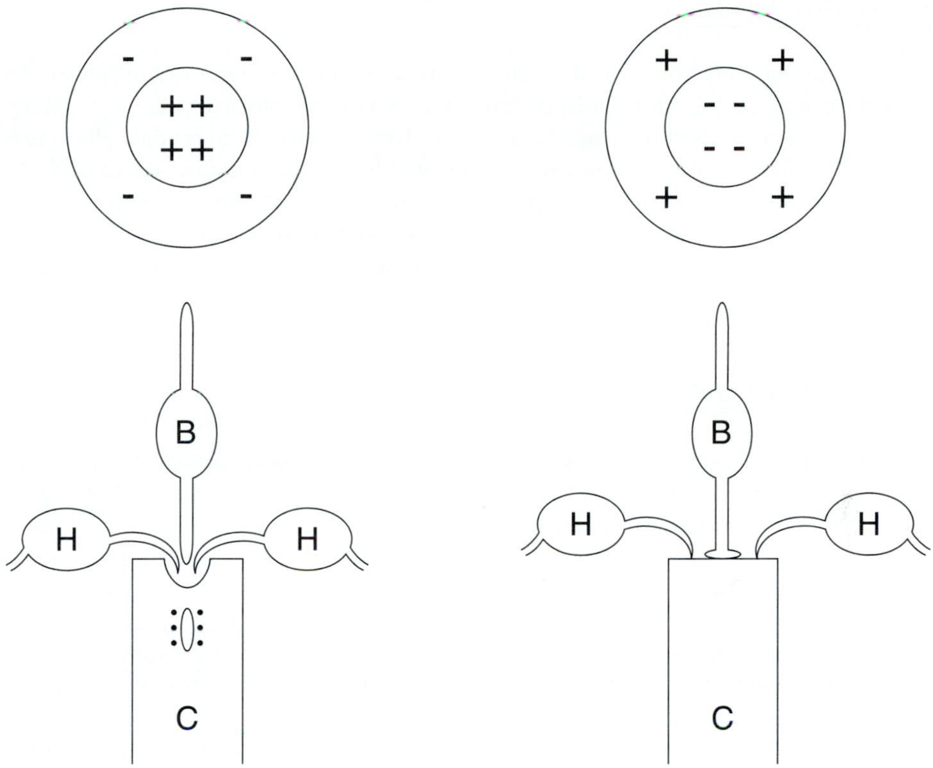


**FIGURE 12–10.** On-center bipolar cells (left) make an invaginating synapse at a triad. Off-center bipolar cells (right) make a flat synapse with the photoreceptor. (These schematics are not to scale.)

by the photoreceptors, has different effects on the two classes of bipolar cells (Slaughter and Miller, 1985).

Under dark conditions, the photoreceptors continuously release neurotransmitter. Light stimulation causes hyperpolarization of the photoreceptors and a consequent reduction in the release of neurotransmitter. It is thought that for on-center bipolar cells, glutamate is inhibitory. Therefore, a reduction in its release causes a relative excitation (depolarization) of the bipolar cell. For off-center bipolar cells, the same neurotransmitter has the opposite effect; the neurotransmitter is excitatory, and a reduction in its release, secondary to the hyperpolarization of a photoreceptor, causes a relative inhibition (hyperpolarization) of the bipolar cell.

## *AMACRINE CELLS*

Many amacrine cells, like bipolar cells, show a center–surround organization. An important feature that distinguishes amacrine cells from bipolar cells is the time-related characteristics of their neural response. Unlike more distal retinal cells, many amacrine cells tend to respond briefly—transiently—at the stimulus onset and offset. Consequently, these neurons may play a critical role in coding movement.

Amacrine cells are the first retinal neurons to display action potentials. Photoreceptors, horizontal cells, and bipolar cells show graded potentials, not action potentials (Barnes and Werblin, 1986).

## *GANGLION CELLS*

Like bipolar and amacrine cells, ganglion cells show spatial antagonism. Figure 12–11 schematically illustrates the manner in which the receptive field of a ganglion cell is constructed from central photoreceptors that are antagonistic to surrounding photoreceptors. Ganglion cells manifest either an on-center with an antagonistic off-surround or an off-center and on-surround.

Similar to amacrine cells, ganglion cells generate action potentials. This is critical because the axons of ganglion cells must traverse a substantial distance before they reach their primary destination, the dorsal lateral geniculate nucleus (dLGN). Action potentials, unlike graded potentials, do not decay over distance. As the axons of the ganglion cells leave the eye at the disk to form the optic nerve, they become myelinated. The myelin sheath increases the speed of transmission along the nerve.

The size of the receptive fields of ganglion cells increases as retinal eccentricity increases. Foveal ganglion cells have very small receptive field centers. As

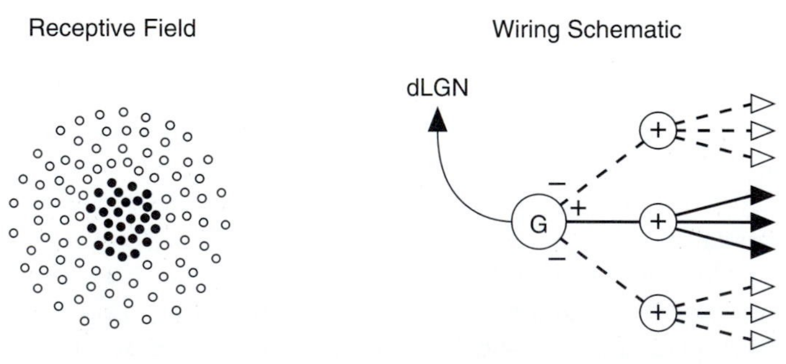


**FIGURE 12–11.** The receptive field of a ganglion cell results from the apposition of central photoreceptors to surrounding photoreceptors. In the case of this on-center ganglion cell, light falling upon the central photoreceptors leads to excitation of the ganglion cell, whereas light falling upon the surrounding photoreceptors leads to inhibition.

few as one cone may contribute to the receptive field center of a foveal ganglion cell, resulting in a high degree of spatial resolution. In comparison, the larger receptive field centers of more peripherally located ganglion cells result from the summation of many cones (Rodieck, 1991).

Ganglion cells can be divided into two primary categories: **magno (parasol)** and **parvo (midget)** cells. These neurons are anatomically distinct, with the magno cells manifesting a much more extensive dendritic tree. As a consequence, magno neurons have larger receptive fields than parvo cells.

As we will discuss in the following chapter, magno and parvo cells show numerous differences in the manner that they respond to light. One difference is the time course of their responses to a flash of light. Magno ganglion cells show a transient response to this stimulus, while parvo ganglion cells manifest a sustained response (see Fig. 13–5) (DeMonasterio and Gouras, 1975). This difference in the temporal response properties of magno and parvo ganglion cells may be due to the nature of the amacrine cell input they receive. Magno ganglion cells presumably receive substantial input from transient amacrine cells, whereas parvo ganglion cells have a large input from sustained amacrine cells (Werblin and Dowling, 1969).

The axons of parvo and magno ganglion cells constitute two major pathways that leave the retina and synapse at the dLGN. After the dLGN, these two pathways maintain various degrees of independence through the striate cortex, visual area 2, and specialized higher cortical centers (see Fig. 14–16) (Livingstone and Hubel, 1988).

The receptive field properties of ganglion cells reflect the collective properties of the neurons that precede them. A primary focus of contemporary retinal research is directed toward determining the precise synaptic connections that result in the receptive field properties of ganglion cells and of other retinal neurons. The roles of the myriad neurotransmitters associated with these synapses are of great interest.

## CLINICAL CONSIDERATIONS

Retinal function is often assessed clinically with gross electrical potentials. In this methodology, the combined electrical activity of a large number of neurons is recorded. Retinal gross potentials, such as the electrooculogram and the electroretinogram, can be obtained through noninvasive procedures. These gross potentials and their clinical application are described in Chapter 16.

## SUMMARY

The photoreceptors have simple requirements for activation: diffuse light falling on their receptive field elicits a response. At more proximal locations within the retina, the requirements for neural activation are more stringent. Ganglion cells, for example, are responsive only to stimuli that manifest spatial contrast.

From a teleological point of view, the retina is largely designed to extract contrast information from the visual world. This is consistent with the singular role that spatial contrast plays in our visual experience.

# Self-Assessment Questions

1. In Chapter 7, we discussed the concept of the visual system as a Fourier analyzer. Explain how the receptive field properties of ganglion cells could be considered consistent with this hypothesis.

2. Foveal visual acuity is 20/20, whereas peripheral visual acuity is on the order of 20/200. How can this be explained in terms of the receptive field properties of ganglion cells?

3. Under dark-adapted conditions, the human visual system shows greater spatial summation than when light adapted. This has been demonstrated in psychophysical experiments. How could the receptive fields of ganglion cells change to account for this psychophysical finding?

# 13

# Parallel Processing

Figure 13–1 shows a coronal section of the dorsal lateral geniculate nucleus (dLGN) of a monkey. The axons of most retinal ganglion cells synapse on the neurons that constitute this laminated structure. In turn, the dLGN sends its primary projection to the visual cortex.

A striking feature of the dLGN is its division into two distinct sections. The two most ventral layers consist of large neurons referred to as **magno cells,** and the dorsal four layers consist of small neurons referred to as **parvo cells.**

Parvo and magno cells have very different visual sensitivities (Schiller and Malpeli, 1978). For example, extracellular recordings from parvo cells reveal that these cells are selective for color, but not sensitive to fast movement. In comparison, magno cells are colorblind and very sensitive to movement. Because of their anatomic segregation and different visual sensitivities, parvo and magno cells can be considered to be portions of separate visual pathways.

The division of the visual system into parvo and magno pathways is most apparent at the level of the dLGN; however, this division is also found in the retina and, to a lesser extent, in the striate cortex and higher cortical areas (DeMonasterio and Gouras, 1975; Livingstone and Hubel, 1987, 1988). One can think of the parvo and magno pathways as forming parallel retinocortical visual pathways. The parvo pathway is a detail-oriented color pathway, whereas the magno pathway is a movement-sensitive, alerting pathway. In this chapter, we discuss the experimental development of this model and its clinical implications.

## *What the Frog's Eye Tells Its Brain*

The concept of parallel processing received much impetus from an experiment performed in the late 1950s by Lettvin and colleagues. Using extracellular techniques, these investigators found that individual frog ganglion cells are specialized for specific tasks (Lettvin et al, 1959).

Frogs prey on small, airborne bugs. Curiously, one class of frog ganglion cells responds best to small black spots of the same visual characteristics as an airborne bug. These cells are specific for this stimulus and do not respond well

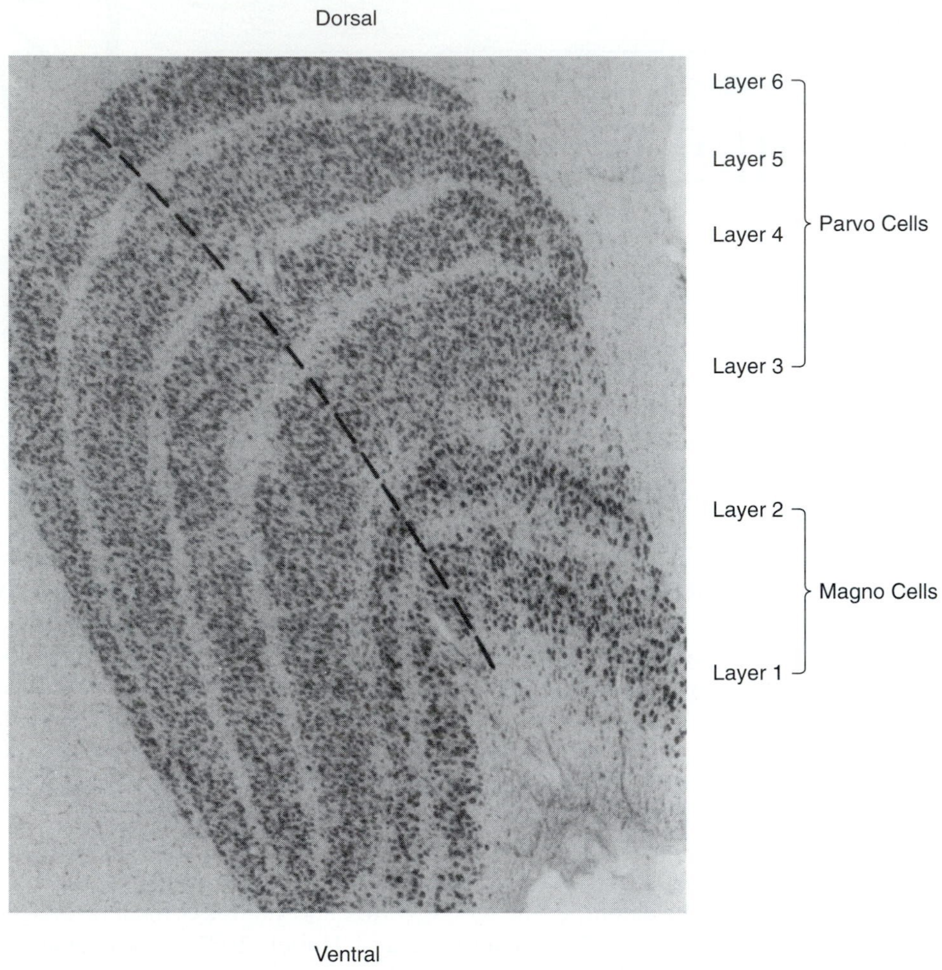


**FIGURE 13–1.** Coronal section of a monkey dorsal lateral geniculate nucleus. Note the division into two ventral magnocellular layers (bottom layers) and four dorsal parvocellular layers (upper layers). The dashed line represents a microelectrode track. (*From Hubel DH.* Eye, Brain, and Vision. *New York: Scientific American Library; 1988. Reprinted with permission of Dr. David Hubel.*)

to other stimuli. They are called bug detectors. Another class of ganglion cells has receptive fields that respond best to large moving shadows. These cells are well adapted to signal the presence of a predator, such as a hawk.

It appears that ganglion cells in the frog's retina have evolved to detect specific features; these cells are commonly referred to as **feature detectors.** Feature detection is a manifestation of **parallel processing;** specific aspects of visual information are processed along specialized visual pathways or channels.

## *X AND Y-CELLS*

In a classic experiment, Enroth-Cugell and Robson (1966) determined the manner in which cat ganglion cells respond to spatial stimuli, specifically sine wave gratings. Their experiment was done at a time when sine wave gratings and linear system analysis (Fourier analysis) were first being used to study the human visual system (see Chap. 7). A requirement for the application of linear system analysis is that the system must be spatially linear. Enroth-Cugell and Robson (1966) used sine wave gratings to determine if cat retinal ganglion cells are spatially linear or nonlinear. They found that some cells are spatially linear and, surprisingly, other cells are nonlinear. Linear cells are labeled X-cells and nonlinear cells are labeled Y-cells.

To obtain a better understanding of spatial linearity, refer to Figure 13–2. For an X-cell, the spatial grating can be positioned within the cell's receptive field such that no response is elicited. At this position, referred to as the null position, excitation and inhibition are linearly summed and cancel each other. The excitation is equal to the inhibition.

The nonlinear Y-cell behaves very differently. A null position cannot be found for this neuron. No matter where the grating is positioned, the cell responds. The lack of a null position indicates that this cell does not sum spatial information in a linear fashion.

On the basis of differences in linearity and other distinctions, it is clear that X and Y-cells play different roles in vision. One can think of them as forming parallel visual pathways.

## *PARVO AND MAGNO PATHWAYS*

Based on the results found in cats, scientists have studied the primate visual system looking for comparable findings (DeMonasterio and Gouras, 1975; Dreher et al, 1976; Schiller and Malpeli, 1978; Shapley, 1990). The experiments have been performed largely on rhesus monkeys. These Old World monkeys manifest essentially the same visual capabilities as humans and serve as a valuable animal model (DeValois et al, 1974).

It is apparent that beginning in the retina, the primate retinocortical visual system is organized into two major pathways, the parvo and magno pathways. This organization into parvo and magno pathways is found in the retina, dLGN, and, to a lesser extent, in the striate cortex and higher cortical areas (see Fig. 14–16). The neurons that constitute these pathways manifest different sensitivities to chromatic, temporal, and spatial stimuli.

The properties of parvo and magno cells are typically determined under photopic conditions. These experimental conditions lead to the saturation of rods; consequently, rods probably do not contribute to the properties of parvo or magno cells as discussed in this chapter.

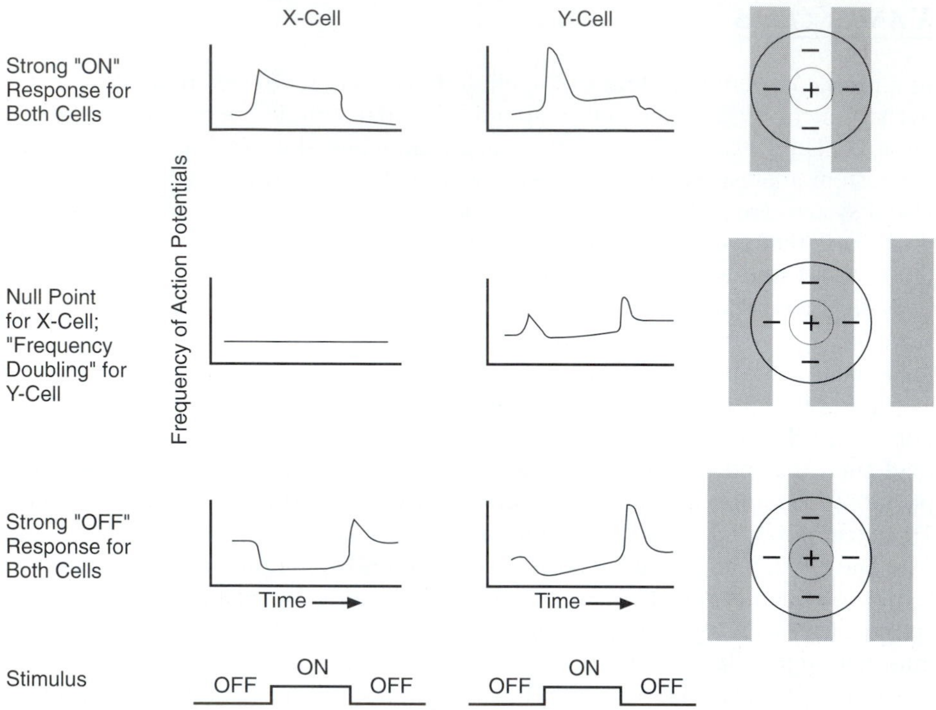


**FIGURE 13–2.** A spatial grating can be positioned within the receptive field of an X-cell such that a null position is located (left). This indicates that X-cells manifest linear spatial summation. For a nonlinear Y-cell (right) a null position is not found. (*Adapted from Enroth-Cugell C, Robson JG. The contrast sensitivity of retinal ganglion cells of the cat.* J Physiol. *1966;187:517–552.*)

The following discussion concerns parvo and magno cells located in both the primate retina and dLGN. Parvo cells in the retina manifest essentially the same properties as parvo cells located in the dLGN. Likewise, magno cells located in the retina and dLGN share similar properties. Features of these neurons are summarized in Table 13–1.

A fundamental difference between parvo and magno neurons concerns color coding capabilities. Parvo neurons display color opponency. Stimuli of certain wavelengths excite a parvo neuron, whereas other wavelengths cause it to be inhibited (Fig. 13–3). The sign of the response (excitatory or inhibitory) presumably serves as a basis for coding the wavelength of the stimulus (DeValois et al, 1966; Wiesel and Hubel, 1966). Because parvo neurons show color opponency, it is thought that they play a large role in color perception.

**TABLE 13–1. CHARACTERISTICS OF PARVO AND MAGNO NEURONS LOCATED IN THE PRIMATE RETINA AND DORSAL LATERAL GENICULATE NUCLEUS**

| Characteristic | Parvo Neurons | Magno Neurons |
|---|---|---|
| Color coding | Color opponent | Weak or no color opponency |
| Temporal responsiveness | Sustained | Transient |
| Speed of transmission | Slow | Fast |
| Spatial linearity | Linear | Linear or nonlinear |
| Retinal distribution | Central | Peripheral |
| Spatial sensitivity | High frequencies | Low frequencies |
| Response to increasing contrast | Weak | Saturates |
| Cortical projection (V1) | 4A, 4C$\beta$ | 4C$\alpha$ |

In comparison, magno neurons show little or no color opponency. Regardless of the stimulus wavelength, these cells give a response of the same sign (Fig. 13–4). These cells are essentially monochromatic (see Chap. 5) and are not capable of contributing to wavelength-based discriminations. They play little or no role in chromatic discrimination.

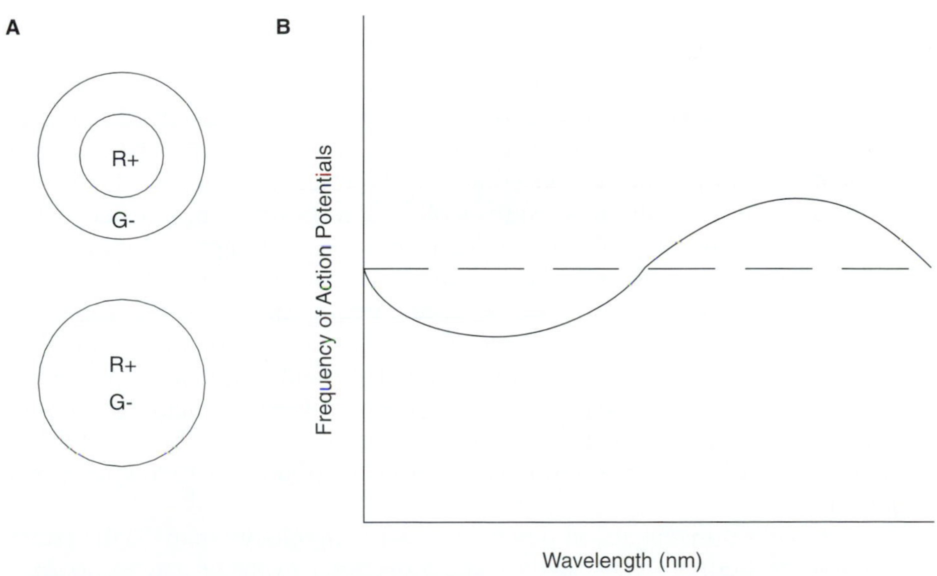


**FIGURE 13–3. A.** The receptive fields of parvo cells show color opponency. The color opponent regions can be spatially segregated (top) or spatially coincident (bottom). **B.** Short wavelengths inhibit this color opponent neuron, whereas longer wavelengths cause excitation.

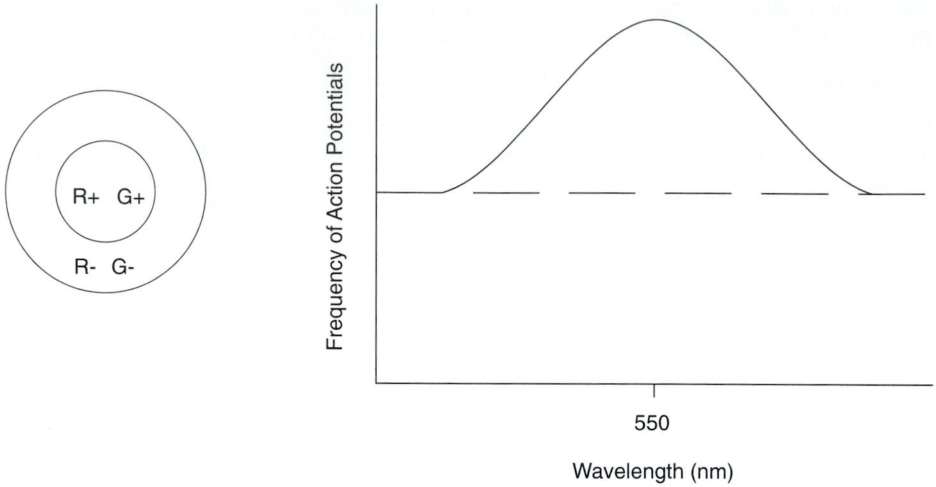


**FIGURE 13–4.** Magno neurons show approximately the same spectral sensitivity in their center and surround. Consequently, although this neuron manifests spatial antagonism, it does not display color opponency. As all wavelengths cause this neuron to increase its rate of firing, it is essentially monochromatic.

Another feature that distinguishes parvo and magno neurons is the time course of their neural response (Fig. 13–5). Parvo neurons show a sustained response when presented with a long-duration stimulus. The neuron responds to the stimulus for a relatively long period of time.

Magno neurons show a different response to the same stimulus. They respond in a transient fashion; only a brief burst of activity is displayed at stimulus onset and offset. The transient nature of magno neurons may be due to a substantial input from transient amacrine cells (Werblin and Dowling, 1969).

The differences in the time courses of their responses implies that parvo and magno neurons play different roles in processing temporal information. Transient neurons quickly respond to rapid changes in illumination; consequently, they are able to resolve high temporal frequency stimuli (see Fig. 8–6). Sustained neurons respond to a stimulus for a longer period of time. Therefore, sustained neurons are better able to code low temporal frequencies. Temporal modulation transfer functions (TMTFs) for parvo and magno neurons support this model (Lee et al, 1990). These TMTFs show that magno cells respond best to high temporal frequencies and parvo neurons respond best to low temporal frequencies.

Magno cells transmit action potentials at a faster velocity than do the parvo cells. Cable properties dictate that the larger diameter axons of magno neurons transmit action potentials faster than the smaller diameter axons of parvo neurons. Parvo cells have smaller receptive fields than magno cells. Consequently, parvo cells manifest higher spatial frequency resolution.

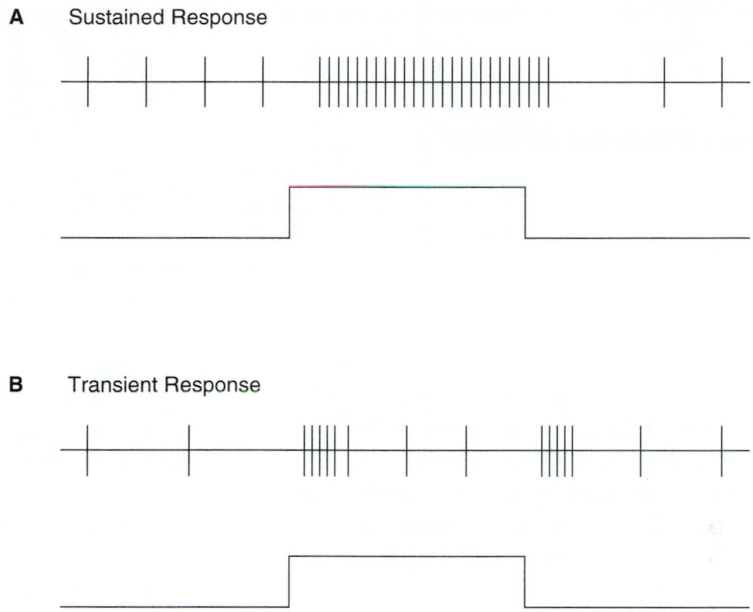


**FIGURE 13–5. A.** This parvo neuron responds throughout the duration of the stimulus. **B.** In comparison, this magno neuron responds only to the onset and offset of the stimulus.

The concentration of magno cells located outside the fovea is constant across the retina. Magno cells represent about only 10 percent of nonfoveal ganglion cells, whereas parvo cells account for about 90 percent of nonfoveal ganglion cells (Lennie et al, 1990).

## CORTICAL SEGREGATION OF PARVO AND MAGNO PATHWAYS

The segregation of the visual system into parvo and magno pathways continues into the striate cortex and higher cortical areas (Livingstone and Hubel, 1987, 1988). Because of the complexity of the cortex, it is challenging to determine the details of this organization. A simplified model is presented in Figure 14–16 and discussed in the following chapters on the cortex.

## FUNCTIONS OF THE PARVO AND MAGNO PATHWAYS

Given the anatomic segregation of parvo and magno neurons and their different visual sensitivities, it is reasonable to suspect that these neurons play different roles in visual perception. Evidence to support this notion comes from animal studies in which lesions are made in these pathways and from human psychophysical investigations.

### *Behavioral Studies in Monkeys*

When a lesion is made in the parvocellular region of the dLGN of a monkey, the animal's vision is altered in a dramatic, yet predictable, manner (Merigan, 1989; Schiller et al, 1990a,b). These animals display a substantially reduced ability to make wavelength-based discriminations. In addition, they manifest poor contrast sensitivity for high spatial frequency gratings. Other visual attributes, such as the detection of high-frequency flicker, remain unaltered.

Lesions in the magno pathway have very different effects (Merigan and Maunsell, 1990; Schiller et al, 1990a,b). Monkeys with these lesions retain normal wavelength-based discrimination and normal contrast sensitivity to high spatial frequencies; however, they manifest a profound reduction in their ability to resolve high-frequency flicker. Moreover, these animals display a reduction in contrast sensitivity for low spatial frequencies.

The preceding results are consistent with the notion that the parvo system mediates color discrimination and analyzes high spatial frequency information. It can be thought of as a highly evolved system that processes those visual capabilities that are so well developed in primates, abilities to detect color contrast and spatial details (high resolution acuity tasks).

The magno system can be thought of as a more primitive alerting system. It transmits high temporal frequency information, such as rapid movement. It is more sensitive to large stimuli (low spatial frequencies) than spatial details (high spatial frequencies).

Some have suggested that the magno system serves as a **"where"** system, and the parvo system as a **"what"** system (Livingstone and Hubel, 1987, 1988). By this it is meant that the magno system alerts us that a visual event has occurred. Most visual events that deserve attention are associated with movement. The magno system, being sensitive to high temporal frequencies, detects this movement. Because the magno system is fast, this information rapidly reaches the cortex. The details of the alerting visual event are then analyzed by the "what" parvo system. This system processes that information the magno system does not code, such as color and spatial detail.

At the risk of oversimplifying this issue, consider a monkey being stalked by a leopard. The "where" magno system alerts the monkey to the danger. The "what" parvo system allows the monkey to identify the danger.

### *Psychophysical Studies in Humans*

The basic visual capabilities of rhesus monkeys and humans are essentially the same (DeValois et al, 1974). Moreover, the anatomic characteristics of the rhesus monkey and human visual system are very similar. Therefore, it is assumed that the human visual system has parallel parvo and magno pathways.

It is of interest to isolate these pathways in humans using psychophysical procedures. These experiments help determine the precise functions of the pathways. Moreover, such psychophysical isolation has important clinical applications.

How do we go about psychophysically isolating these pathways? One approach is to use suprathreshold **isoluminant stimuli** to isolate the parvo pathway. An example of this type of stimulus is an isoluminant spatial grating (Fig. 13–6). These gratings are uniform in their luminance, yet vary in their chromaticity. They consist of bars of various hues; all of these bars are of the same luminance.

Magno neurons manifest spectral sensitivity functions that are similar to the photopic luminance function (see Chap. 5). Therefore, it is thought that only parvo cells are activated by the chromatic borders present in an isoluminant stimulus (Livingstone and Hubel, 1987, 1988). The magno pathway is "silenced" by these stimuli.

This strategy is controversial because, among other factors, the spectral sensitivity of magno cells varies slightly from cell to cell. This makes it unlikely that isoluminant stimuli silence all magno neurons. Consequently, perceptions obtained using isoluminant stimuli may reflect a predominantly parvo system, but they do not represent this system in isolation (Cavanagh, 1991; Logothetis et al, 1990).

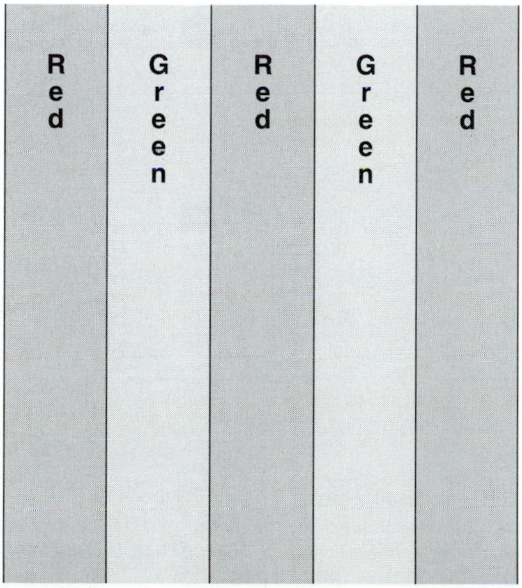


**FIGURE 13–6.** The red and green bars that constitute an isoluminant grating have equal luminance.

Another strategy to isolate the parvo and magno pathways involves the determination of increment spectral sensitivity functions (Fig. 13–7). Spectral increments are presented on a white background and the increment is temporally modulated at a high rate (25 Hz). For each wavelength, two thresholds are determined, a threshold for flicker detection (solid curve) and a threshold for color detection (dashed curve). At some wavelengths (e.g., 440 nm) sensitivity is greater for detection of color. Only after the stimulus intensity is increased beyond the color threshold is a flicker threshold reached. At other wavelengths (e.g., 580 nm) the opposite effect is noted: sensitivity is greater for flicker than for color.

Discrete thresholds for color and flicker suggest the existence of two independent physiologic pathways (Schwartz, 1993). Presumably, the color curve represents thresholds for the color coding, sustained parvo pathway, and the flicker curve represents thresholds for the transient magno pathway.

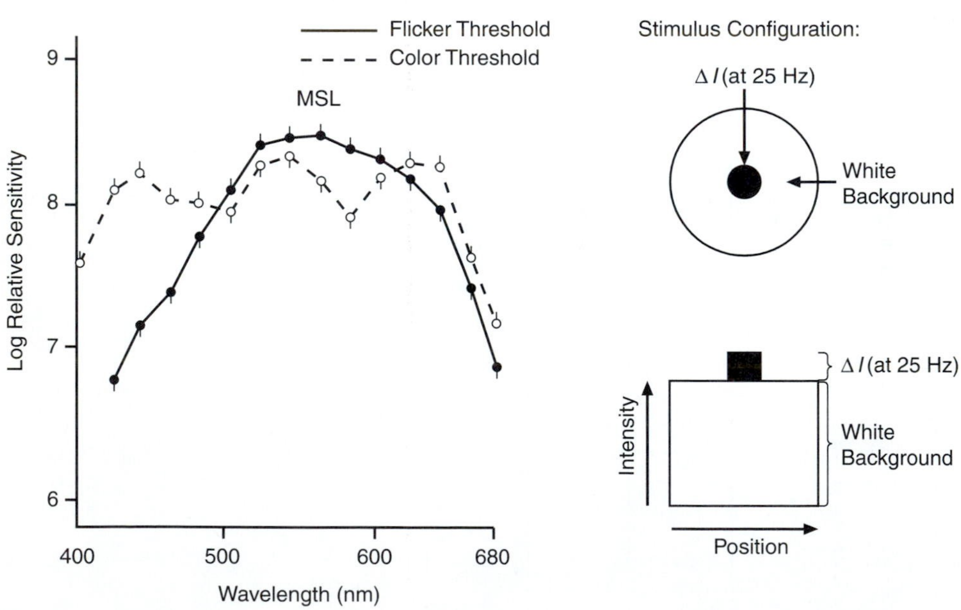


**FIGURE 13–7.** Increments, modulated at 25 Hz, are used to obtain color and flicker spectral sensitivity functions. The dashed curve represents thresholds for color detection, and the solid curve represents thresholds for flicker detection. (*Adapted from Schwartz SH. Colour and flicker thresholds for high frequency increments.* Ophthalmic Physiol Opt. *1993;13:299–302.*)

## CLINICAL CONSIDERATIONS

### Glaucoma

In this chapter we have learned that visual information is transmitted along two major retinocortical pathways. These pathways are, to a large extent, anatomically segregated and show different physiologic sensitivities.

It is reasonable to suggest that certain eye diseases may be selective in the damage they cause to the pathways. For example, certain diseases may affect primarily the parvo pathway, whereas other diseases affect primarily the magno pathway. If this is the case, noninvasive psychophysical procedures that isolate the pathways could be useful for the early and differential diagnosis of certain eye diseases.

Although work in this area is in its early stages, there are encouraging results. Consider the example of glaucoma. Primary open angle glaucoma (POAG) is a condition in which an elevation in the intraocular pressure typically, but not always, precedes optic nerve damage. The disease is progressive and can lead to blindness. The diagnosis is usually made on the basis of visual field loss and the appearance of the optic nerve head. Unfortunately, these diagnostic procedures are of limited effectiveness. At the time of diagnosis, a substantial proportion of the optic nerve fibers have been destroyed (Quigley et al, 1982). It would be preferable to make the diagnosis earlier in the disease process so that treatment could be initiated. Early treatment may prevent subsequent visual loss.

There are data suggesting that in POAG, axons of large neurons tend to be damaged prior to axons of smaller neurons (Quigley et al, 1987). Based on the knowledge that magno neurons have larger axons than parvo neurons, it is reasonable to hypothesize that glaucoma may affect the magno system prior to the parvo pathway.

Given the preceding information, psychophysical studies have been performed on glaucoma patients and glaucoma suspects (persons with ocular hypertension) using stimuli that are intended to reveal magno function. One procedure is based on **frequency doubling,** which presumably results from the nonlinearities of certain magno neurons (Maddess and Henry, 1992). To demonstrate this phenomenon, a patient views a flickering sine wave grating. As the temporal rate is increased, the patient notes that the apparent *spatial frequency* of the grating doubles, hence the term, frequency doubling.

If frequency doubling is mediated by the magno pathway, and the magno pathway is most susceptible to glaucomatous damage, this procedure may be useful for the early diagnosis of POAG. Early data suggest that this is the case; frequency doubling appears to be abnormal in the early stages of POAG.

Experiments of this nature highlight the potential benefits of applying basic science knowledge to clinical problems. Tremendous progress has been made over the past three decades in understanding the visual system. Yet, application of basic knowledge to clinical conditions has occurred at a slow pace. Consider that the only psychophysical thresholds measured in many eye exams are associated with visual acuity and visual fields; these procedures are more than 100 years old.

Currently, there is an emphasis on turning our basic knowledge into useful clinical tools. Knowledge regarding parvo and magno pathways seems particularly well suited for this application.

### *Reading Disability*

Developmental dyslexia is defined as a selective impairment of reading skills in spite of normal intelligence, vision, hearing, instruction, and motivation. The origins of this condition remain controversial. Some believe it is due to defects of the visual system, while others consider it to be primarily a cognitive disorder.

There are data suggesting that developmental dyslexics manifest deficits in the processing of temporal information (Lovegrove et al, 1990). In particular, individuals with this condition display abnormalities in flicker fusion rates and the ability to temporally resolve two consecutive stimuli (Slaghuis and Lovegrove, 1985; Brannan and Williams, 1988).These and other findings have led certain investigators to propose that developmental dyslexia is associated with a defect in the pathway most responsible for processing high frequency temporal information, the magnocellular pathway (Livingstone et al, 1991).

## SUMMARY

A fundamental characteristic of the human visual system is its organization into parallel magno and parvo pathways. These pathways play different roles in visual perception. The magno system apparently is an alerting "where" system, whereas the parvo system is a detail-oriented "what" system.

The discovery of these separate pathways may offer an important clinical opportunity. Disease processes, such as glaucoma, are believed to preferentially affect one of the pathways. By designing psychophysical tests to isolate a pathway, it may be possible to diagnose certain eye diseases at an earlier stage. Although this research is still in an early phase, such methodologies hold substantial promise.

# Self-Assessment Questions

1. Provide an example of a commonly encountered animal that appears to have an exceptionally well-developed "where" system and a less developed "what" system. Justify your choice.

2. A disease is thought to have a predilection for the parvo system. What would you expect the increment threshold functions (see Fig. 13–7) to look like for a patient with this disease?

3. If glaucoma does indeed affect primarily the magno pathway, what effect would you expect early stages of this disease to have on visual acuity. Explain.

4. Isoluminant gratings are thought by some to "silence" the magno pathway. As all the bars are of equal luminance, they are thought not to activate magno neurons. Present an argument against this hypothesis.

# 14

# The Striate Cortex

The most highly evolved portion of the human brain is the cortex. It is within the cortex that visual information is organized and combined with memory and other senses to produce visual perception as we experience it. Visual perception, in its ultimate expression, is visual consciousness. The neural processes that lead to visual consciousness are complex, and we are only in the early stages of understanding these processes.

The first stage of cortical processing of visual information occurs in the striate cortex, the primary target site for projections from the dLGN. Fundamental aspects of visual analysis occur within the striate cortex. From the striate cortex, visual information is disseminated throughout the cortex to both exclusively visual centers and other areas where it is integrated with memory and other senses. Before discussing the striate cortex, let us review the basic organization of the cortex.

## *The Basic Organization of the Cortex*

As illustrated in Figure 14–1, cortex tissue consists of superficial gray matter (cell bodies) and underlying white matter (myelinated axons). Although the gray matter is rather thin (about 2 mm thick), the cortical surface area is enormous, on the order of 1400 $cm^2$. This tremendous surface area can fit within the skull because the tissue is folded into gyri (ridges) and sulci (furrows). The extensive surface area of the cortex presumably contributes to the computational (i.e., processing) capacities of the cortex. The human cortex contains about $10^{10}$ cells with $10^{15}$ synapses and 2000 miles of axonal connections (Tovée, 1996; Young and Scannel, 1993).

The cortex is traditionally considered to consist of four lobes: the frontal, parietal, temporal, and occipital lobes (Fig. 14–2). These lobes are separated from one another by particularly deep sulci. The striate cortex is located within the occipital lobe.

Upon gross inspection, the tissue of the cortex (except the striate cortex) generally appears to be uniform. However, neurophysiologic studies, anatomic

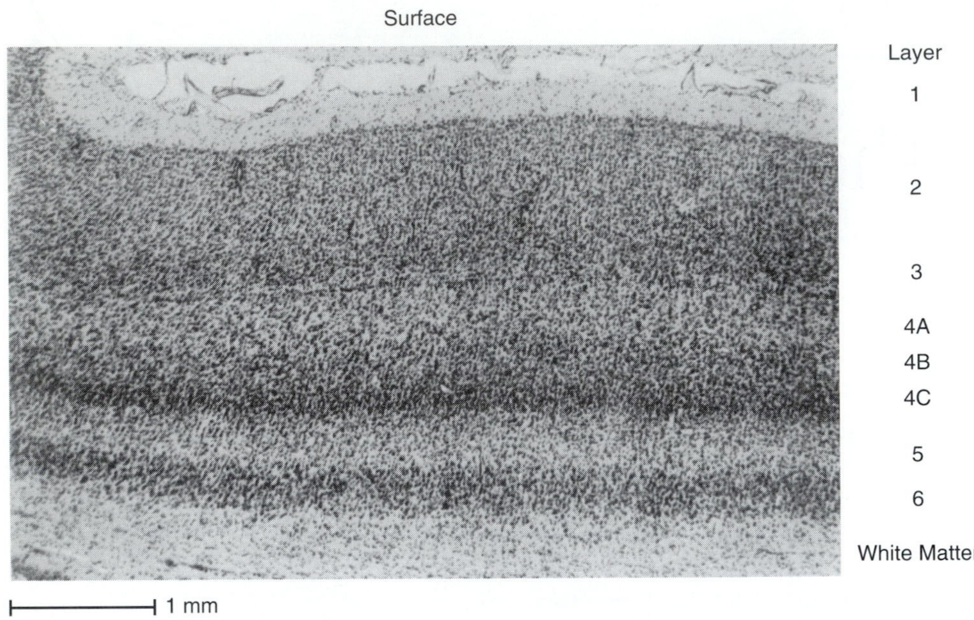


**FIGURE 14–1.** Cross section of the monkey striate cortex showing its layered nature. The surface of the cortex is at the top of the picture. Axons from the dorsal lateral geniculate nucleus tend to synapse in the middle layers of the cortex. (*Reprinted with permission from Hubel DH, Wiesel TN. Functional architecture of the macaque monkey visual cortex.* Proc R Soc Lond [Biol]. *1977;198:1–59.*)

tracings, and brain imaging studies reveal that each of the lobes is organized into many different functional areas. Certain of these areas (approximately 20) are predominantly devoted to analyzing visual information (DeYoe and Van Essen, 1988; Van Essen et al, 1992).

The striate cortex is so named because of the dense plexus of geniculate axons that forms a distinctive striae, referred to as the **line of Gennari,** in layer 4B. Striate cortex is commonly referred to as primary visual cortex, visual area 1, V1, and Brodmann's area 17. As is the case for all cortical tissue, the striate cortex is a layered structure (Fig. 14–1).

The striate cortex projects to the **extrastriate cortex,** the region of visual cortex that is not distinguished by the line of Gennari. Among the extrastriate areas that we will refer to are visual area 2 (V2); visual area 4 (V4); inferotemporal cortex (IT); and visual area 5 (V5), also referred to as middle temporal cortex or (MT).

Figure 14–3 shows the basic flow of information within the cortex. In general, visual information in the cortex can be thought to travel along two path-

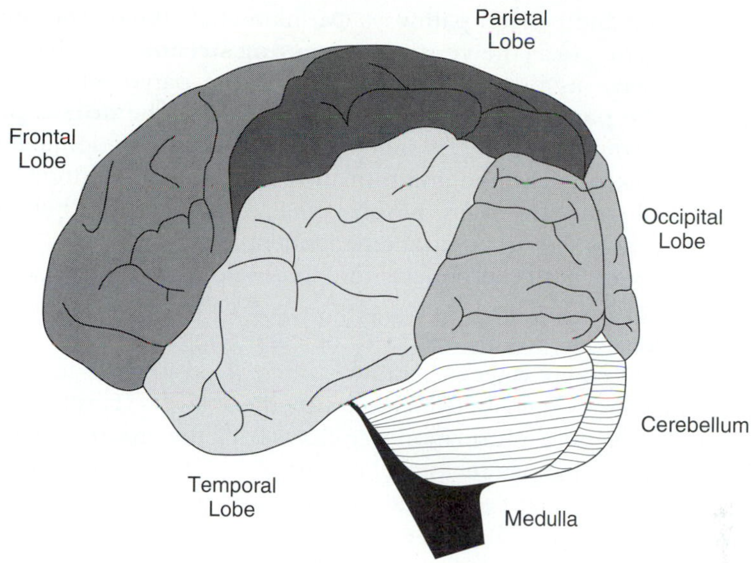


**FIGURE 14–2.** The cortex is divided into the frontal, parietal, temporal, and occipital lobes. Striate cortex is located in the occipital lobe. (*Adapted from Wandell BA.* Foundations of Vision. *Sunderland, Massachusetts: Sinauer 1995.*)

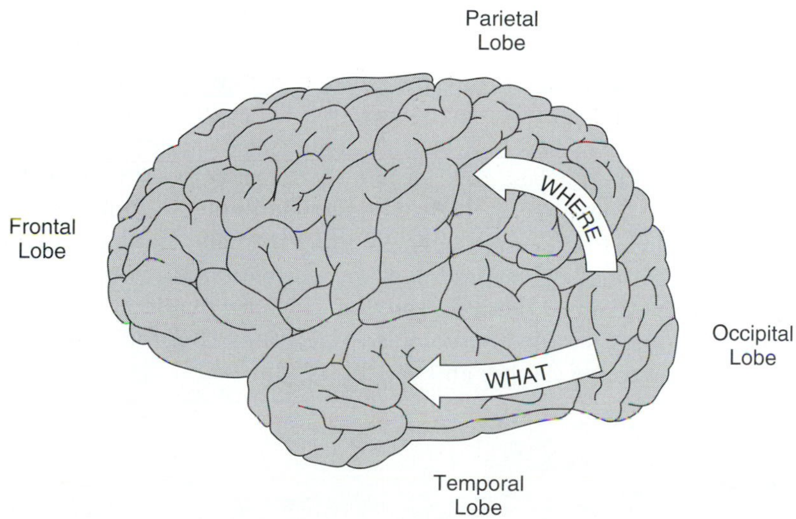


**FIGURE 14–3.** The temporal (also referred to as the ventral or what) and parietal (also referred to as the dorsal or where) processing streams emanate from striate cortex (*Adapted from Mishkin M, Ungerleider LG, Macko KA. Object vision and spatial vision: two cortial pathways.* Trends Neurosci. *1983;6:414–417.)*

ways, the temporal and parietal pathways (Mishkin et al, 1983). The **temporal** pathway (also referred to as the **ventral processing stream,** or "what" system) is thought to receive its predominant input from the parvo retinogeniculate pathway, while the **parietal** pathway (also referred to as the **dorsal processing stream,** or "where" system) is thought to receive its predominant input from the magno pathway. Although information is parceled out along the temporal and parietal pathways, there is substantial communication between the two pathways; the two systems are not independent.

The striate cortex not only projects to extrastriate cortex, but also sends a major reciprocal projection back to the dLGN. As a general rule, projections to lower visual centers (i.e., dLGN, superior colliculus) originate from the deeper layers of the striate cortex (layers 5 and 6), whereas projections to the higher level extrastriate cortex originate from more superficial layers (Lund et al, 1979). It is important to note that information also flows back toward the striate cortex from the extrastriate cortex via reciprocal pathways (i.e., feedback loops). These are analogous to the retinal centrifugal pathway and the reciprocal projection from the striate cortex to the dLGN (see Chap. 2).

This chapter will concentrate on the striate cortex. The subsequent chapter will emphasize visual processing distal to the striate cortex in regions of the extrastriate cortex frequently referred to as higher cortical areas.

## SIMPLE AND COMPLEX CELLS

For quite some time, scientists were baffled by the striate visual cortex. It had been known that concentrically organized cells are located in the retinas of mammals. Yet, when scientists probed the striate cortex using stimuli appropriate for concentric receptive fields (small spots of light), they came up empty handed.

Things changed in the late 1950s when David Hubel and Tortsen Wiesel, working at Harvard University, noted an unexpected finding while making extracellular recordings from single cells in the cat striate cortex (Hubel and Wiesel, 1959, 1962). They discovered neurons that were most sensitive to elongated stimuli, such as bars and edges. Hubel and Wiesel divided these cells into two general categories: simple and complex cells. They later found comparable cells in the monkey cortex (Hubel and Wiesel, 1968).

### Simple Cells

Simple cells are most sensitive to a light or dark edge, or bar, of a specific orientation (Fig. 14–4). Different cells are sensitive to different orientations. The stimulus, if a bar, must be of a specific width. Moreover, the bar or edge must be properly positioned within the cell's receptive field.

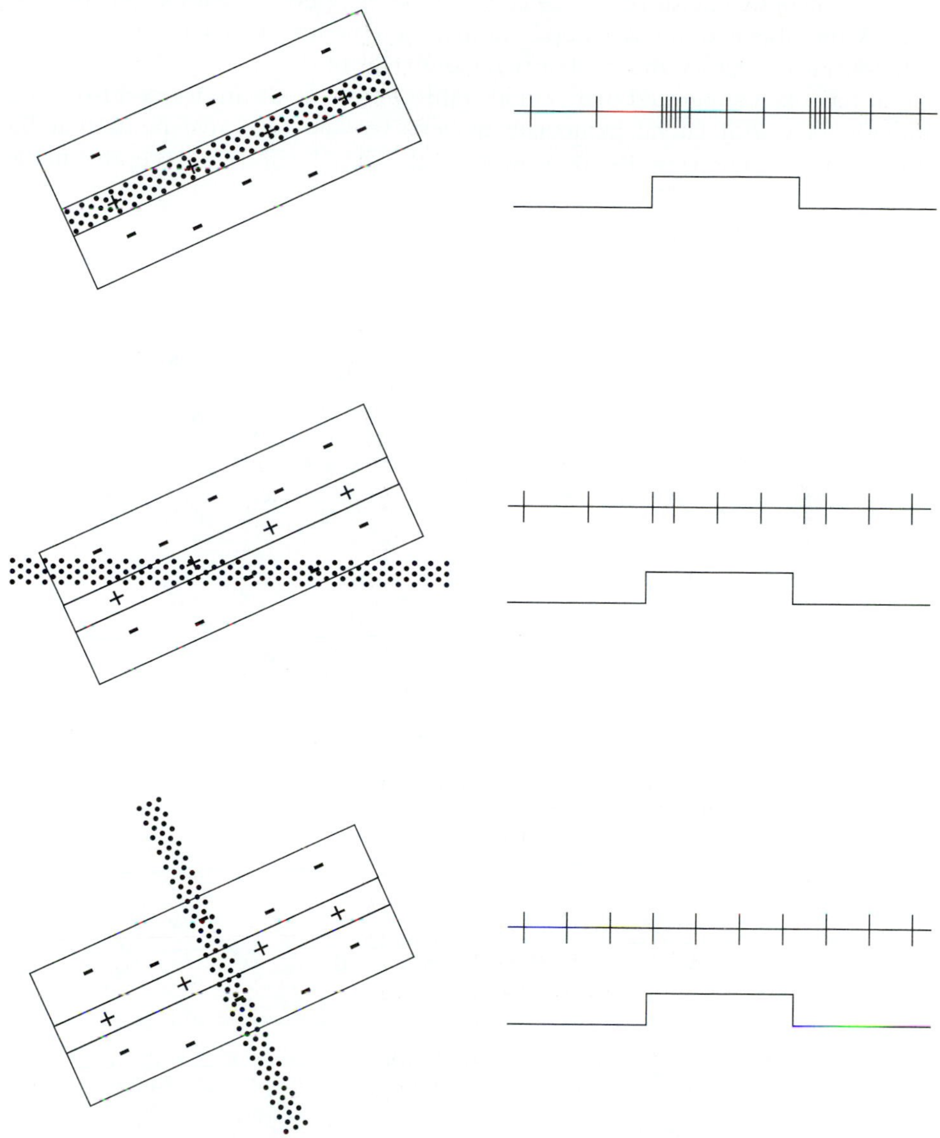

**FIGURE 14–4.** This simple cell is maximally sensitive to a bar of light. The bar must be at a specific orientation to activate the neuron maximally (top diagram). When the stimulus is presented at other orientations, as indicated in the bottom two diagrams, the response is diminished.

The receptive fields of simple cells can be mapped out with small spots of light. When this is done, it is apparent that the receptive fields are divided into antagonistic excitatory and inhibitory regions (Fig. 14–5).

It has been suggested that simple cell receptive fields are formed from the addition of dorsal lateral geniculate nucleus (dLGN) receptive fields that lie along a straight line (Fig. 14–6). Neurons in the dLGN with their receptive fields

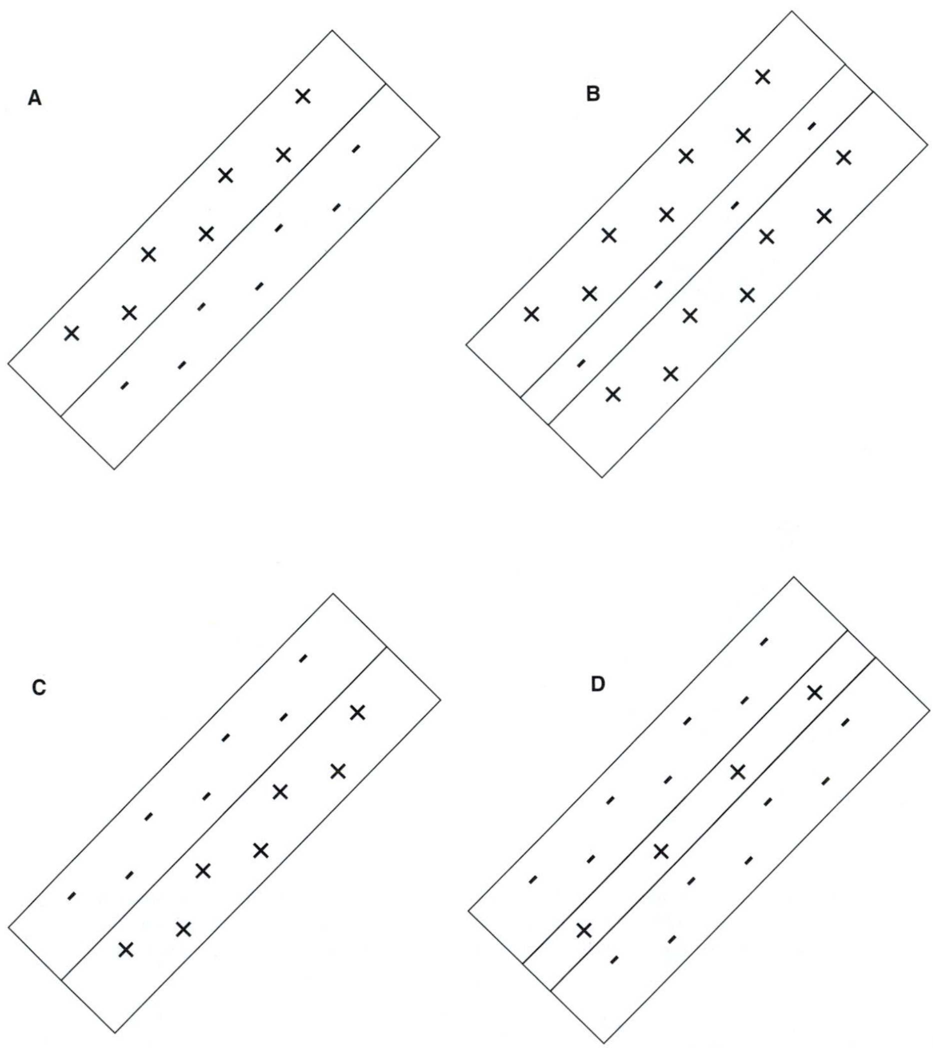


**FIGURE 14–5.** The receptive field of a simple cell is divided into separate excitatory and inhibitory regions. Some cells are maximally sensitive to dark or light bars **(B** and **D);** others respond best to edges **(A** and **C).**

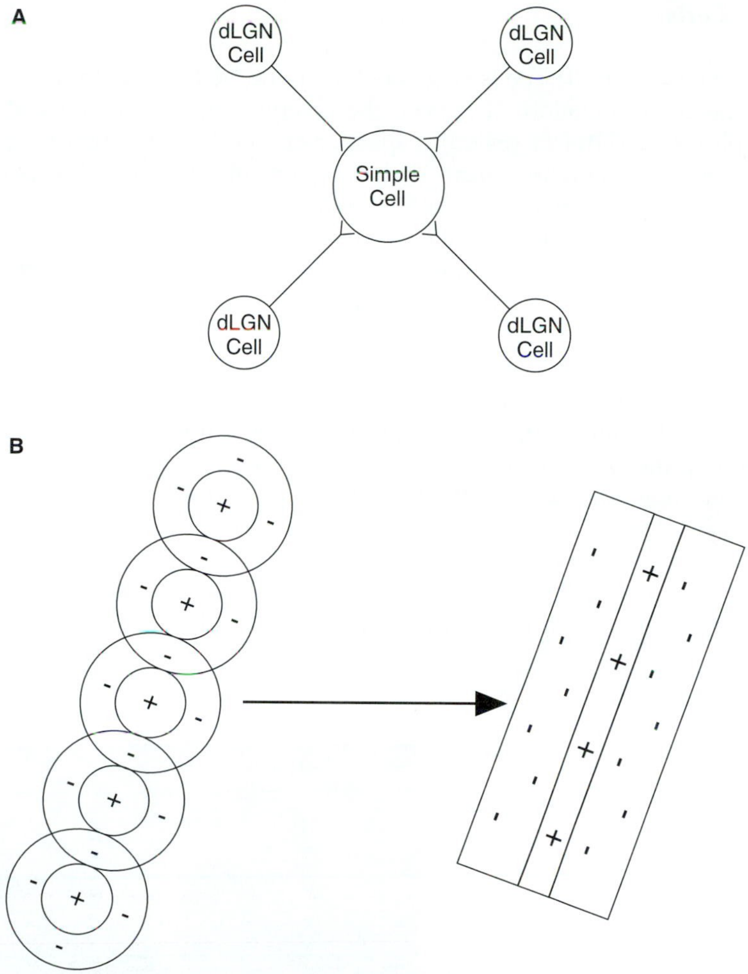


**FIGURE 14–6.** The receptive field of a simple cell is thought to represent a linear arrangement of dorsal lateral geniculate nucleus cell receptive fields. (*Adapted from Hubel DH, Wiesel TN. Receptive fields, binocular interaction and functional architecture in the cat's visual cortex.* J Physiol. *1962;160:106–154.*)

configured in this manner synapse on a simple cell. The building up of more complicated receptive field arrangements (e.g., simple cells) from less complicated arrangements (e.g., concentric dLGN cells) is referred to as **serial** or **hierarchical processing** (Hubel and Wiesel, 1962, 1965a). This is the same process that occurs in the retina. The receptive fields of distal retinal elements (i.e., photoreceptors, horizontal cells, bipolar cells, and amacrine cells) are combined to form the receptive fields of ganglion cells.

## *Complex Cells*

Like simple cells, complex cells (Fig. 14–7) respond best to an elongated stimulus of a specific orientation. However, the receptive field properties of simple and complex cells differ in several respects. For simple cells, stimulus position within the receptive field is critical. With complex cells, the stimulus can be positioned anywhere within the neuron's receptive field.

Many complex cells are characterized by direction selectivity; they are sensitive to a stimulus moving in a specific direction. A stimulus moving in the opposite direction, even if of the proper orientation, does not elicit a response (Fig. 14–8).

The receptive fields of simple cells consist of discrete excitatory and inhibitory regions (Fig. 14–5). In comparison, the receptive fields of complex cells cannot be divided into separate excitatory and inhibitory regions. It has been suggested that the receptive fields of complex cells are the result of hierarchical processing (Hubel and Wiesel, 1962, 1965a). Just as dLGN cells combine their outputs to produce a simple cell's receptive field, simple cells are thought to combine their outputs to produce a complex cell's receptive field. The manner in which simple cells combine to produce a complex cell receptive field is not understood. If there were linear addition of simple cells, complex cells would

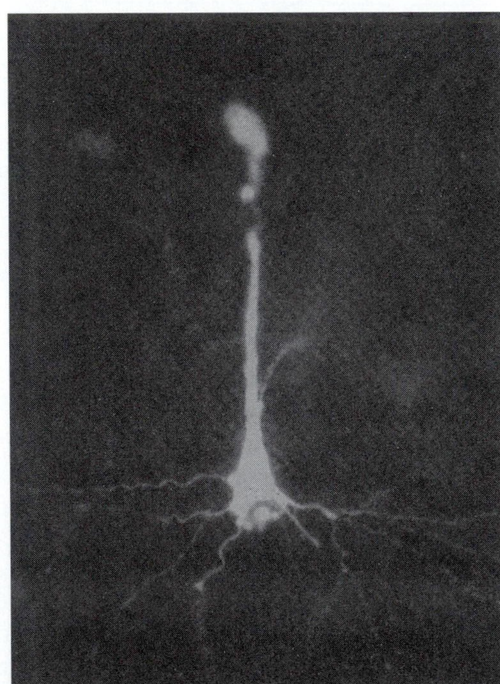

**FIGURE 14–7.** Complex cell located in cat striate cortex. Following intracellular recording, this pyramidal neuron was filled with procyon yellow dye. (*Photograph by Dr. David Van Essen and Dr. James Kelly. From Hubel DH.* Eye, Brain, and Vision. *New York: Scientific American Library; 1988*).

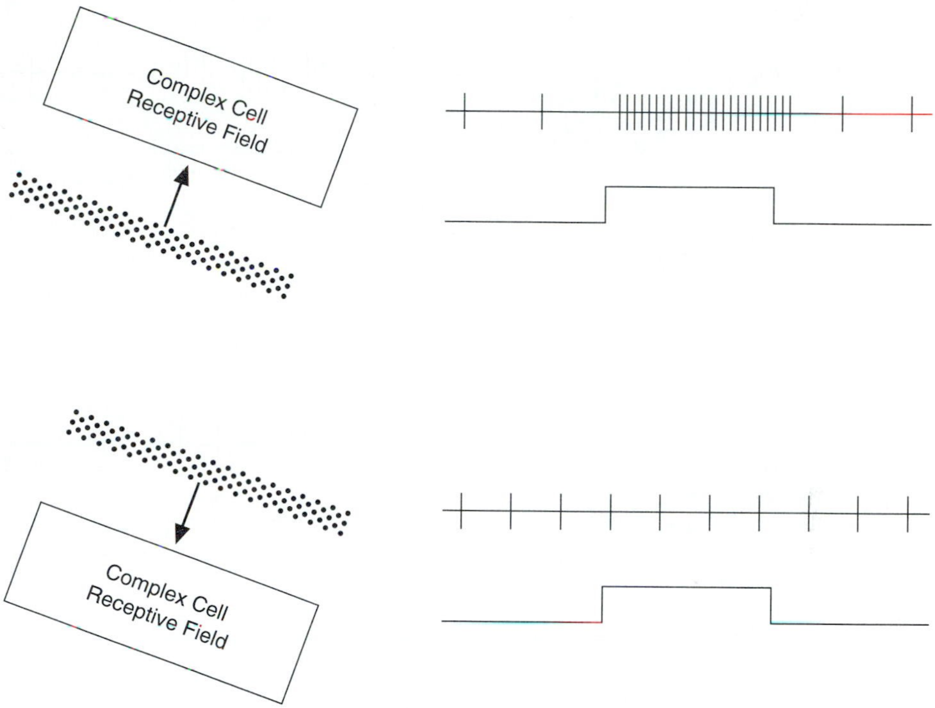


**FIGURE 14–8.** (Top) A complex cell is maximally stimulated by a bar of light moving in a specific direction. (Bottom) When moving in the opposite direction, the stimulus is not effective at driving the complex cell.

manifest separate excitatory and inhibitory areas. This is not the case. Perhaps the summation is nonlinear. Or perhaps nonlinear dLGN cells (magno cells) play a larger role in the formation of the receptive fields of complex cells than they do for simple cells (Hoffman and Stone, 1971; Stone et al, 1979).

Hubel and Wiesel (1965a) found that certain cortical neurons are sensitive to the length of the stimulus (Fig. 14–9). These **end-stopped neurons** were originally classified as **hypercomplex cells.** Subsequent examination of the visual cortex reveals that sensitivity to stimulus length is a feature common to many cortical cells (Schiller et al, 1976; Gilbert, 1977). Consequently, hypercomplex cells do not constitute a separate category of cortical neurons.

The work of Hubel and Wiesel highlights the importance of hierarchical processing. Models of hierarchical processing propose that the receptive fields of higher neurons are constructed from those of preceding neurons. Consequently, at progressively higher stages in the visual system, receptive fields become more specific in their requirements. A cone responds to diffuse light, a ganglion cell to a spot of light of a specific diameter, a simple cell to a bar of light

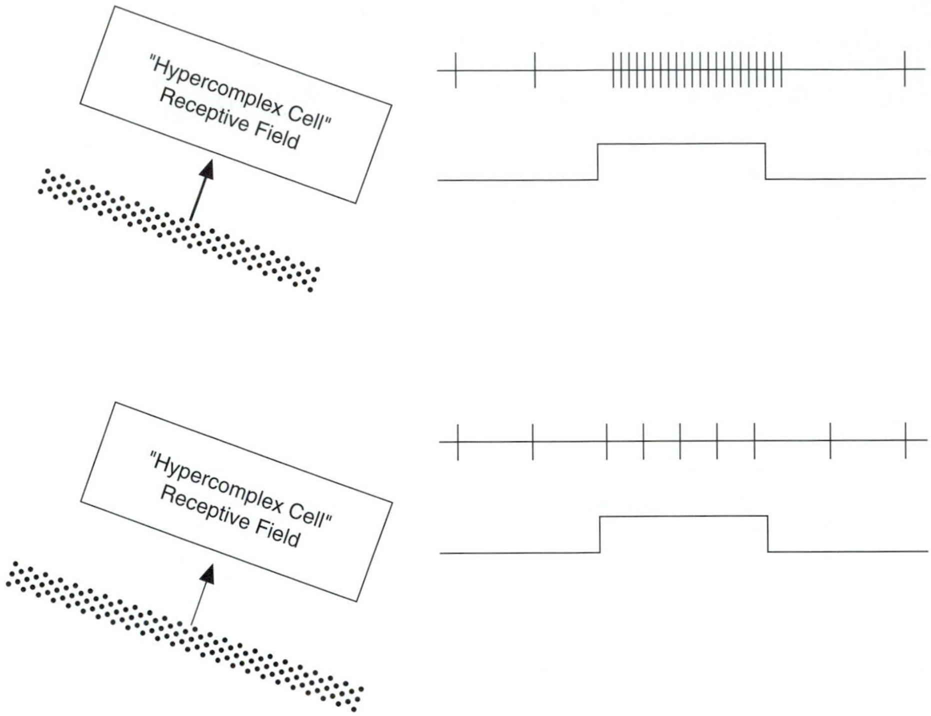


**FIGURE 14–9.** (Top) End-stopped cortical neurons show a maximal response to a bar of light of a specific length. (Bottom) A stimulus longer than this optimal length elicits less of a response.

of a specific orientation, and a complex cell to this same bar of light moving in the proper direction. The higher up in the visual system, the more stringent are the requirements to drive a visual neuron.

In the previous chapter, we developed the concept of parallel processing. The concepts of parallel processing and hierarchical processing are compatible. Hierarchical processing occurs along each of the parallel pathways. For example, the first elements in the parvo pathway are cones, which are followed by color opponent horizontal cells, followed by spatially and chromatically antagonistic bipolar cells, and so forth. Likewise, hierarchical processing also occurs along the magno pathway.

## *EDGES OR SPATIAL FREQUENCIES?*

Neurons in the striate cortex are sensitive to bars or edges of a specific orientation. This implies that the striate cortex signals the edges of objects, and from this information a percept is constructed.

DeValois et al (1982) presented an alternative model of cortical processing. These investigators studied the receptive field properties of cortical cells using sine wave spatial gratings, rather than bars and edges. They found that cortical neurons respond well to sine wave gratings and are selective for a particular spatial frequency. For example, one cell may be finely tuned to stimuli of 3 cycles/degree whereas another cell is tuned to 6 cycles/degree. This finding is consistent with the hypothesis that the visual system performs a Fourier analysis of the visual world (see Chap. 7); however, these data do not prove that the primary operating principle of the visual cortex is that of a Fourier analyzer. This issue remains unresolved.

## STRIATE CORTICAL ARCHITECTURE

Many cortical neurons are binocular: they receive input from both eyes. This can be demonstrated by recording from a cortical cell while stimulating one eye and subsequently recording from the same cell while stimulating the other eye. The proper stimulus, presented to either eye, will activate a binocular cortical neuron.

Binocular cortical cells may mediate stereopsis (see Chap. 10). The receptive fields of many binocular cells, when determined at a fixed distance, are in slightly different positions for each eye. They do not overlap (Fig. 14–10). This permits the coding of disparity because the receptive fields do overlap at a critical distance from the eyes (at point D in Fig. 14–10). A stimulus located at this critical distance maximally activates the neuron because the inputs from the two eyes are summed. As a result, the stimulus distance is encoded. This presumably provides the physiologic basis for stereopsis (Barlow et al, 1967).

Let us return to the primary focus of this section, striate cortical architecture. Although the majority of cortical neurons are binocular, most cortical cells are dominated by one eye or the other. Stimulation of the so-called **dominant eye** causes a stronger response than stimulation of the other eye. In the striate cortex, ocular dominance is laid out in a regular pattern of alternating right and left ocular dominance slabs, sometimes called ocular dominance columns ("R" and "L" in Fig. 14–11 and 14–14; also see Fig. 14–12) (Hubel and Wiesel, 1965b, 1968).

How does the ocular dominance of cortical neurons vary if an electrode penetration is made perpendicular to the surface of the cortex and the ocular dominance of all encountered cells is determined? Consider electrode 1 in Figure 14–11, which penetrates the cortex perpendicular to its surface. The answer is that all encountered neurons show the same ocular dominance. They are dominated by either the left or the right eye. This is because the slabs run through the substance of the cortex, perpendicular to the cortical surface.

When an electrode penetration is made perpendicular to the cortical surface, it is also found that orientation sensitivity remains constant (Hubel and Wiesel, 1962, 1974). As the electrode penetrates perpendicular to the surface, all neurons it encounters are tuned for the same orientation. If the electrode is

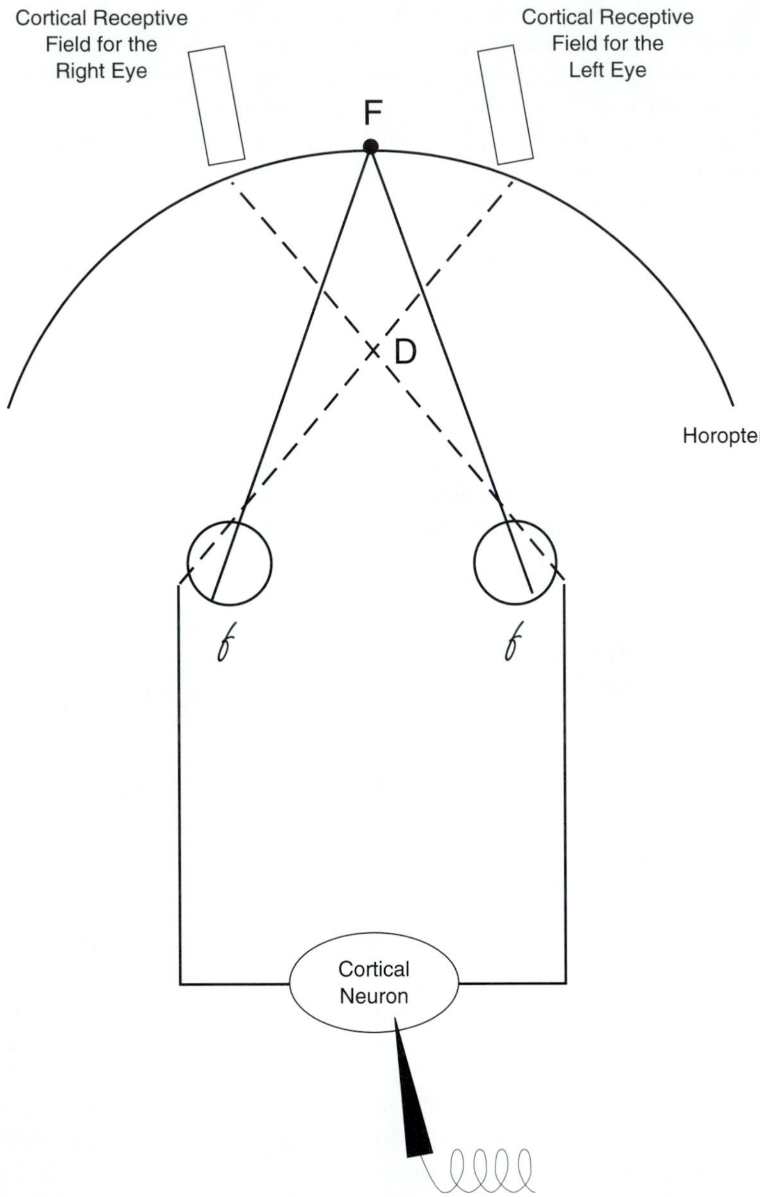


**FIGURE 14–10.** When measured at the fixation distance, the monocular receptive fields of this cortical cell do not overlap. They do overlap, however, at point D. Stimuli presented binocularly at this distance maximally excite this cortical cell. This is the physiologic mechanism whereby stimulus distance is encoded by cortical cells and is the basis for stereopsis. The solid curve represents the Veith–Müller horopter (see Chap. 10).

withdrawn and reinserted perpendicular to the surface at another location, it is found that all neurons encountered in this penetration are tuned to a different orientation. If, however, a penetration is made parallel to the cortical surface, it is found that the orientation sensitivity of encountered neurons systematically progresses from one orientation to another orientation (see electrode 2 in Fig. 14–11; also see Fig. 14–13). This shows that the striate cortex is organized into orientation slabs as well as ocular dominance slabs.

A complete set of ocular dominance columns (both eyes) and orientation columns (all orientations) form a **hypercolumn** (Figs. 14–11 and 14–14) (Hubel and Wiesel, 1977; Hubel et al, 1978). Each hypercolumn has dimensions of approximately 1 × 1 mm.

Normal cortical architecture is dependent on normal visual input early in life (Hubel and Wiesel, 1965b). Cortical architecture can be altered by environmental manipulations, such as the occlusion of one eye early in life (see Chap. 17).

## *PARVO AND MAGNO PATHWAYS*

The segregation of the visual system into parvo and magno pathways continues into the striate cortex and beyond (Livingstone and Hubel, 1987, 1988). Staining the cortex for cytochrome oxidase reveals an irregular pattern of **blobs** within the superficial layers of striate cortex (Fig. 14–14) and a regular pattern of stripes in adjoining visual area 2 (Wong-Riley, 1979). The blobs in the striate cortex are rich with concentrically organized, double-color opponent neurons (Fig. 14–15) (Ts'o and Gilbert, 1988). Blobs are connected in an organized manner to certain stripes in visual area 2; this constitutes a continuation of the color-sensitive parvo pathway.

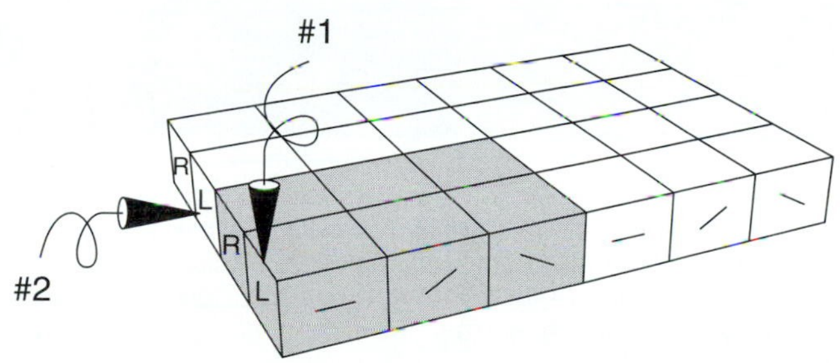


**FIGURE 14–11.** The striate cortex is organized into ocular dominance slabs (R and L) and orientation slabs. All cells encountered in an electrode penetration of an ocular dominance slab, *perpendicular* to the cortical surface, are of the same ocular dominance (electrode 1). Likewise, all cells in an orientation slab manifest the same orientation sensitivity. An electrode penetration *parallel* to the cortical surface reveals a systematic organization of the orientation slabs (electrode 2). The shaded region shows a hypercolumn. A hypercolumn consists of a complete set of orientation columns for each eye.

A

B

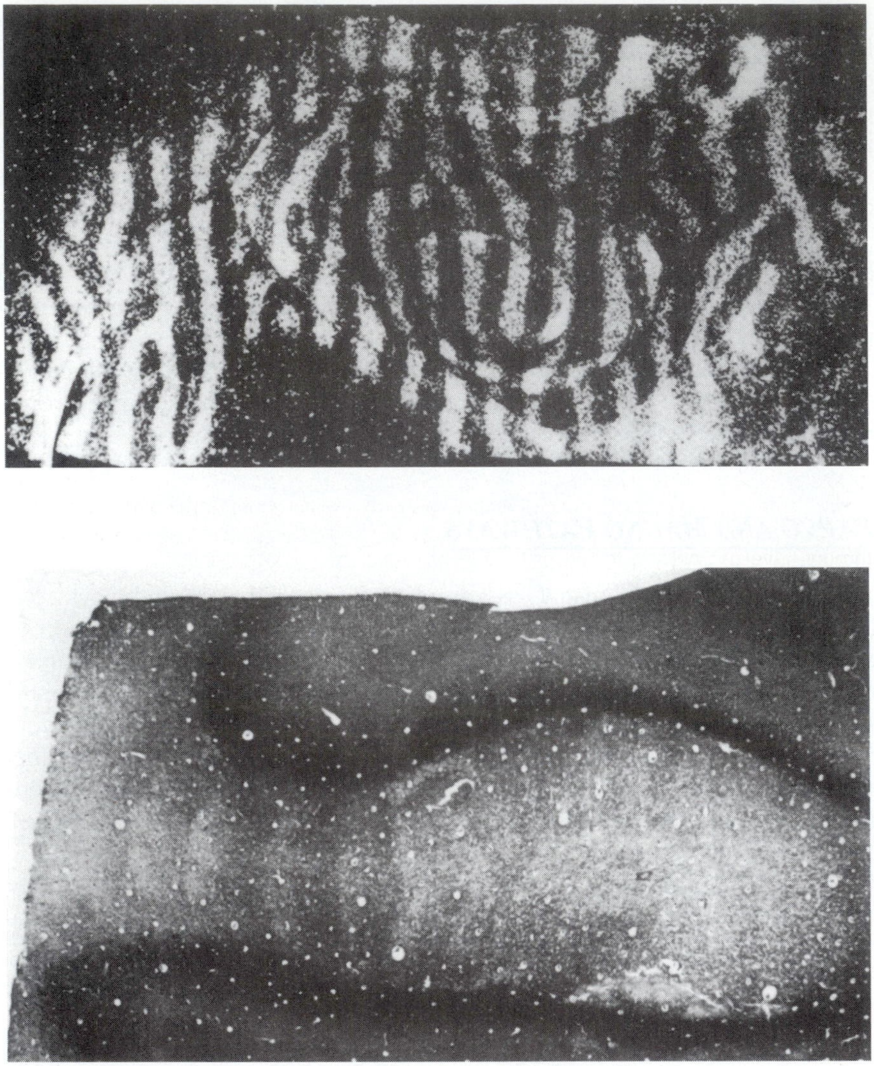

**FIGURE 14–12. A.** Ocular dominance columns in the striate cortex of a monkey. (*Reprinted with permission from Hubel DH, Wiesel TN. Functional architecture of macaque monkey visual cortex.* Proc R Soc Lond [Biol]. *1977;198:1–59.*) **B.** Ocular dominance columns in the human striate cortex. (*Reprinted with permission from Hitchcock PF, Hickey TL. Ocular dominance columns: Evidence for their presence in humans.* Brain Res. *1980;182:176–179. Photograph kindly provided by Dr. Peter F. Hitchcock.*)

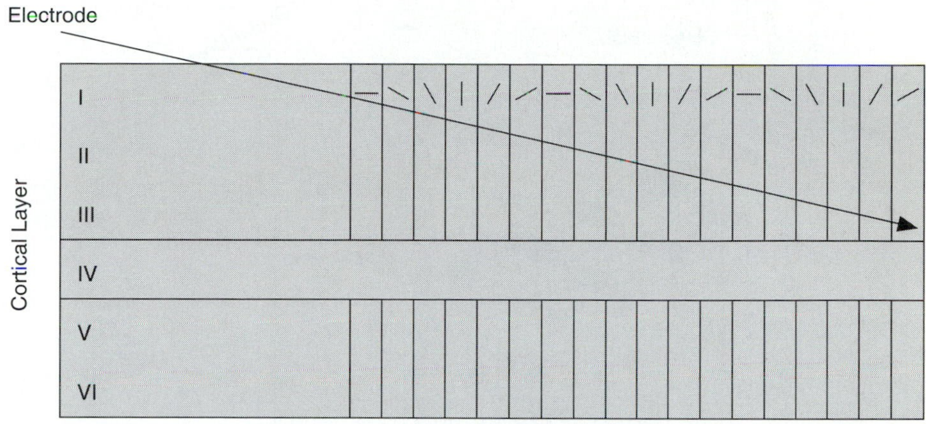


**FIGURE 14–13.** As an electrode (indicated by the arrow) transverses the orientation columns in striate cortex, the orientation selectivity of the encountered neurons systematically changes. In this case, there is a systematic shift in the clockwise direction. Orientation columns do not extend through layer IV; cells in this layer tend to have a center-surround organization. (*Adapted from Hubel DH, Wiesel, TN. Functional architecture of macaque visual cortex.* Proc R Soc Lond [Biol]. *1977;198:1–59.*)

The superficial region of the striate cortex between blobs, the **interblob** region, also appears to be a portion of the parvo pathway. The magno pathway apparently bypasses the blob and interblob regions of the striate cortex by synapsing within deeper layers of the striate cortex.

The parvo blob and interblob pathways and the magno pathway send organized projections to the stripes in visual area 2, and these stripes project to the higher cortical centers. The blob and interblob system apparently projects to the visual area 4, a color area, whereas the magno pathway projects to the visual area 5 (middle temporal cortex), a motion area. Livingstone and Hubel (1988) have characterized the parvo pathway as a detail-oriented "what" system and the magno system as an alerting "where" system (see Chap. 13). A basic scheme of parvo and magno organization, from the retina to higher cortical areas, is given in Figure 14–16. Higher cortical areas are discussed in detail in the following chapter.

## CLINICAL CONSIDERATIONS

Of particular relevance to this chapter is the phenomenon of **blind sight.** This phenomenon occurs in patients with occipital lesions that destroy all of the striate cortex. These patients present as totally blind.

Suppose that such a patient is confronted with a forced choice task. A stimulus is flashed on one of two spatially adjacent panels, and the patient is forced

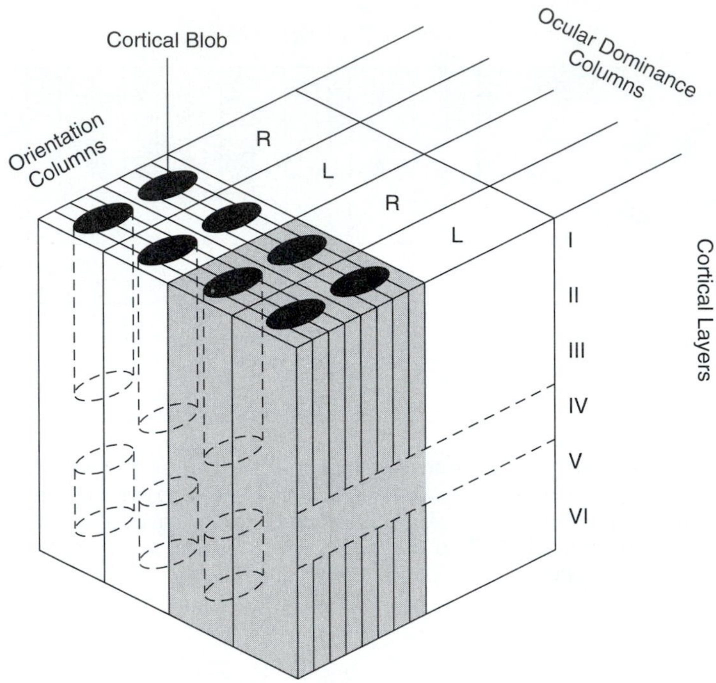


**FIGURE 14–14.** This simplified diagram shows the relationship of the cytochrome oxidase blobs to the functional architecture of striate cortex. Note that the orientation columns do not extend through layer IV. The lightly shaded area is a cortical hypercolumn. (*Adapted from Hubel DH, Weisel TN, Stryker MP. Anatomical demonstration of orientation columns in macaque monkey.* J Comp Neuro. *1978;77:361–380.*)

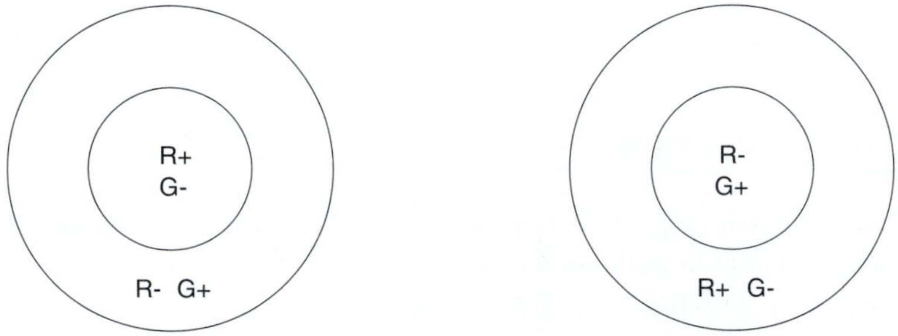


**FIGURE 14–15.** Examples of double color opponent neurons found in the blobs in striate cortex.

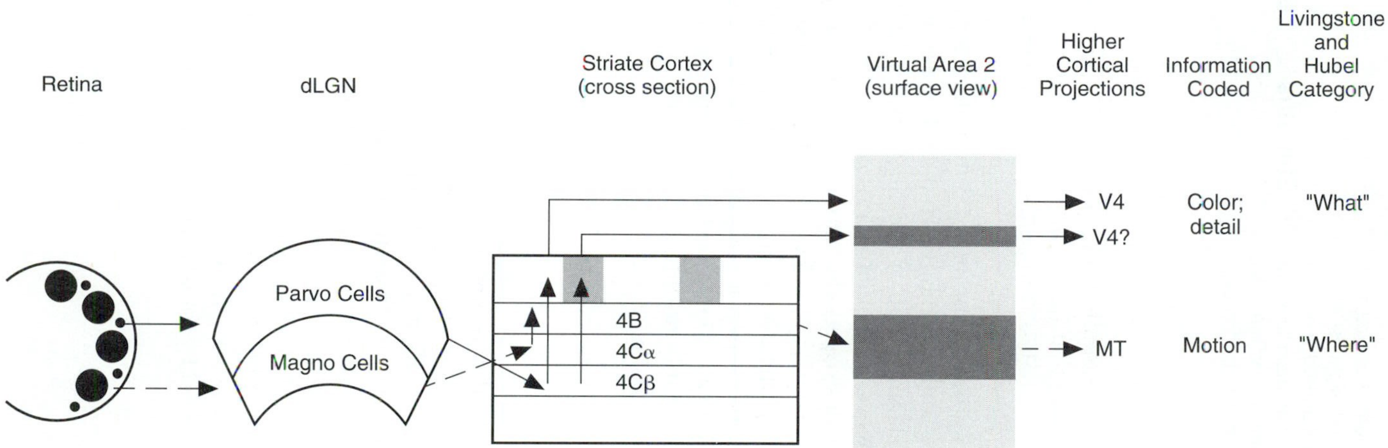


**FIGURE 14–16.** Schematic diagram showing the organization of the parvo and magno pathways from the retina to the cortex. Axons from magno neurons in the dorsal lateral geniculate nucleus (dLGN) synapse in layer 4C$\alpha$ of the striate cortex. Cells in this cortical layer send their axons to layer 4B, which projects to the thick dark stripes in visual area 2. The thick dark stripes project to the middle temporal (MT) region. This magno pathway forms a "where" system. In comparison, the dLGN parvo neurons project to layer 4C$\beta$, which projects to the blobs and spaces between the blobs (interblobs). The blob system sends its axons to the thin dark stripes in visual area 2; these thin dark stripes project to visual area 4 (V4). The interblob system projects to the pale stripes in visual area 2; the pale stripes also project to V4. The parvo blob and interblob pathway constitutes a "what" system. (*Adapted from Livingstone MS, Hubel DH. Segregation of form, color, movement, and depth: Anatomy, physiology, and perception.* Science. *1988;240:740–749.*)

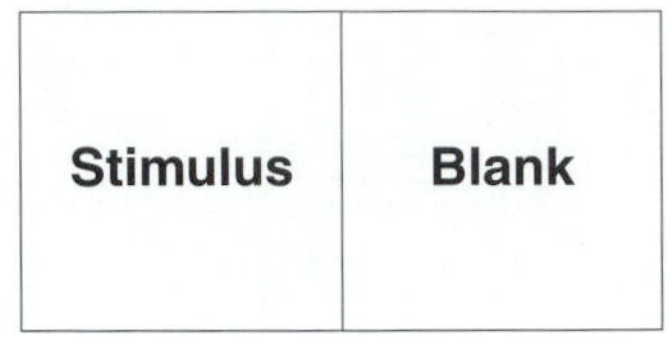


**FIGURE 14–17.** In a two-alternative forced choice task, the performance of a patient with blind sight is above chance. Although the patient is by all standard measurements blind, he or she can use visual information to locate a target. Presumably, this visual discrimination is mediated through subcortical pathways which results in "nonconscious vision."

to choose which panel contains the stimulus (Fig. 14–17). The patient will object to performing this task, claiming that he or she is blind and not able to tell where the stimulus is located. Nonetheless, the patient is encouraged to choose the panel that contains the stimulus.

This experiment produces an interesting result. The patient's performance in choosing the location of the stimulus is above chance. Even though the patient cannot consciously see the stimulus, he or she can locate it on the basis of visual cues. This is blind sight (Weiskrantz, 1986).

Because the striate cortex is destroyed, the patient is unable to *consciously* see the stimulus. She or he is, however, able to visually detect the stimulus presumably because of subcortical pathways, such as the retinotectal pathway. (The retina sends a projection to the superior colliculus, which is referred to as the retinotectal pathway. This pathway is important for coding eye movements.) As subcortical pathways are presumably not involved in consciousness, the patient has no visual awareness of the stimulus.

## SUMMARY

The receptive fields of striate cortical neurons are more complicated than those of neurons encountered earlier in the visual system. There is an increasing specificity of the requirements necessary to activate higher cortical cells. This is due largely to the hierarchical processing of visual information.

The visual cortex is a structured tissue. Ocular dominance and orientation slabs are important features of striate cortex architecture. The parvo and magno pathways are regularly organized within the striate cortex.

The striate cortex projects to higher cortical areas (extrastriate cortex) that appear to be specialized to analyze specific visual attributes. The manner in which visual information is processed by these higher cortical areas is discussed in the following chapter.

# Self-Assessment Questions

1. Ocular dominance columns are not present at birth. Rather, they develop early in life secondary to normal visual experience. Devise an experiment that would allow you to determine the time course of development of ocular dominance columns in an animal model such as the cat.

2. Describe the stimulus that would maximally excite each of the double color opponent cells in Figure 14–15.

3. Beginning with photoreceptors, draw the receptive fields of all subsequent visual neurons up through complex cells.

# 15

# Information Streams and Extrastriate Processing

Our visual capabilities are exceedingly complex and extend far beyond the recognition of edges and other simple spatial patterns for which the striate cortex is so well suited. While the striate cortex plays a fundamental role in basic analysis of visual information, considerably more processing must occur to produce the rich visual world that we perceive. This analysis is largely performed by visual areas outside of the striate cortex, collectively referred to as the extrastriate cortex.

## *INFORMATION DIVERGES BEYOND THE STRIATE CORTEX*

Beyond the level of the striate cortex there is a great divergence of information (see Figs. 2–11 and 14–3). The striate cortex sends projections to neighboring cortical areas, which in turn send projections to numerous other **higher visual areas** and so forth (Van Essen et al, 1992). In addition to this feed-forward distribution of information to many different regions of the brain, there is feedback (reciprocal connections) from the higher cortical areas to lower areas.

At the present time, we know of at least 20 distinct visual areas. By visual area, we mean a region of the brain that contains a map of the visual field (also called a **retinotopic map**). The reasons that the visual field is mapped out at least 20 different times (in 20 different cortical areas) are not fully understood, but it suggests that each of the visual areas is specialized to play a different role in processing visual information.

Visual information appears to be organized into distinct, but not independent, processing streams (Mishkin et al, 1983; Maunsell and Newsome, 1987; Merigan and Maunsell, 1993). One of these streams (variously referred to as the **temporal, ventral,** or **"what"** stream) appears to be critical for identifying and recognizing objects, while the other major stream (the **parietal, dorsal,** or **"where"** stream) plays a central role in motion perception and localization in visual space (see Fig. 14–3). Although the ventral and dorsal processing streams are adapted to analyze different aspects of visual information, there is some communication between the two pathways. The ventral and dorsal processing streams are commonly considered to be extensions of the parvo and magno pathways, respectively (see Chap. 13).

## *HIGHER VISUAL AREAS HAVE SPECIALIZED FUNCTIONS*

Numerous lines of evidence support the notion that certain higher visual areas are specialized to analyze specific attributes of our visual world (Fig. 15–1). Extracellular recordings in the macaque **visual area 4 (V4)** reveal an abundance of cells with chromatic sensitivities, making this area well adapted to play an important role in color perception (Zeki, 1983). Cells in the **inferotemporal cortex (IT)** respond to complex forms, including faces, indicating a role in form perception (Gross, 1973; Tovée and Cohen-Tovée, 1993; Rolls and Tovée, 1995). Both V4 and inferotemporal cortex are considered part of the ventral processing stream. Cells in **V5** (also called **middle temporal cortex,** or **MT),** a component of the dorsal processing stream, are well-suited for the encoding of motion (Rodman and Albright, 1989).

Additional compelling evidence for cortical specialization comes from recent brain imaging studies involving human subjects. It is now possible to monitor activity in the *human* brain while a participant is performing a task (such as looking at a moving object) (Posner, 1993; Ungerleider, 1995). In **positron emission tomography (PET),** a radioactive tracer (radioactively labeled water) allows observation of changes in blood flow that are indicative of increased metabolism due to cortical activity. A newer technique, **functional magnetic resonance imaging (fMRI),** works by detecting the level of blood oxygenation.

Brain imaging reveals that the region of the brain that is most active depends on the participant's task (Corbetta et al, 1990). If a human subject views an array of variously colored, moving objects (for example, red and green objects) and is asked to attend to the green object, V4 shows the most activity. In comparison, when the person views the same array, but is asked to pay attention to the movement of the objects, V5 shows the most activity. When the shape (or form) of the object becomes the participant's focus, the activity is greatest in the ventral processing stream. The areas of the brain that are most active depend on the aspect of the object array (i.e., color, motion, or form) to which the individual is paying attention.

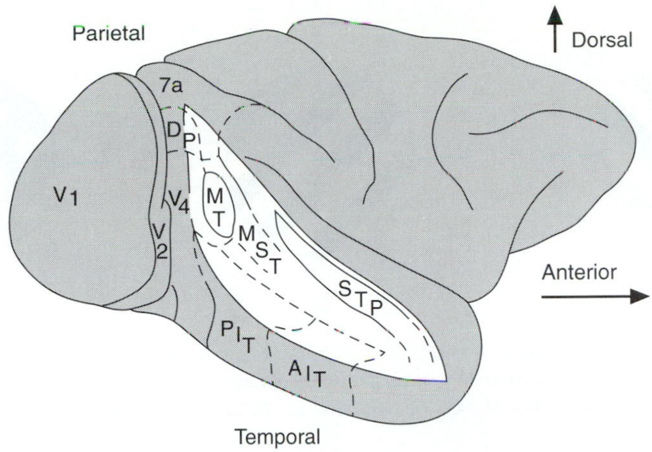


**FIGURE 15–1.** In this lateral view of the right hemisphere of the macaque cortex, the superior temporal sulcus (unshaded region) has been opened to reveal visual areas that are normally hidden from view, such as MT. Other labeled areas discussed in the book are V1 (striate cortex), V2, V4, and inferotemporal cortex (AIT and PIT). Note that there are numerous other visual areas. (*Adapted from Maunsell JHR. The brain's visual world: representation of visual targets in cerebral cortex.* Science. *1995;270:764–768.*)

## *VISUAL AREA 5 PROCESSES MOTION INFORMATION*

A visual area that is comparatively well studied and apparently better understood than other higher visual centers is visual area 5. Cells in this area presumably receive substantial input from the magno pathway and have properties that enable them to perform a comparatively sophisticated analysis of motion information (Albright, 1984; Maunsell et al, 1990).

Consider the dilemma posed by the stimulus illustrated in Figure 15–2C (Adelson and Movshon, 1982; Stoner and Albright, 1996). This stimulus, which is perceived as a plaid moving in the indicated direction, is composed of two drifting gratings as illustrated in A and B of the figure. Whereas each of the two component drifting gratings would appear to move in the directions indicated, the plaid (a **global stimulus** composed of two components) appears as a single object moving in an intermediate direction.

Extracellular recordings in rhesus monkeys reveal that direction selective neurons in the striate cortex tend to respond best to the movement of the individual grating components of the plaid (Fig. 15–2) (Movshon et al, 1985). They do not respond well to the movement of the plaid itself. In comparison, certain cells in V5 respond best to the movement of the plaid as a whole. The neurons in V5 are coding what we perceive (i.e., the integrated movement of the plaid rather than the individual grating components) and apparently play an important role in global motion perception.

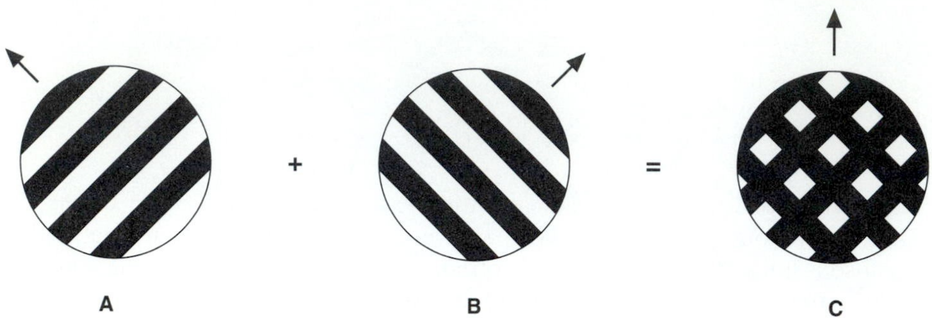


**FIGURE 15–2.** The gratings in **A** and **B** are combined to produce the plaid in **C.** The plaid can be perceived as a unified figure moving in the indicated direction. (*Adapted from Stoner GR, Albright TD. The interpretation of visual motion: Evidence for surface segmentation mechanisms.* Vision Res. *1996;36:1291–1310.*)

Global motion perception has also been examined in V5 in monkeys using random dot kinematograms (see Fig. 9–3). Extracellular recordings show that certain of the neurons that constitute this region manifest coherence thresholds that are very similar to those of the monkey itself. The neuron's coherence thresholds are comparable to those measured psychophysically in the same animal (Newsome and Paré, 1988).

Additional evidence for the role of V5 in motion perception comes from PET and fMRI studies on humans. V5 is more active when a human subject views a moving object than when he or she views a stationary object (Watson et al, 1993).

## Activity in Visual Area 5 Is Linked to the Perception of Motion

An interesting question regards the level of activity in V5 while participants are experiencing **motion aftereffects (MAEs).** MAEs are illusions of motion that occur in the absence of motion. One commonly experienced MAE is the waterfall illusion, which is induced by staring at the downward rushing water of a waterfall for several minutes. Looking from the waterfall to the surrounding landscape, the landscape appears to rise.

MAEs are presumably due to the adaptation of direction-specific motion detectors. The adapting stimulus reduces sensitivity to the direction that is adapted, and subsequently viewed stationary stimuli appear to move in the opposite direction. It has been suspected that the motion detectors are located in the cortex, the first site of substantial interaction between the two eyes, because adaptation of one eye elicits a MAE in the other eye (Mitchell et al, 1975).

Is V5 active when we are experiencing a MAE? This question has been answered by adapting human subjects to concentric rings that were moving in an outward direction (Fig. 15–3). As we have learned, these moving rings will activate V5. What happens in V5 when the rings are suddenly made stationary and the individual experiences the aftereffect (i.e., the illusion of the stationary rings moving inward)? The answer is that V5 is active, as demonstrated by fMRI, when the individual is experiencing the aftereffect (Tootell et al, 1995). The rings are stationary, yet V5 is active. This is an important and interesting finding because it links the perception of motion, in the absence of a moving stimulus, to the activity within a specific area of the coetex.

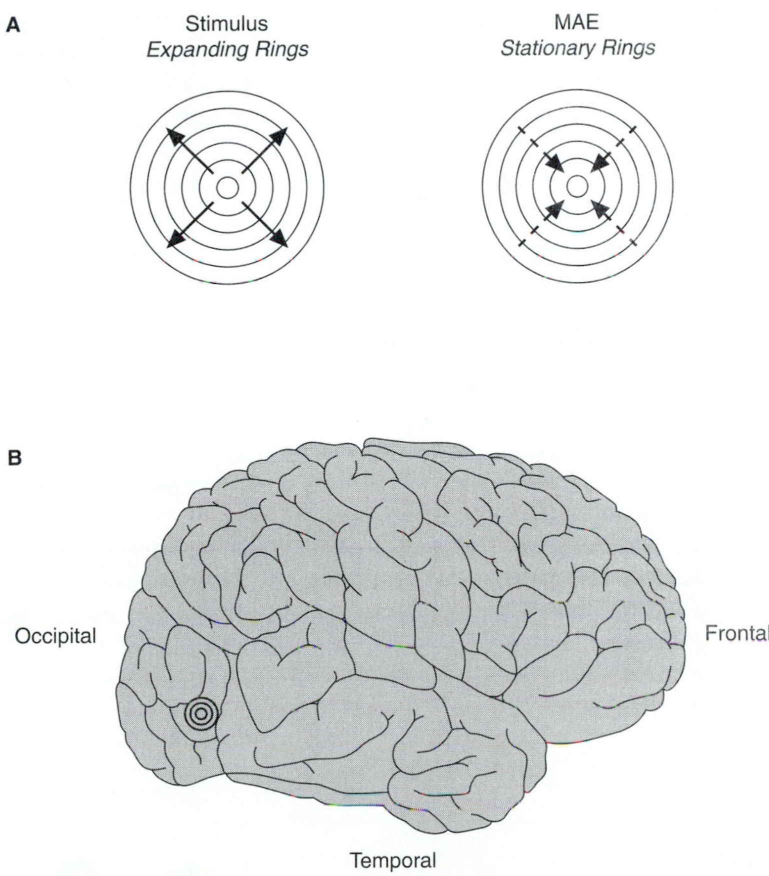


**FIGURE 15–3. A.** Prior adaptation to outwardly moving concentric rings leads to a MAE in which stationary rings appear to move inwards. **B** While a human subject is experiencing the MAE, f MRI reveals activity in the visual area MT. In this schematic, the activity is indicated by the concentric circles. (*Adapted from Tootell et al. Visual motion aftereffect in human cortical area MT revealed by functional magnetic resonance imaging.* Science. *1995;375:139–141.*)

## *VISUAL AREA 4 AND INFEROTEMPORAL CORTEX PROCESS COLOR AND FORM INFORMATION*

Visual area 4 (V4) and inferotemporal cortex (IT) belong to the ventral processing stream and contain cells that are responsive, respectively, to color and sophisticated forms. Although a simplification, V4 is sometimes said to analyze color information (Zeki, 1983), while IT is thought to analyze form information (Fuster and Jervey, 1981; Tanaka et al, 1991).

The receptive fields of cells in IT are large, thereby providing the basis to integrate information over an extensive area. This is necessary to analyze complex patterns. Certain of the shapes to which cells in IT respond are given in Figure 15–4. While cells in the striate cortex respond best to bars, edges, and gratings, cells in IT respond best to comparatively sophisticated, albeit basic, shapes (e.g.,circles, squares, and ovals). These basic forms could serve as building blocks to construct even more complex forms (Gallant et al, 1993). Interestingly, there is evidence that IT is involved in the recognition of faces, a form analysis task of considerable importance (Gross, 1973; Rolls and Tovée, 1995).

IT and V4 are in close proximity to each other. Consequently, patients who suffer from **prosopagnosia** (the inability to recognize faces) frequently manifest achromatopsia, the inability to distinguish hues (Tovée, 1996).

## *VISUAL AGNOSIAS SUPPORT THE NOTION OF CORTICAL SPECIALIZATION*

The specialization of the cortex, which has been elucidated with extracellular recordings and brain imaging studies, has long been suspected based on the distinctive visual deficits that are manifested by patients with circumscribed brain lesions such as localized brain injuries, infarcts, or tumors. Whereas lesions in the striate cortex produce simple blind spots (scotomas), certain extrastriate lesions can lead to the inability to recognize objects, **visual agnosia** (Damasio et al, 1980). This condition can take many different forms, as indicated in Table 15–1, depending on the area of the brain that is compromised.

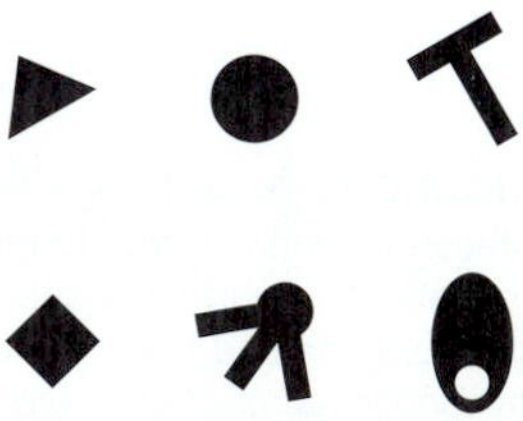

**FIGURE 15–4.** Certain neurons in IT respond well to these basic shapes. These shapes could serve as the building blocks to construct even more complex forms. (*Adapted from Tanaka K. Inferotemporal cortex and higher visual functions.* Curr Opinion Neurobiol. *1992;2:502–505.*)

**TABLE 15–1. VISUAL AGNOSIAS**

| Classification | Deficiency |
|---|---|
| ***Form and Pattern*** | |
| Object agnosia | Recognition of real objects |
| Agnosia for drawings | Recognition of drawn objects |
| Prosopagnosia | Recognition of faces |
| ***Color*** | |
| Color agnosia | Association of colors with objects |
| Color anomia | Naming colors |
| Achromatopsia | Distinguishing hues |
| ***Depth and Movement*** | |
| Visual spatial agnosia | Stereoscopic vision, topographical relations |
| Akinetopsia | Motion perception |

Adapted from Kolb B, Whishaw IQ. *Fundamentals of Human Neuropsychology.* San Francisco: Freeman; 1980.

Lesions in the dorsal processing stream can lead to **visual neglect.** For instance, a patient with a lesion located in the left parietal area may shave only the left side of his face and ignore the right side (Bisiach and Rusconi, 1990; Tovée, 1996). The neglect is apparently accentuated when a patient is presented with objects in both the affected and nonaffected regions of his or her visual field. It is for this reason that clinicians, when performing a confrontation visual field test, sometimes present objects to both the patient's left and right visual fields (Newman, 1992). Presentation of an object in the normal visual field *extinguishes* visualization of the object in the field affected by the parietal lesion, thereby facilitating detection of the abnormality.

## *ARE THERE GRANDMOTHER CELLS?*

When thinking about specialized higher cortical centers and the hierarchical processing that results in these centers, it is important not to fall into a conceptual trap. It is not reasonable to assume that visual information is continuously processed until it reaches an ultimately high cortical cell with activity that results in visual consciousness as we know it. In this scenario, there might be a cell so specialized that it responds only to the face of your grandmother; a so-called **grandmother cell.**

Brain imaging studies are inconsistent with the existence of grandmother cells. When participants are asked to visualize a specific object (e.g., visualize your spouse's face), activity is distributed over a fairly wide expanse of cortex.

Interestingly, the activity does not seem to be confined to the higher cortical areas, but also occurs in the lower centers including the striate cortex (Kosslyn and Oschner, 1994). Apparently, the visualization of a remembered object results in a pattern of activity that is similar to that elicited by actually viewing the object (Ishai and Sagi, 1995).

Information from the various cortical areas must be integrated to result in an integrated percept (Schiller, 1993). For instance, to perceive a red automobile that is traveling along a highway, the motion and position information that is processed along the dorsal stream must be integrated with color and form information that is processed along the ventral stream. Information from these two streams must be combined with memory. This integration apparently is coordinated in the **prefrontal cortex,** an area that has long been thought to play a role in cognition (Rao et al, 1997).

## DOES THE ACTIVITY OF NEURONS IN HIGHER CORTICAL AREAS REFLECT A SUBJECT'S PERCEPTIONS?

Consider the stimuli displayed in Figure 15–5A. If the left-tilted bars are viewed by only the left eye and the right-tilted bars only by the right eye, the observer, at any one instance, will perceive either the left or right-tilted bars. The observer's perception will alternate between the left and right-tilted bars, but he or she never fuses the disparate stimuli. This alternating perception of nonfusible images is referred to as **binocular rivalry.**

Macaque monkeys perceive binocular rivalry and can be trained to indicate (by pushing a button) which stimulus they see (i.e., the left or right-tilted bars). An important question regards the responses of single cortical neurons in the striate cortex and higher cortical areas to bars that elicit binocular rivalry. Does the activity of these neurons correspond to the stimulus that is falling within their receptive fields or does their activity reflect the animal's perception?

To answer the question posed above, Leopold and Logothetis (1996) made extracellular recordings from neurons in striate cortex and V4 while monkeys were experiencing binocular rivalry. The animals indicated which stimulus they saw (left or right-tilted bars) by depressing a button. For most orientation selective cells in striate cortex, the important factor was the orientation of the bars. If a cell was optimally tuned to left-tilted bars, the cell would respond to the left-tilted bars regardless of the animal's perception. The animal could report that they were *seeing* the right-tilted bars, yet this striate cell (that was tuned to left-tilted bars) would respond as long as the left-tilted bars fell within its receptive field.

A different story emerged for area V4. While many orientation selective cells responded the same as those in striate cortex, other cells only responded when the animal reported seeing a stimulus of a given orientation. For instance, such a cell would respond when the monkey reported that it was seeing the left-tilted bars, but would not fire when the monkey reported seeing the right-

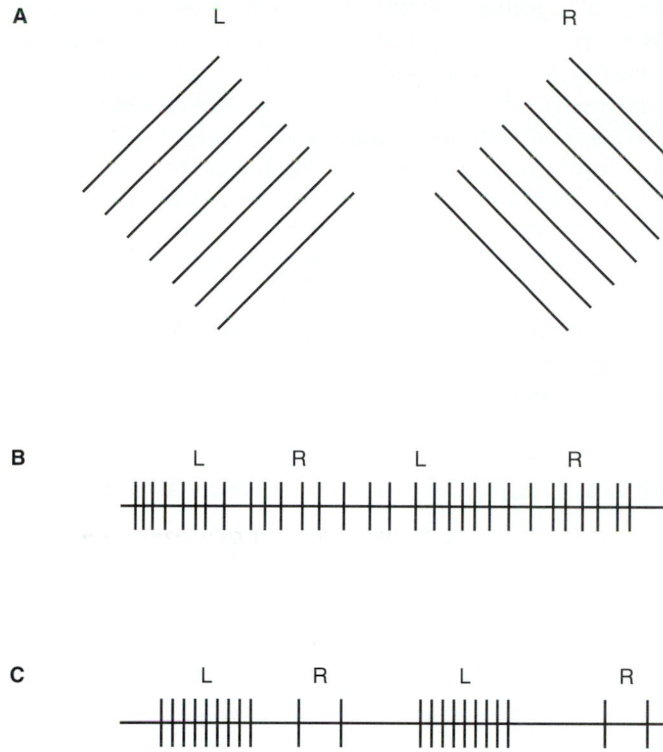


**FIGURE 15–5. A.** Stimulus used to induce binocular rivalry. When left-tilted gratings are viewed by the left eye and right-tilted gratings by the right eye, the observer experiences an alternating perception of left and right-tilted gratings: one of the gratings (e.g., the left-tilted grating) is seen, followed by the right-tilted grating, followed by the left-tilted grating, and so forth. **B.** Idealized recording from a neuron in a macaque monkey's striate cortex taken while the animal is experiencing binocular rivalry. This neuron is tuned (optimally sensitive) to left-tilted gratings. The "L" and "R" designate which orientation (left or right-tilted) the animal *experiences.* Note that the neuron continues to fire regardless of whether the animal is perceiving a left or right-tilted grating. **C.** Idealized recording from a neuron located in V4 measured under the same conditions. Note that this neuron's response is modulated; it only responds when the animal reports that it is perceiving a left-titled grating. Other neurons show a response that is linked to perception of a right-tilted grating. Although modulated neurons are found in both striate cortex and V4, a higher percentage of neurons in V4 show modulated responses than is the case for striate cortex (Leopold and Logothetis, 1996.)

tilted bars. Keep in mind that the stimulus did not change; what changed was the monkey's perception. Leopold and Logothetis (1996) showed that cells in higher cortical areas are more likely to code what the animal is actually seeing than are cells in lower visual areas (i.e., striate cortex).

A similar explanation may hold for certain ambiguous figures that produce bistable percepts, such as the **Necker cube** and **Rubin's face-vase** reversible figure (Leopold and Logothetis, 1996) (Fig. 15–6). Cells in lower visual areas may respond to the physical characteristics of the stimulus, while activity in the higher centers may reflect which of the two equally plausible perceptions the observer experiences. This hypothesis awaits empirical investigation.

Binocular rivalry and ambiguous figures are sometimes said to be manifestations of **bottom-up** visual attention. The untrained observer presumably does not choose which perception he or she experiences. A more classic example of bottom-up attention is an observer's response to a novel stimulus, such as a flash of light or motion that is detected in the periphery of the visual field. The attention that is induced by these stimuli is not voluntary or conscious, and can be considered as resulting from bottom-up processes (Steinman and Steinman, 1998; Steinman et al, 1995). This form of attention is to be contrasted with **top-down** visual attention, which is our next topic.

## *DO THOUGHTS INFLUENCE THE ACTIVITY OF INDIVIDUAL NEURONS?*

It is common experience that we perform better on certain tasks when we are attentive to the demands of these tasks. If you are a batter in a baseball game and you suspect that the pitcher is about to throw you a curve ball, you are more likely to hit the pitch than if you were not attending to this likelihood.

Do cortical cells reflect this conscious choice of attention, a process sometimes referred to as top-down attention? This question can be addressed by performing extracellular recordings from cortical visual neurons while a monkey chooses to attend to a specific aspect of a stimulus.

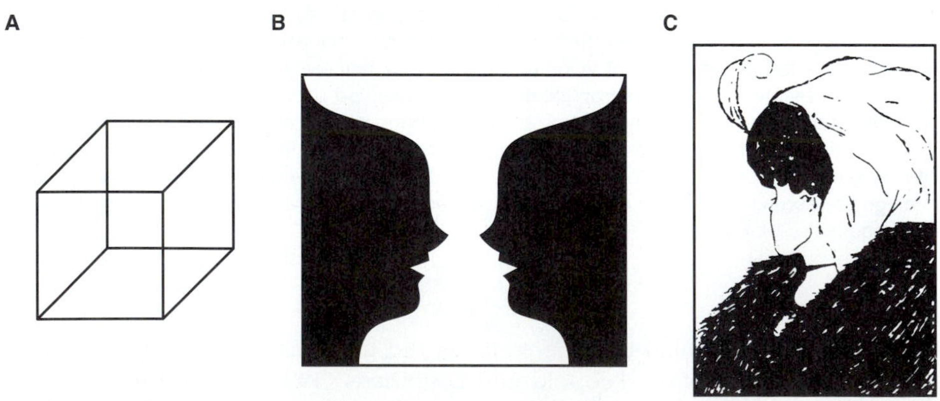


**FIGURE 15–6.** Examples of ambiguous figures. **A.** The Necker cube is seen as either projecting into or out of the page. **B.** The Rubin face–vase figure is perceived as either two faces or a vase. **C.** This ambiguous figure is seen as either an older or younger woman. You may need to stare at this figure for a few minutes to visualize both images.

Consider the stimulus array in Figure 15–7. This array, which consists of a red and green bar, is positioned so that it falls within the receptive field of a red-sensitive neuron in V4. (Neurons in higher visual centers tend to be larger than those in lower centers, making it possible to study them with large, complex stimulus arrays.) When the animal is required to attend to the red stimulus, the neuron responds vigorously. However, when the animal is required to attend to the green stimulus, the response is diminished (Moran and Desimone, 1985; Motter, 1994). Note that the stimulus (and the monkey's eye position) are precisely the same under both conditions. The only thing that has changed is the animal's focus of attention. The monkey's choice of which object to attend to within the cell's receptive field affects the response of the cell. Since the choice of which object to attend comes from higher areas within the brain, perhaps the prefrontal cortex, this is an example of top-down visual attention (Desimone and Duncan, 1995).

In comparison to the results found in V4, cells in the striate cortex apparently do not demonstrate top-down attentional influences (Moran and Desimone, 1985). This suggests that there is a filtering of visual information from the striate cortex to V4 that is at least partially dependent on the stimulus to which the animal is attending.

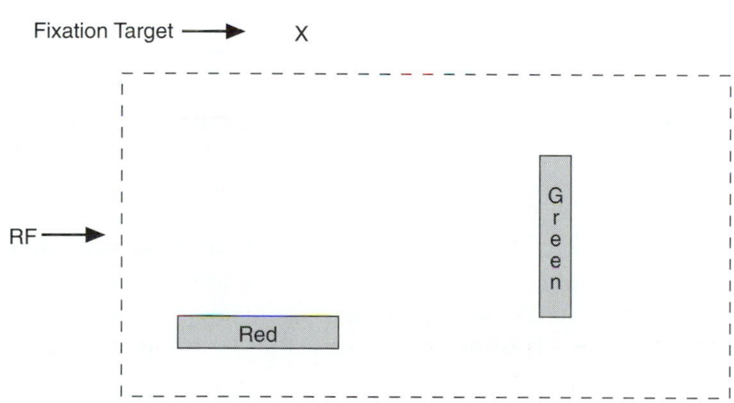


**Figure 15–7.** To study top-down attention, red and green bars are presented within the receptive field (RF) of a neuron located in V4. The activity of certain neurons depends on the bar to which the animal is paying attention. For instance, a neuron may only respond when the animal is attending to the red bar. The same neuron may not respond when the animal attends to the green bar although neither the stimulus nor the animal's eye position (i.e., fixation) have changed. (*Adapted from Moran J, Desimone R. Selective attention gates visual processing in extrastriate cortex.* Science. *1985;229:782–784.)*

## CAN VISION BE TRAINED?

It has been common practice among certain eye care practitioners to train the vision of their patients. This visual training is often directed at improving performance in particular visual skills, such as awareness of the peripheral field of vision. Although there have been numerous anecdotal reports of the efficacy of this form of visual skill training, the underlying mechanisms have not been elucidated.

Advances in our understanding of the mechanisms underlying attention provide some insight regarding the possible basis for improvement in visual skills that results from visual training. We know that top-down attention leads to temporary modifications in the receptive field sensitivities of visual neurons. With practice, it is possible (but not yet demonstrated) that these changes in receptive field properties become ingrained, leading to improved task performance. Another way of stating this is that improvement in visual performance may be attributable to learning by individual neurons within the visual pathways. This is a testable hypothesis.

Psychophysical studies reveal that the visual performance of adults can be improved with practice. The learning of certain tasks appears to be stimulus specific (e.g., specific to a learned orientation), suggesting that the neural learning occurs early in the visual system (Fiorentini and Berardi, 1980; Ball and Sekuler, 1982). The learning of other tasks, however, is generalizable (Beard et al, 1995; Levi et al, 1997). A vernier acuity task that is practiced at one orientation leads to improved performance at other orientations and for other tasks (i.e., Snellen acuity). The generalizable nature of the learning indicates that it occurs in higher visual centers.

There is ample evidence that lower level neurons have different requirements for activation than do higher level neurons. Recall that cells in the striate cortex respond well to lines of a specific orientation, while cells in inferotemporal cortex respond best to more global forms (i.e., basic forms such as circles and squares). This observation has implications for the site of learning within the visual system. Perhaps very specific tasks require learning at lower visual areas, whereas more generalizable tasks involve learning at higher levels.

A recently proposed model of visual learning suggests that higher visual centers direct the learning of tasks to the relevant lower visual areas (Ahissar and Hochstein, 1997). According to this reverse hierarchy model, learning is facilitated when there is exposure to generalizable tasks prior to more specific tasks.

## A WORD OF CAUTION

Our understanding of cortical physiology is limited by the available technology. As technology becomes more sophisticated, our comprehension of cortical physiology becomes more informed.

For decades, insights regarding cortical function were driven by experiments in which activity was recorded from single neurons. Such experiments continue to enrich our understanding of cortical physiology. These experiments are, however, limited because they do not tell us how information is integrated across populations of cortical neurons.

Consider the processing of color information in the striate cortex. Color opponent neurons are not commonly encountered when recording from single neurons in the striate cortex (Lennie et al, 1990). This has lead to the belief that the striate cortex does not play a major role in processing color information.

A different picture emerges when the striate cortex is studied using *f*MRI. This technique reveals the activity of a large area of cortex containing many neurons. When examined with *f*MRI, it appears that the striate cortex (as a whole) manifests significant color opponency (Engel et al, 1997). Few individual neurons in the striate cortex manifest color opponency, but a collection of many striate cortical neurons displays color opponency. Consequently, it is important to examine not only the activity of individual neurons, but the activity of neural networks spanning many neurons or visual areas.

The finding of color opponency in the striate cortex with *f*MRI suggests caution in finalizing our thinking with regard to processing of information by the cortex. As technology advances, previously held theories will be modified (or debunked) and replaced by new theories. While the past decades have seen great leaps in our understanding of cortical functioning, we still have much to learn about this most complex of organs. Further progress is likely to coincide with advances in technology.

## SUMMARY

Given the enormous quantity of visual information that is processed by the cortex, it is not surprising that this organ manifests a significant degree of specialization. Cortical areas within the ventral processing stream, including V4 and IT, apparently play a large role in object recognition and can be thought of as constituting a "what" pathway. Areas that constitute the dorsal stream, including MT, appear to be important for motion analysis and spatial localization and can be thought of as being part of a "where" pathway. Integration of information from the two systems may be coordinated by prefrontal cortex.

It is important to keep in mind that the ventral and dorsal processing streams are not independent from each other; there is significant communication between the two systems. Nonetheless, the ventral and dorsal pathways do appear to have distinct functions.

The activity of neurons in higher visual centers corresponds more closely with our perceptions than does the activity of neurons in the striate cortex. Higher level neurons manifest changes in sensitivity depending on the attentional status of the animal and may be important for learning generalizable visual tasks.

# Self-Assessment Questions

1. Subsequent to viewing a grating tilted to the left, human subjects note that a vertical grating appears tilted to the right. This is referred to as the tilt-aftereffect. Devise a psychophysical experiment that enables you to answer the following hypothesis: the tilt-aftereffect is mediated by binocular cortical neurons.

# 16

# Gross Electrical Potentials

Gross electrical potentials represent the summed electrical activity of a large number of neurons. Because these potentials can be recorded by noninvasive methods, they are of clinical value. The gross potentials discussed in this chapter are the electrooculogram (EOG), the electroretinogram (ERG), and the visually evoked potential (VEP).

## ELECTROOCULOGRAM

For the purpose of understanding the EOG, think of the eye as a battery. As illustrated in Figure 16–1, the front of the eye has a positive charge relative to the back of the eye. This standing (or resting) potential of the eye is the basis of the EOG. It is the largest of the gross potentials we will discuss and is on the order of 6 mV (Arden and Barrada, 1962).

### Clinical Measurement

To determine the EOG, electrodes are attached to the inner and outer canthi as illustrated in Figure 16–2. These electrodes are connected to an amplifier that feeds into a chart recorder. The patient is instructed to alternately view fixation points such that the eyes move from extreme left gaze to extreme right gaze. The result is an EOG trace showing the eyes' standing potential for left and right gaze (Fig. 16–1).

The EOG is substantially larger under light-adapted conditions than under dark-adapted conditions (Arden et al, 1962). In a typical recording session, the EOG is first recorded under dark-adapted conditions and then under light-adapted conditions (Fig. 16–3). It reaches its minimum value **(dark trough)** af-

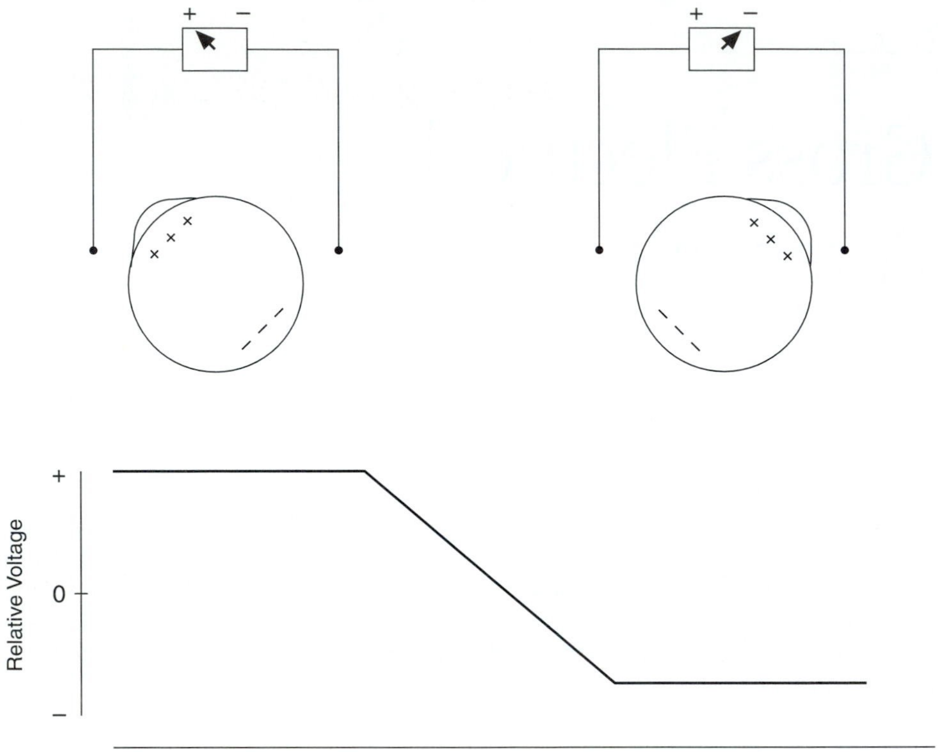


**FIGURE 16–1.** The electrooculogram can be thought of as a standing potential of the eye. The measured polarity of the response changes as the gaze is shifted. This is indicated by the voltmeters in the top diagram and the schematic trace on the bottom.

ter about 8 minutes of dark adaptation. The maximum value **(light rise)** is obtained following approximately 10 to 15 minutes of light adaptation (Berson, 1992).

For clinical purposes, it is useful to determine the ratio of the light rise to the dark trough (Arden et al, 1962). This ratio, expressed as a percentage, is referred

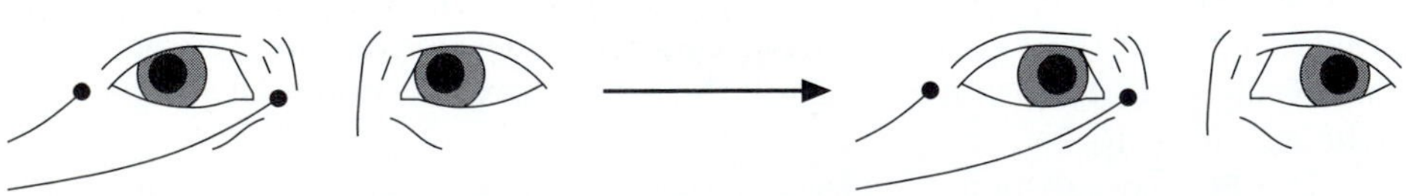

**FIGURE 16–2.** The electrooculogram is measured with electrodes attached to the inner and outer canthi. The patient shifts his or her gaze from extreme rightward to extreme leftward to cause the change in polarity displayed in Figure 16–1.

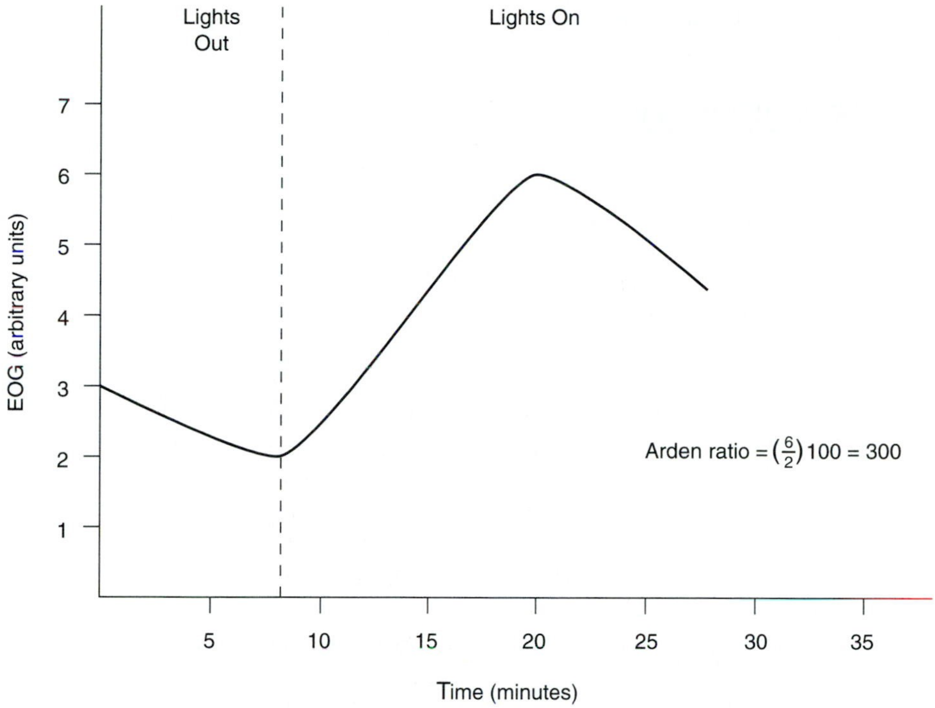


**FIGURE 16–3.** The electrooculogram reaches a minimum (dark trough) after about 8 minutes of dark adaptation and a maximum (light rise) following approximately 10 to 15 minutes of light adaptation. The Arden ratio represents the ratio of the light rise to the dark trough. This diagram is a schematic.

to as the **Arden ratio.** Values lower than about 165 percent to 180 percent are considered abnormal.

## *Origins and Clinical Applications*

The origin of the dark-adapted EOG is most likely the retinal pigment epithelium (RPE) (Brown and Wiesel, 1961). The increased value of the EOG under light-adapted conditions (the light rise) appears to be due primarily to rod activity, although cones do play a role in its genesis (Gouras and Carr, 1965).

Although the EOG is occasionally used for the diagnosis of outer retinal disease, it has largely been replaced by the electroretinogram (ERG). It is, however, useful in the diagnosis of the following four conditions that may not affect the ERG, but often result in a reduced Arden ratio: butterfly-shaped dystrophy of the fovea, fundus flavimaculatus, advanced drusen, and vitteliform dystrophy (Best's disease) (Berson, 1992).

## ELECTRORETINOGRAM

### *Standard ERG*

The standard ERG, also referred to as a flash ERG, is a retinal potential elicited by a brief flash of light. A typical standard ERG is illustrated in Figure 16–4A. This potential, unlike the EOG, is not continuously present; it must be elicited

A

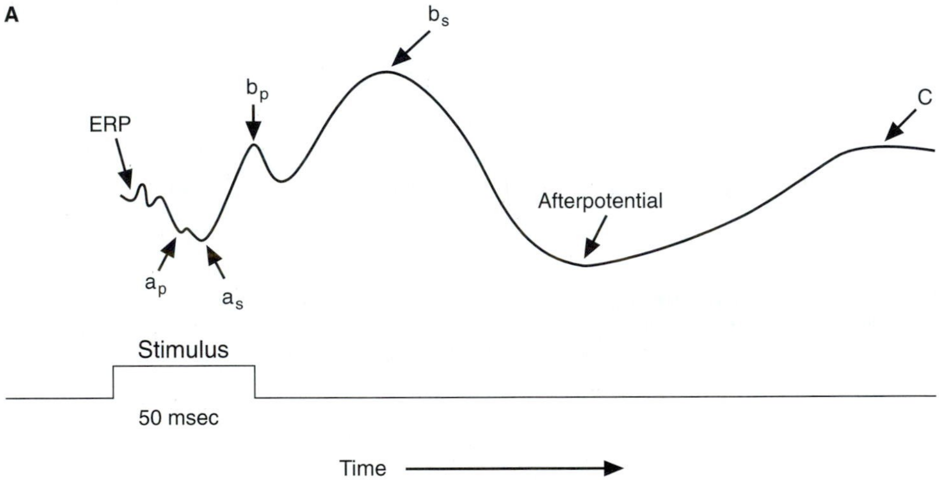


B

| WAVE | PRESUMED ORIGINS |
|---|---|
| ERP | Outer segments of photoreceptors, primarily cones |
| a-wave | Photoreceptors |
| b-wave | Muller cells |
| c-wave | RPE? |

**FIGURE 16–4. A.** Schematic of a standard flash electroretinogram. Note that the a and b-waves are composed of scotopic ($a_s$, $b_s$) and photopic ($a_p$, $b_p$) components. **B.** Presumed origins of the various waves that constitute the standard flash electroretinogram (Armington, 1974; Dowling, 1987; Berson, 1992).

by a visual stimulus. The ERG is a smaller potential than the EOG and is on the order of 1 mV.

The standard ERG is composed of a number of different waves (Einthoven and Jolly, 1908). The first wave is a biphasic wave referred to as the **early receptor potential (ERP).** This is followed by the negative **a-wave** and the positive **b-wave.** The b-wave is the largest ERG component. It is followed by the **afterpotential** and the **c-wave.**

The origins of the various component waves of the flash ERG have received considerable attention. It is believed that the standard ERG is derived largely from the outer retina (Armington, 1974). The presumed origins of the component waves are given in Figure 16–4B.

Note that the a-wave and the b-wave of the ERG in Figure 16–4A each consist of two components: a scotopic component ($a_s$, $b_s$) and a photopic component ($a_p$, $b_p$). This is because the illustrated ERG was produced with stimulus conditions that elicit activity in both rods and cones. The scotopic or the photopic component, however, can be made to dominate the ERG by the proper choice of stimulus conditions. This ability to separate the scotopic and photopic aspects of the ERG has important clinical value for assessing rod and cone function.

A scotopic-dominated ERG is obtained by dark adapting the patient prior to stimulation with a dim, low-wavelength (e.g., 505 nm) stimulus. To obtain a photopic-dominated ERG, a light-adapted patient is exposed to a relatively bright stimulus consisting of a wavelength to which the photopic system is maximally sensitive, approximately 555 nm.

Schematic scotopic and photopic ERGs are given in Figure 16–5A. Note that the scotopic ERG is both larger and slower than the photopic ERG. This can also be seen by observing an ERG that has both scotopic and photopic components (Fig. 16–4A).

A photopic-dominated ERG can also be obtained with the use of a stimulus presented at a high temporal rate ($\geq$ 30 Hz) (Armington, 1974). Such a stimulus would appear to flicker. A temporal rate of equal to or greater than 30 Hz is followed (resolved) by the cones, but not by the rods. The schematic flicker ERG given in Figure 16–5B represents photopic activity.

### *Focal Electroretinogram*

The ERG represents the summed activity of the retinal tissue exposed to the stimulating flash of light (Armington, 1974). In the case of a full-field flash ERG, the flash of light covers the entire retina; consequently, the measured ERG represents the summed activity for the entire retina.

On occasion, it is clinically useful to determine the functional status of a limited area of the retina. For example, it may be necessary to determine the functional status of the macular area. A full-field ERG is not an appropriate test in this instance because it is not sufficiently sensitive to a macular lesion. The macula represents only a small fraction of the retinal area and contributes rela-

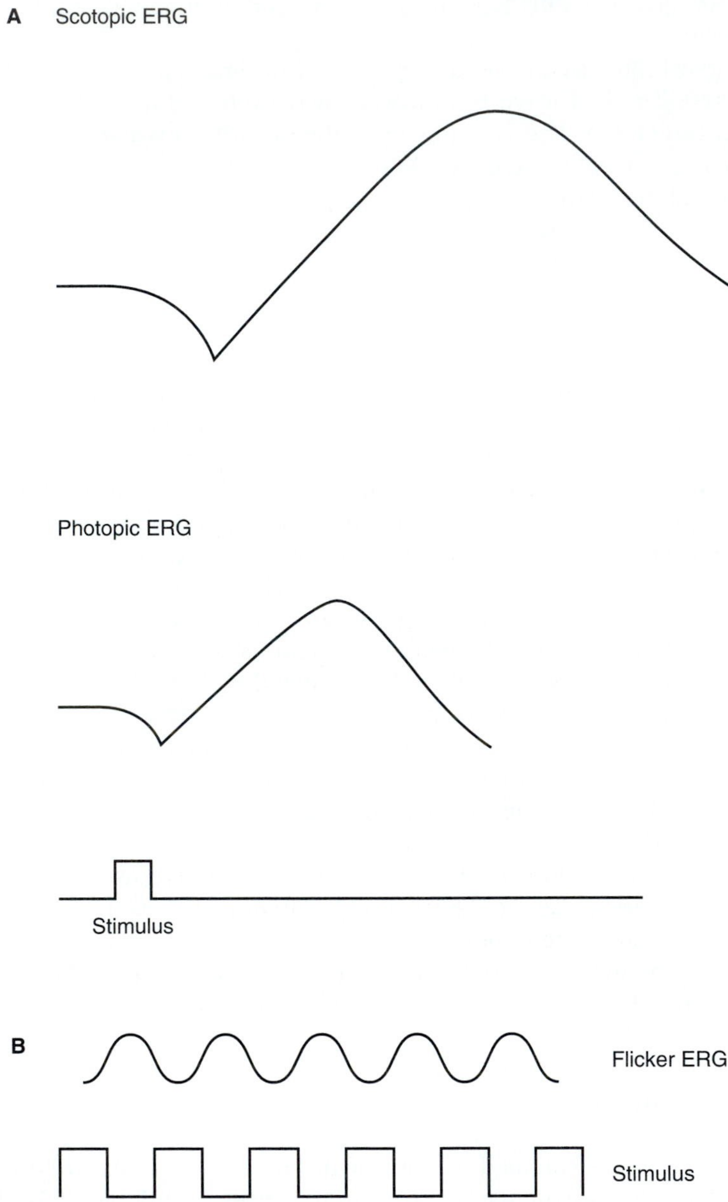


**FIGURE 16–5. A.** Schematics of standard scotopic and photopic flash electroretinograms (ERGs). Note that the scotopic ERG is larger in amplitude and slower than the photopic ERG. **B.** A flicker ERG can be produced with a high temporal frequency (~30 Hz) square-wave stimulus.

tively little to a full-field ERG. Therefore, a macular lesion has little effect on a full-field flash ERG.

Focal retinal lesions, such as a macular lesion, can be examined using a focal ERG. A focal ERG is obtained by limiting the stimulus to the affected retinal area; therefore, it tests the responsiveness of this specific area. Figure 16–6 shows schematic focal and full-field flicker ERGs for a patient with a macular lesion. Note that the focal ERG is greatly reduced, whereas the full-field ERG is unaffected.

## *Multifocal ERG*

The multifocal ERG, a relatively new technique, enables ERGs to be recorded for many different retinal locations in a brief period of time (about 4 minutes) (Sutter and Tran, 1992). The patient is presented with a stimulus array consisting of about 240 hexagons, half of which are illuminated at any one instance. Each hexagon is modulated independently according to a binary sequence (Fig. 16–7). ERGs for various retinal loci are derived with an algorithm that links recorded electrical activity to the location of a specific hexagon.

An important advantage of the multifocal ERG is that unlike a full-field ERG, it permits the evaluation of specific regions of the retina. Figure 16–7B presents a

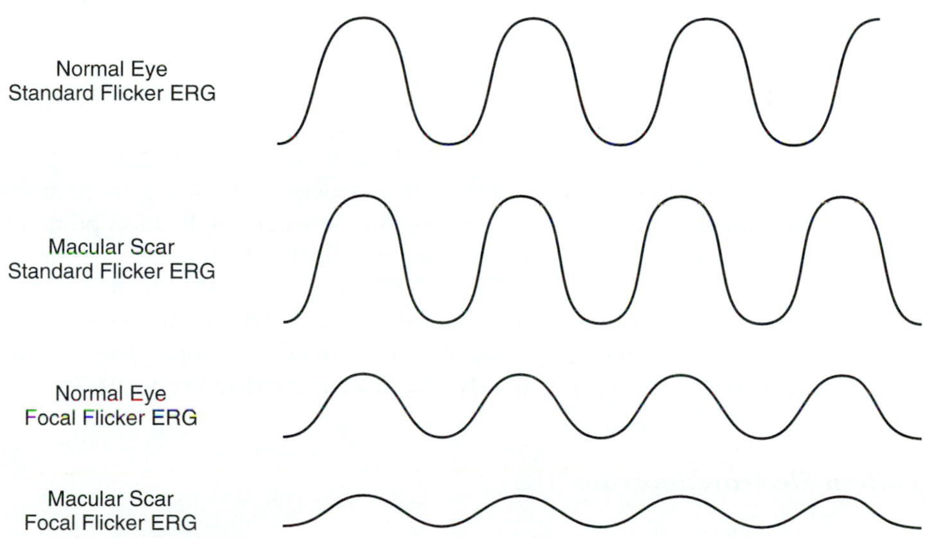


**FIGURE 16–6.** A macular scar does not have a substantial effect on a standard (full-field) flicker electroretinogram (ERG). As indicated in the bottom trace, however, a focal ERG confined to the macular area manifests a reduced amplitude.

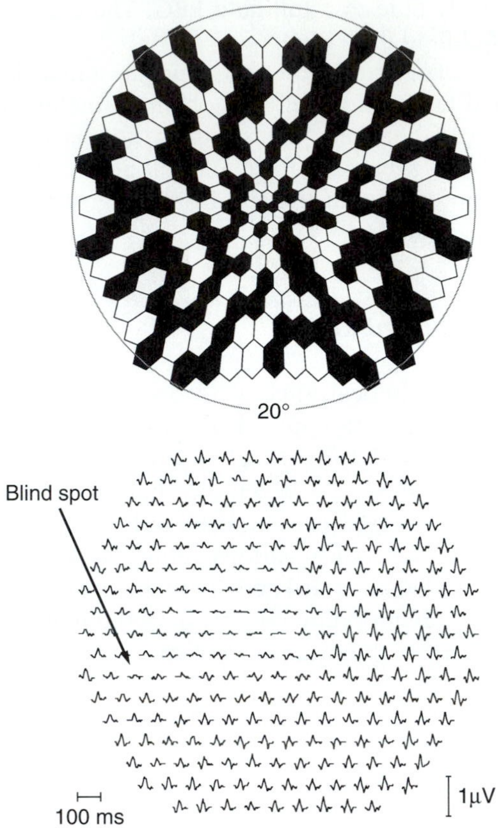


**FIGURE 16–7. A.** Stimulus array utilized to generate a multifocal ERG. **B.** Multifocal ERG for the left eye of 29 year-old male with suspected central serous retinopathy. Note the abnormal ERGs nasal to the blind spot. (*This figure was kindly provided by Marcus A. Bearse, PhD and Erich E. Sutter, PhD of the Smith-Kettlewell Eye Research Institute.*)

multifocal ERG for a 29-year-old patient with suspected central serous retinopathy, who presented with a small scotoma located between the fixation point and blind spot. A full-field ERG is normal, yet the multifocal ERG reveals a region between fixation and the blind spot where the ERG waves are abnormal. The multifocal ERG is not only useful in the diagnosis of localized retinal abnormalities, but it might allow the earlier diagnosis of more generalized retinal disease, such as retinitis pigmentosa and glaucoma (Bearse et al, 1996; Hood et al, 1997).

### *Pattern Electroretinogram*

The pattern electroretinogram (PERG) is obtained with a patterned stimulus with an overall luminance that does not change (Johnson et al, 1966). Either a grating or checkerboard pattern is typically used (Fig. 16–8A and B). This pattern is phase-shifted by 180 degrees at a moderate temporal rate. In essence, the posi-

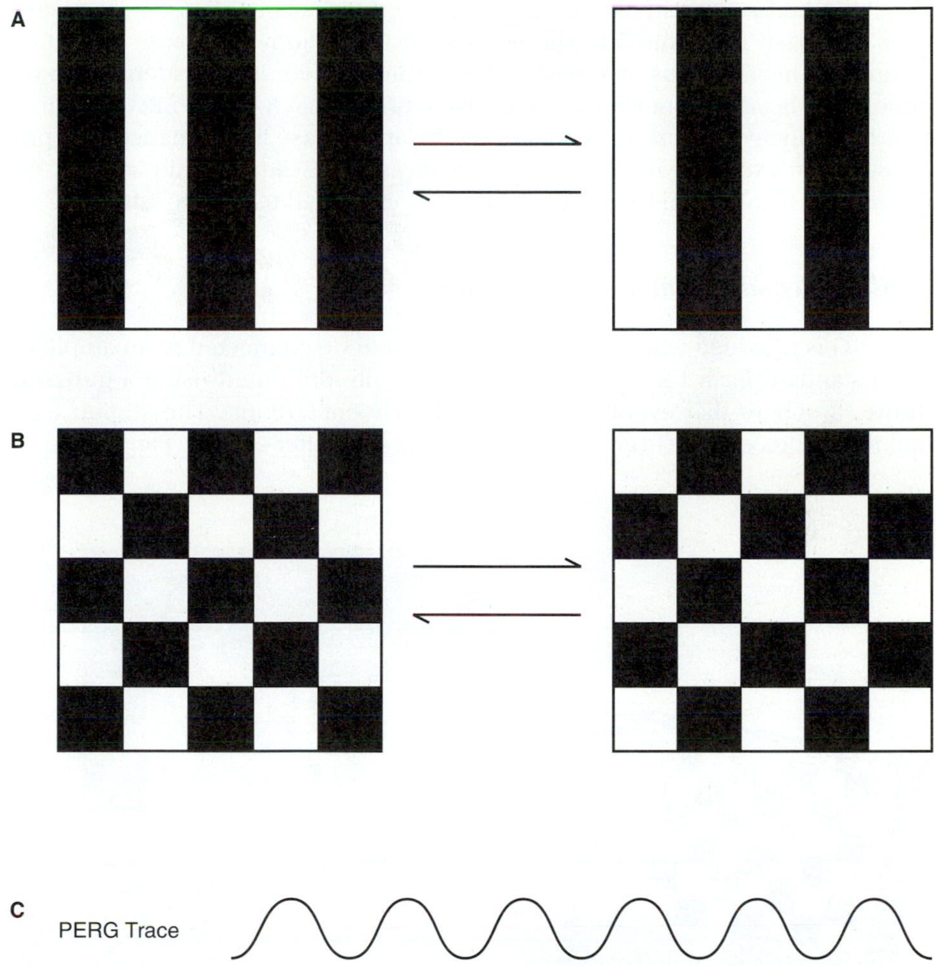


**FIGURE 16–8. A.** A pattern electroretinogram (PERG) can be obtained with a grating that undergoes a 180-degree phase shift. **B.** A checkerboard pattern that undergoes a 180-degree phase shift also elicits a PERG. **C.** A PERG is a modulated response that follows the phase shift of the stimulus.

tions of the white and black components of the pattern are continuously exchanged (counterphase modulation). Therefore, the PERG is elicited by a phase shift in contrast rather than an overall increase in luminance.

An idealized PERG is given in Figure 16–8C. Although similar in form to a standard flicker ERG, the PERG apparently has different retinal origins. The standard flicker ERG, as well as the flash ERG, are generated by the outer retina, whereas the PERG apparently has its origins in the inner retina. In particular, the retinal ganglion cells may play a large role in the genesis of the PERG.

A flashed stimulus has the disadvantage of producing retinal light scatter. Even if a flash is confined to the nonresponsive optic nerve head, an ERG is recorded. This is because the flashed light scatters when it is incident upon the optic nerve head and stimulates responsive retinal areas. A *focal* PERG minimizes this disadvantage because it is not elicited by an increase in luminance; it is produced by an exchange of contrast. This reduces light scatter within the eye. For this reason, focal retinal lesions are sometimes examined using a focal PERG.

### *Clinical Measurement and Applications*

The ERG is recorded with a corneal contact electrode connected to an amplifier. For a standard flash ERG, the stimulus is typically presented using a **ganzfeld dome,** a sphere that evenly illuminates the patient's retina. The stimuli for a multifocal ERG or PERG can be presented on a computer screen (Fig. 16–9).

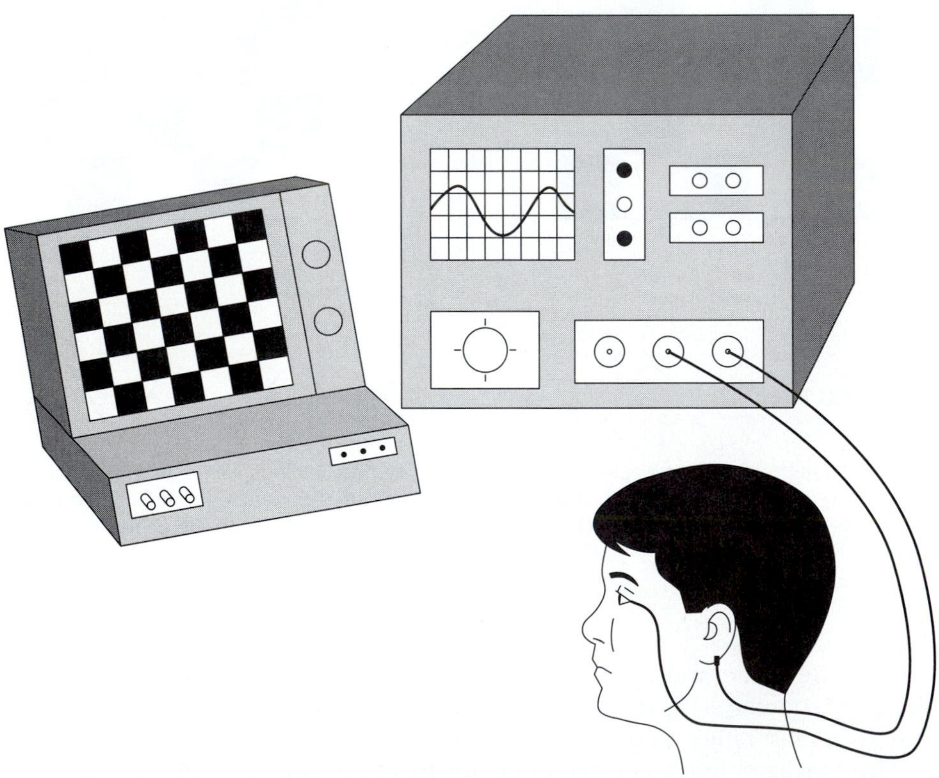

**FIGURE 16–9.** The PERG is measured with a corneal contact electrode that feeds into an amplifier. The stimulus is a checkerboard that undergoes a 180-degree phase shift. The same stimulus can be used to elicit a steady-state visually evoked potential when electrodes are appropriately attached to the scalp.

The flash ERG (standard, flicker, or multifocal) is frequently used in the diagnosis of outer retinal disease, such as rod–cone degenerations. It is particularly useful in the diagnosis of retinitis pigmentosa (RP). RP is an inherited retinal degeneration that affects the metabolism of rod and cone outer segments. Rod function is apparently affected first, with patients often demonstrating night blindness in the early stages of the disease. Subsequently, the disease can affect photopic vision; visual fields frequently show a ring scotoma which can progress, resulting in blindness.

The fundoscopic characteristics typical of RP include superficial bone spicule pigmentation, narrowed arterioles, and optic atrophy (Fig. 16–10). Fundoscopic appearance alone, however, may not be sufficient for a diagnosis as other conditions show similar presentations. Electrodiagnostic testing is often required to make an accurate diagnosis.

Figure 16–11 shows schematic ERGs typical of the early stages of RP. Note that both the photopic and scotopic ERGs are reduced in amplitude. Also of diagnostic value is the increased latency or, as it is sometimes referred to, the delayed **implicit time.**

The delayed implicit time is of important diagnostic value because certain retinal conditions that mimic RP (sector RP, stationary night blindness) may manifest reduced amplitudes but show normal implicit times (Berson, 1992). These

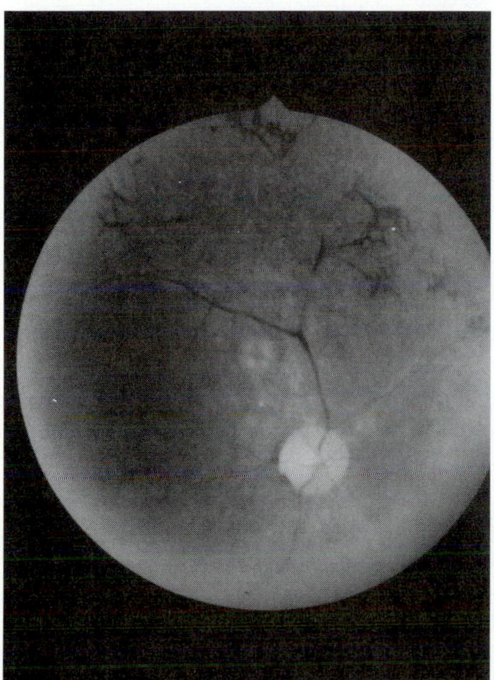

**FIGURE 16–10.** Fundus of a 26-year-old black female with retinitis pigmentosa. Note the bone spicule pigmentation (superior retina) and narrowing of arterioles. (*Photograph is courtesy of Dr. Karla Hefty and Dr. Mohammad Rafieetary.*)

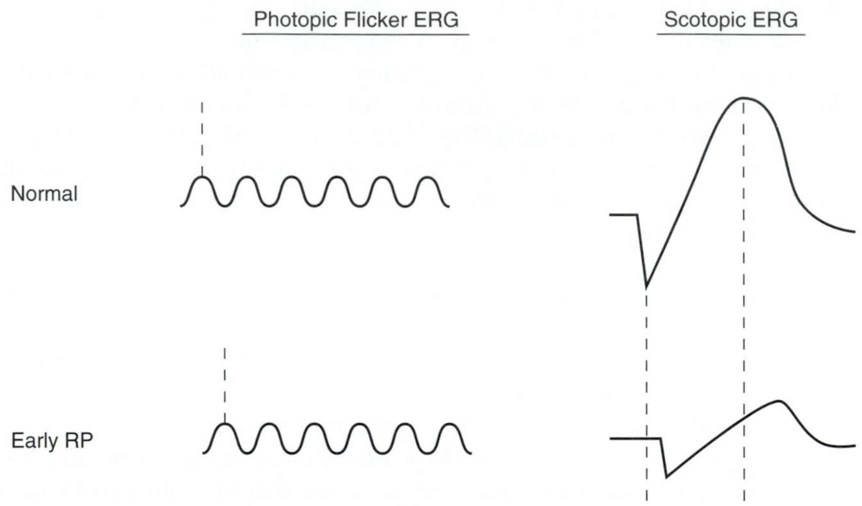


**FIGURE 16–11.** Schematic photopic flicker and scotopic electroretinograms for a healthy eye and an eye with early retinitis pigmentosa. Note the delayed implicit times in early retinitis pigmentosa.

conditions are typically nonprogressive. RP, which manifests a delayed implicit time, is typically progressive.

Whereas the standard ERG is useful in the diagnosis of outer retinal disease, the PERG may be helpful in the assessment of inner retinal function (Maffei and Fiorentini, 1981). PERGs can be abnormal in glaucoma, a disease that affects the nerve fiber and ganglion cell layers of the retina (Trick, 1985).

## VISUALLY EVOKED POTENTIALS

Visually evoked potentials (VEPs), also referred to as evoked potentials (EPs), visually evoked cortical potentials (VECPs), or visually evoked responses (VERs), are very small cortical potentials elicited by visual stimuli. These small potentials, which are on the order of 5 μV, are embedded in the large-amplitude, randomly fluctuating electroencephalogram (EEG). The EEG has an amplitude of about 60 μV.

Prior to the introduction of computer technology, it was not possible to reliably record VEPs. This is because these small potentials must be detected against the background of the high-amplitude random noise of the EEG. The use of an averaging computer obviates this problem. Electrodes are positioned on the scalp and the stimulus is presented multiple times. The computer stores and sums the responses to produce a readable VEP.

### *Flash Visually Evoked Potentials*

Flash VEPs, sometimes called transient VEPs, are elicited by flashes of light similar to those used to elicit a standard ERG. The flash VEP is a complex waveform composed of numerous component waves (Fig. 16–12A) (Regan, 1989). It is thought that these individual waves represent the activity of different regions of the brain, particularly the cortex.

### *Steady-state Visually Evoked Potentials*

A steady-state VEP is obtained with stimuli similar to those used to elicit the PERG, a spatial pattern that undergoes phase reversal (see Fig. 16–9). Consequently, the steady-state VEP represents a response to contrast reversals rather than to changes in overall luminance. An example of a steady-state VEP is given in Figure 16–12B.

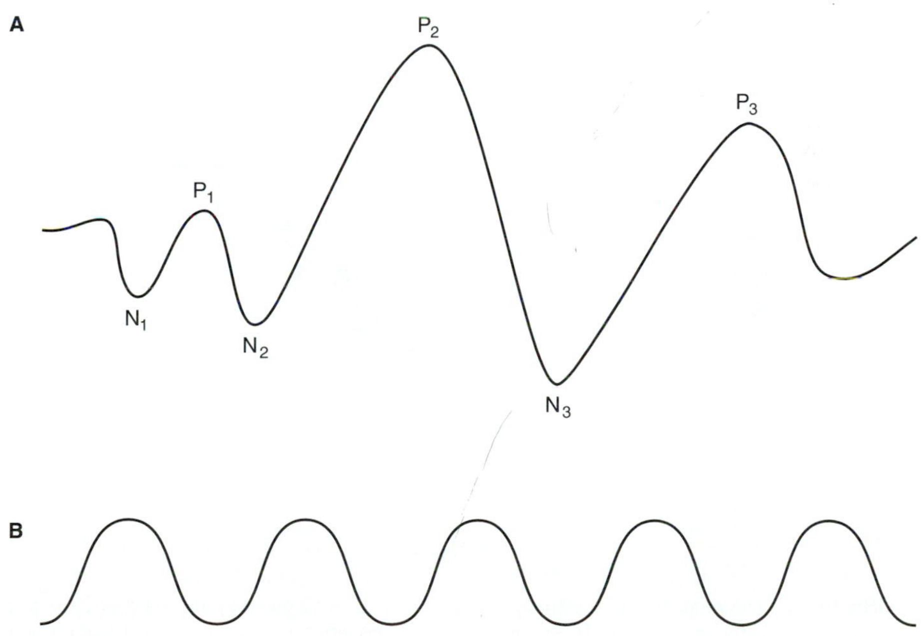


**FIGURE 16–12. A.** Flash (transient) visually evoked potential. **B.** Steady-state visually evoked potential. Both traces are schematics.

### *Effect of Contrast on the Amplitude of Visually Evoked Potentials*

If the patterned stimulus used to elicit a steady-state VEP is of high contrast, the amplitude of the VEP is larger than if the stimulus is of low contrast (Campbell and Maffei, 1970). This correlation of VEP amplitude and stimulus contrast has been used as a basis to assess contrast sensitivity and visual acuity.

Figure 16–13 shows a plot of VEP amplitude as a function of grating contrast for a given spatial frequency. By obtaining VEPs for a sample of moderate and high-contrast stimuli, it is possible to extrapolate the data to a zero-amplitude response. The grating contrast that is predicted to elicit this zero-amplitude response typically corresponds well with the psychophysically measured threshold contrast. Consequently, VEPs allow an objective determination of threshold contrast. Likewise, visual acuity can be estimated by presenting high-contrast stimuli of increasing spatial frequency and extrapolating to the zero-amplitude response.

The preceding has important implications with respect to assessing visual function in nonresponsive patients. The contrast sensitivity and visual acuity of malingerers, hysterics, the mentally retarded, infants, and other noncooperative

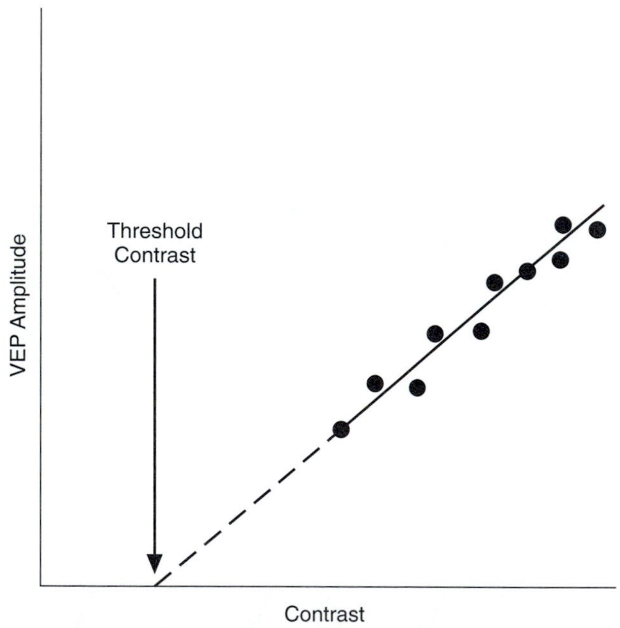


**FIGURE 16–13.** The amplitude of a visually evoked potential, for a given spatial frequency, is proportional to the stimulus contrast. Threshold contrast is obtained by extrapolation (dashed line) from data obtained at higher contrast levels (circles). (*Adapted from Campbell FW, Maffei, L. Electrophysiological evidence for the existence of orientation and size detectors in the human visual system.* J Physiol. *1970;207:635–652.*)

patients can be objectively assessed using VEPs. It should be noted, however, that VEPs produce higher estimates of visual acuity in infants than do behavioral procedures such as forced-choice preferential looking (Norcia et al, 1986; Teller and Movshon, 1986). This is discussed in Chapter 17.

### *Importance of the Fovea in Visually Evoked Potentials*

The vast majority of the striate cortex is devoted to analyzing foveal vision. Because of this *cortical magnification of foveal vision,* the VEP is largely a foveal phenomenon. Approximately two thirds of the VEP is due to foveal and macular input (Riggs and Wooten, 1972; Berson, 1992).

The importance of the fovea in generating the VEP is illustrated in Figure 16–14, which shows idealized PERGs and VEPs expected for three different stimuli: a stimulus that covers both the foveal and parafoveal area, a stimulus that covers only the fovea, and a stimulus that covers only the parafoveal re-

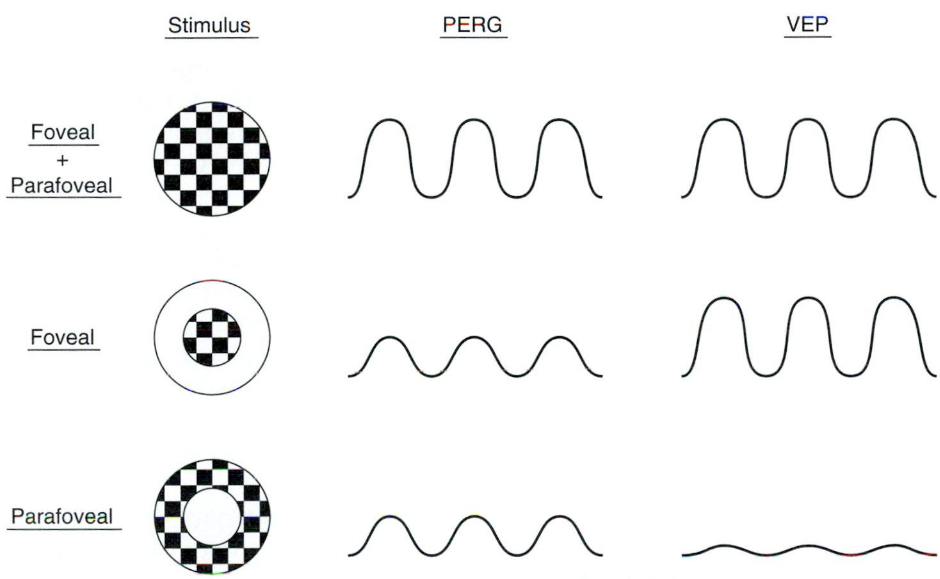


**FIGURE 16–14.** The amplitude of the pattern electroretinogram (PERG) is proportional to the area of the retina stimulated. Reducing the stimulus size in half, as is done in the bottom two PERG traces, reduces the PERG amplitude in half. It does not make any difference that one stimulus is foveal and the other is parafoveal. For the visually evoked potential (VEP), however, the area of the retina stimulated is not the critical issue. The VEP is a foveal response; consequently, a parafoveal stimulus does not elicit a significant response. (*Adapted from Carr RE, Siegel JM.* Visual Electrodiagnostic Testing: A Practical Guide for the Clinician. *Baltimore: Williams and Wilkins; 1982.*)

gion. The bottom two stimuli represent the same area, and each is half the area of the top stimulus.

Note that the PERG amplitude is reduced by half for both the foveal and parafoveal stimuli. This is because the PERG amplitude is primarily dependent on the area of retina stimulated. Reducing the stimulated retinal area by half reduces the PERG amplitude by half. The fact that a stimulus stimulates the fovea does not result in a disproportionately large PERG.

The results for the VEP are very different. The foveal stimulus produces a strong VEP, whereas the parafoveal stimulus elicits a weak VEP. This demonstrates the importance of the fovea in generating VEPs.

For the reasons discussed here, it is critical to ensure that patients are fixating the stimulus during a VEP measurement. Malingerers have been known to avert their gaze from the stimulus, thereby reducing the amplitude of the VEP.

### *Clinical Considerations*

Visually evoked potentials provide an objective method to assess contrast sensitivity and visual acuity. Although the results obtained with VEPs are well correlated with psychophysical data, there are occasions when VEPs do not tell the entire story. For example, VEPs overestimate infant acuity (Teller and Movshon, 1986). In addition, certain lesions of higher cortical areas could presumably have profound effects on vision and little effect on VEPs. This is because these lesions may occur in regions that do not significantly contribute to the VEP (Bodis-Wollner et al, 1977). It is also important to keep in mind that the VEP tests primarily central vision; it allows little assessment of noncentral visual function.

Although VEPs can be useful for establishing the existence of a visual deficit, they do not localize the causative lesion. VEPs manifest reduced amplitudes in macular, optic nerve, and cortical lesions. Any lesion of the visual pathway that affects central vision may result in an abnormal VEP.

Visually evoked potentials are frequently used in conjunction with other gross potentials, such as PERGs, to localize a disease process within the visual pathways (Table 16–1). For example, if the VEP is reduced and the PERG is normal, the problem is postretinal. If both the VEP and PERG are reduced, the lesion is retinal.

Amblyopia manifests normal ERGs and reduced VEPs (Sokol, 1990). This is consistent with the notion that amblyopia represents a disorder of cortical development rather than a retinal abnormality (see Chap. 17).

Visually evoked potentials have been used in the diagnosis of multiple sclerosis. Multiple sclerosis, a demyelinating disease, is frequently associated with optic neuritis. During bouts of optic neuritis, the myelin sheath and axons of the optic nerve are damaged. This produces a reduced conduction velocity along the optic nerve. As optic neuritis is typically unilateral, it may produce an increased latency of the VEP for the affected eye relative to the unaffected eye (Halliday et al, 1972).

**TABLE 16–1. EXPECTED STATUS OF GROSS ELECTRICAL POTENTIALS IN VARIOUS DISEASE CONDITIONS**

| Condition | EOG (Arden Ratio) | Standard ERG | Focal PERG | VEP |
|---|---|---|---|---|
| Macular lesion | Normal | Normal | Abnormal | Abnormal |
| Retinitis pigmentosa | Abnormal | Abnormal | Abnormal | Abnormal |
| Optic nerve disease (e.g., glaucoma) | Normal | Normal | Abnormal | Abnormal |
| Amblyopia | Normal | Normal | Normal | Abnormal |
| Hysteria, malingering | Normal | Normal | Normal | Normal |

Adapted from Carr RE, Siegel JM. *Visual Electrodiagnostic Testing: A Practical Guide for the Clinician.* Baltimore: Williams and Wilkins; 1982.

## SUMMARY

Gross electrical potentials represent the summed activity of large numbers of neurons. These potentials are obtained using noninvasive techniques. The appropriate use of these potentials, often in combination with each other, is an important clinical tool for diagnosing certain diseases and disorders of the visual system.

# Q Self-Assessment Questions

1. Malingerers fabricate symptoms to obtain a positive medical diagnosis (i.e., they fake a visual disorder). Most often, these patients claim a reduction in visual acuity. Which single electrodiagnostic test would be most useful in making a diagnosis of malingering? Explain.

2. Discuss a potential pitfall of using electrodiagnostic tests to make a diagnosis of malingering. (*Hint:* Could a patient with severely reduced vision show normal electrodiagnostic test results?)

3. Why must the patient look at the stimulus to obtain a normal evoked potential?

4. The pattern electroretinogram (PERG) and steady-state visually evoked potential (VEP) are obtained with the same stimulus. (This stimulus typically is a checkerboard pattern that undergoes a phase shift.) In amblyopia the PERG is normal, whereas the VEP is abnormal. Explain.

# 17

# Development and Maturation of Vision

The human visual system is not fully developed at birth; rather, it matures over the first several years of life. To mature properly, the visual system must be exposed to a normal visual environment. Disruption of the visual environment during development can have profound consequences for the attainment of normal levels of visual function.

Over recent decades, we have gained substantial insight into the mechanisms of visual development. Clinical procedures have been devised that allow the assessment of the vision of infants. As a result, eye care clinicians are better equipped to effectively diagnose and treat disorders of visual development.

## *DEPRIVATION STUDIES*

Most neurons in the visual cortex receive input from both eyes; they are binocular (see Chap. 14). Most binocular cortical cells do not, however, receive equal input from the two eyes. This is illustrated in Figure 17–1, an **ocular dominance histogram.** This histogram was constructed based on recordings from individual neurons in one hemisphere of the adult cat striate cortex (Hubel and Wiesel, 1962).

Cells in categories 1 and 7 are monocular; category 1 cells receive input from only the contralateral eye, whereas category 7 cells receive input from only the ipsilateral eye. Neurons in category 4 are binocular and receive equal input from both eyes. Cells in the remaining categories are binocular, but dominated by one of the eyes. Neurons in categories 2 and 3 are dominated by the contralateral eye, and those in categories 5 and 6 are dominated by the ipsilateral eye.

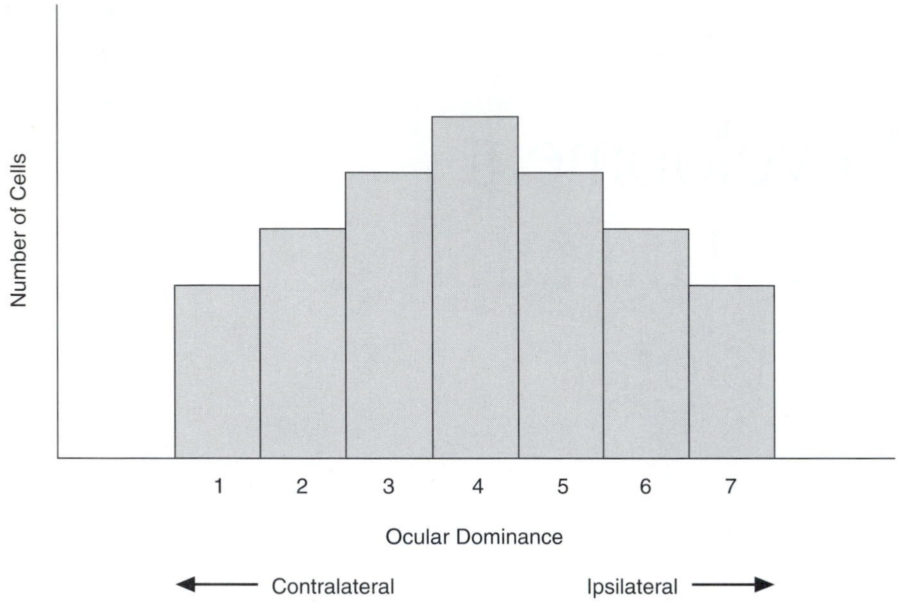


**FIGURE 17–1.** Ocular dominance histogram for neurons located in the striate cortex. Categories 1 and 7 consist of monocularly driven neurons; all other categories consist of binocularly driven neurons. Category 4 neurons receive equal input from the two eyes. (*Adapted from Hubel DH, Wiesel TN. Receptive fields, binocular interaction and functional architecture in the cat's visual cortex.* J Physiol. *1962;160:106–154.*)

In the 1960s, David Hubel and Torston Wiesel, working at Harvard University, asked the following question: what is the effect of **visual deprivation** on the development of ocular dominance? To answer this question, they deprived one eye of a kitten of vision from birth by suturing an eyelid closed, and then recorded from the striate cortex of this animal after it had fully matured (Hubel and Wiesel, 1965b). The striate cortex of this monocularly deprived animal is very different from that of a normal animal (Fig. 17–2). Virtually all cells are monocular and responsive only to the nondeprived eye.

This result leads to an important conclusion. For the striate cortex to develop a normal complement of binocular cells, it is necessary for both eyes to provide input during development. The closure of an eye of an immature animal results in a lack of cortical cells responsive to the deprived eye. If no cortical cells are responsive to stimulation of an eye, we must conclude that the eye provides no useful vision. It is essentially blind (Harwerth et al, 1987). Moreover, since there are no binocular cells, stereopsis is absent.

Suppose a similar experiment is conducted on a mature cat. An eye of a 7-year-old cat is closed for 1 year. At this advanced age, monocular deprivation has no effect; there is a normal complement of cortical neurons. Although the

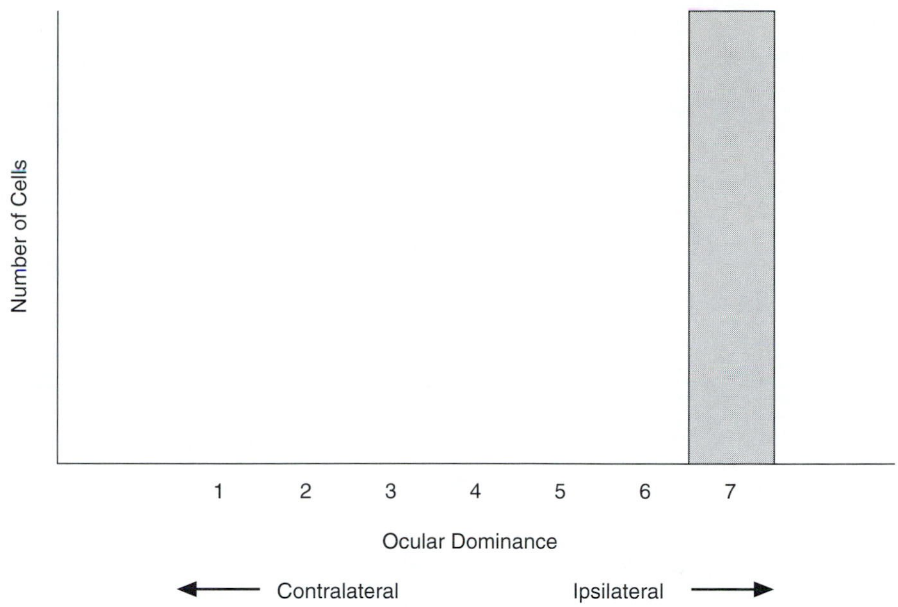


**FIGURE 17–2.** Ocular dominance histogram for the right striate cortex of a mature cat whose left eye was sutured closed at birth. Note that all neurons are driven by the nondeprived right eye. (*Adapted from Wiesel TN, Hubel DH. Single-cell responses in striate cortex of kittens deprived of vision in one eye.* J Neurophysiol. *1963;26:1003–1017.*)

visual system is plastic (malleable) early in life, it becomes hard-wired (inflexible) later in life (Blakemore and Van Sluyters, 1974). The period during which the visual system can be influenced by environmental manipulation is referred to as the **critical** or **sensitive period.**

The duration of the critical period can be determined by reversing an eyelid suture at various ages. If the right eye of a cat is closed for the first 5 weeks of life and the cat's cortex is examined at the end of these 5 weeks, it is found that cells are responsive only to stimulation of the nondeprived left eye. Suppose that the right eye is sutured closed for the first 5 weeks of life and, subsequently the right eye is opened and the left eye closed for the next 5 weeks of life (Fig. 17–3). Stimulation of which eye would now activate cortical neurons? Because the switch occurred early in life, during the critical period, most cortical cells are responsive to stimulation of the right eye.

The flexibility described here apparently is present only during the critical period. For the cat, the critical period ends after 3 months of life (Olson and Freeman, 1980). Consequently, if the suture in the previous experiment had been switched from the right to the left eye at the age of 6 months, cortical cells would still only respond to stimulation of the left eye.

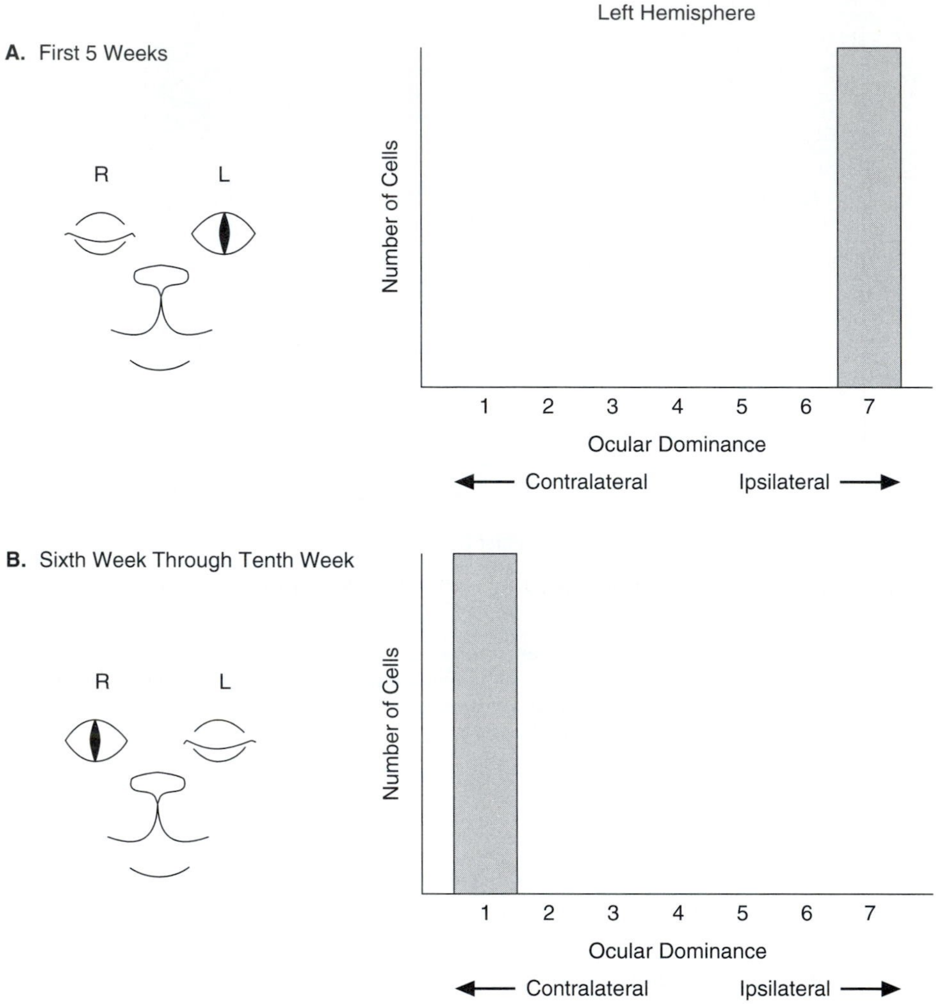


**FIGURE 17–3. A.** As a result of closure of the right eye during the first 5 weeks of life, most of the cortical cells of this adult cat are driven by the nondeprived left eye. **B.** Closure of the right eye for the first 5 weeks of life followed by monocular closure of the left eye for the next 5 weeks results in most cortical cells being driven by the right eye. This result is obtained because the switch from right eye deprivation to left eye deprivation occurred during the critical period.

The human visual system matures at a much slower pace than does the cat visual system. The human visual system is most sensitive to environmental manipulation during the first 2 years of life, with the human critical period over by about 7 to 9 years of age (Vaegan and Taylor, 1980).

The results of Hubel and Wiesel's work suggest that the two eyes compete with each other to dominate cortical neurons (Hubel, 1988). If both eyes have equally clear retinal images during the critical period, then most of the cortical neurons become binocular. One eye might dominate certain neurons, but both eyes provide input to most cortical cells. If, however, one eye is deprived during the critical period, it is at a disadvantage in this binocular competition. The other eye, which has a clear retinal image, wins out in the competition for cortical neurons. As a consequence, cortical neurons are dominated by this eye.

This model assumes that synaptic connections in the cortex are strengthened by neural activity and that lack of neural activity results in the weakening of synaptic connections. As indicated in Figure 17–4, the nondeprived eye provides neural stimulation to a cortical cell, whereas the deprived eye is relatively quiet. Consequently, there is a strengthening of synapses made with the nondeprived eye relative to those made with the deprived eye. For reasons not yet fully understood, this synaptic arrangement becomes permanent at the conclusion of the critical period.

## AMBLYOPIA

Monocularly deprived animals display very poor vision in the deprived eye. Reduction in vision secondary to monocular deprivation during the critical period is referred to as amblyopia (Ciuffreda et al, 1991). It is important to keep in mind that amblyopia is a condition that reflects abnormal cortical development, not an abnormality of the eye itself.

Amblyopia is a commonly encountered clinical condition. The monocular deprivation that produces amblyopia can take several forms. Next we discuss

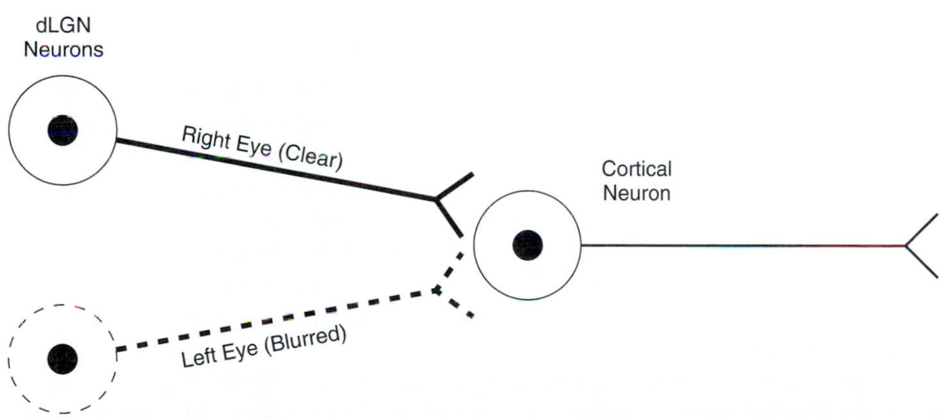


**FIGURE 17–4.** A relatively high level of neural activity strengthens the connection between the eye that has a clear image and a cortical cell. The relative lack of neural activity produces a weakening of the connection between the eye with a poor image and the same cortical neuron. (*Adapted from Hubel DH.* Eye, Brain, and Vision. *New York: Scientific American Library; 1988.*)

amblyopia that is secondary to occlusion, anisometropia, and strabismus. *A diagnosis of amblyopia should only be made if there is a history of one of these factors.*

### Occlusion Amblyopia

Occlusion amblyopia results when an eye is occluded during the critical period. This occlusion can be caused by a monocular congenital cataract, a monocular lid ptosis (the eyelid covers the pupil, either completely or partially), or other monocular blockage of vision.

To minimize permanent visual loss, it is necessary to remove the occlusion. In general, the sooner the occlusion is removed, the better the visual outcome. Consequently, infants with congenital cataracts and ptosis should receive prompt treatment.

### Anisometropic Amblyopia

Anisometropia is a condition in which the two eyes have unequal refractive errors (Levi and Harwerth, 1977; Bradley and Freeman, 1981). Amblyopia develops when one eye has a blurred retinal image at all distances during the critical period and the other eye has a clear retinal image at some distances. This most commonly occurs when one eye manifests a hyperopic refraction and the other eye is less hyperopic (or plano or myopic).

Consider the following hypothetical case of an 8-year-old child who received his first prescription at the age of 7 years:

| | |
|---|---|
| OD | +6.00 DS 20/400 |
| OS | +1.00 DS 20/20 |

Without an optical correction, this patient accommodates 1 diopter to focus the left eye for distance. Because the innervation to accommodation is bilateral and equal, the right eye is always 5 diopters out of focus. This defocused retinal image, if present during the critical period, would result in the right eye losing out in the competition for cortical neurons. Consequently, the right eye develops amblyopia. In addition, because he (presumably) has few binocular cortical neurons, this patient has greatly reduced stereopsis. Much of the patient's visual loss could have been prevented if he had received a prescription for spectacles during the critical period.

It is important to realize that not all anisometropes develop amblyopia. Consider the following hypothetical case of an 8-year-old child who received her first prescription at the age of 7 years:

| | |
|---|---|
| OD | −3.00 DS 20/20 |
| OS | −1.00 DS 20/20 |

If this uncorrected refractive error was present during the critical period, the patient had a clear retinal image in each eye at certain distances. The right eye was in focus at 33 cm; the left eye was in focus at 100 cm. Because each eye had a clear retinal image at some distance, neither eye developed amblyopia.

Although this patient manifests normal monocular acuities, she will most likely demonstrate reduced stereopsis. Because the retinal images of the two eyes were never in focus at the same distance, the patient presumably developed relatively few binocular cortical neurons (i.e., most striate cells are expected to fall into ocular dominance categories 1 and 7) (Holopigian et al, 1986; Movshon et al, 1987). The putative reduction in the number of binocular neurons is expected to result in poor stereopsis.

To prevent vision loss due to anisometropic amblyopia, the first eye exam should occur early in life, preferably during the critical period. Using objective tests, such as retinoscopy, a skilled clinician can readily diagnose anisometropia in a very young child. Consideration should be given to correcting substantial amounts of hyperopic anisometropia.

### *Strabismic Amblyopia*

Constant unilateral strabismus (an eye turn), developed during the critical period, leads to amblyopia in the deviated eye. Figure 17–5B shows a case of constant left esotropia. The right eye views the target of regard while the left eye is deviated inwards. As a consequence of this deviation, the object of regard, a square, does not fall on the left fovea. Instead, the left fovea is exposed to another image, in this case a triangle. If the patient does not make a sensory adaptation for this deviation, he or she will experience diplopia (both a triangle and a square will be seen in the same location as both images fall upon a fovea). To avoid diplopia, patients frequently suppress the deviating eye. This **suppression** presumably leads to amblyopia.

Amblyopia develops in constant unilateral deviations, as frequently occur in esotropia, but not in alternating or nonconstant deviations, as is often the case in exotropia (Fig. 17–6A). Because alternating strabismics view objects alternately with each eye, amblyopia does not develop.

Although alternating strabismics may have normal visual acuity in each eye, these patients frequently suffer profound losses of binocular vision; they have little or no stereoscopic vision (Birch and Stager, 1985). As their visual cortex does not receive normal binocular input during the critical period, there is a presumed paucity of binocular cells capable of mediating stereopsis. This is similar to (but frequently more profound than) the previously discussed example of anisometropia where both eyes are myopic.

The lack of binocular cells in alternating strabismus can be demonstrated in animal models by experimentally inducing this condition with surgery or prisms (Hubel and Wiesel, 1965b; Crawford and von Noorden, 1980). Cells in the stri-

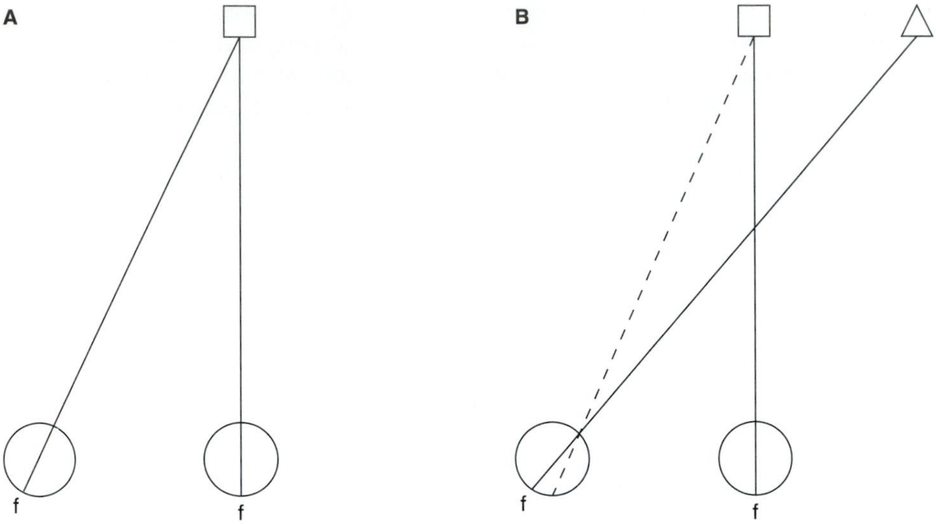


**FIGURE 17–5. A.** Normally, the image of a fixated target (the square) falls on the fovea of each eye. **B.** In esotropia, the fixated target falls on a nonfoveal region of the deviating eye. In this case of constant left eye esotropia, the square falls on a region of the retina nasal to the fovea of the left eye. This would lead to diplopia in the absence of a sensory adaptation, such as suppression.

ate cortex of an animal with alternating exotropia, which is induced during the critical period, are almost exclusively monocular (Fig. 17–6B).

Psychophysical procedures can be used to demonstrate the lack of binocular cells in adult human strabismics. This is accomplished by determining the extent of the interocular transfer of the tilt aftereffect (Banks et al, 1975). Figure 17–7 shows the stimuli used for this experiment.

The participant views the tilted grating monocularly. After viewing this grating for several minutes, the participant views the vertical grating with the other eye. Normal nonstrabismic patients report that the vertical grating appears tilted in a direction opposite to that of the original grating.

Interocular transfer of the tilt aftereffect is mediated by binocular cortical neurons. If no such neurons are present, then interocular transfer does not occur. This is the case for patients who develop strabismus during the critical period; interocular transfer is virtually absent. If, however, the strabismus develops later in the critical period, some residual transfer is noted.

## *MERIDIONAL AMBLYOPIA*

In Chapter 14 we learned that most striate cortical neurons are orientation selective. On the basis of this observation, some have suggested that the develop-

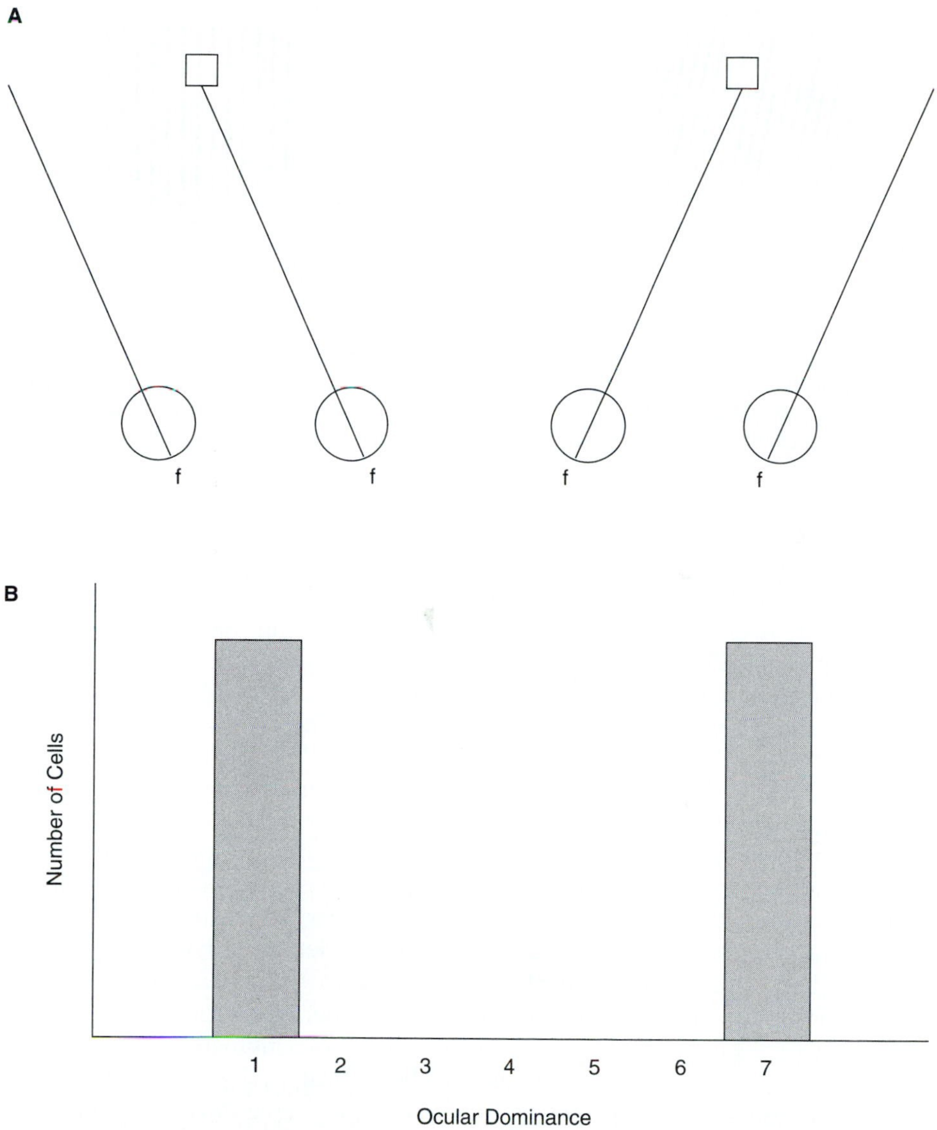


**FIGURE 17–6. A.** In alternating exotropia, one eye views the target at a time. **B.** As a consequence of this alternate viewing, cortical neurons do not receive binocular input. Consequently, most cortical neurons are monocular and fall into categories 1 and 7. (*Adapted from Hubel DH, Wiesel TN. Binocular interaction in striate cortex of kittens reared with artificial squint.* J Neurophysiol. *1965b;28:1041–1059.*)

**FIGURE 17–7.** To demonstrate interocular transfer of the tilt aftereffect, view the tilted grating for 1 minute with your left eye. Next, view the vertical grating with your right eye. An appearance of the vertical grating tilting to the right is evidence of interocular transfer of the aftereffect. (The interocular transfer effect is subtle and is not noticed by all normal observers. Most observers are able to experience a monocular tilt after effect. Cover one eye and move your eye across the length of the horizontal bar for one minute. Next, view the dot with the same eye and note that the vertical lines appear tilted. This is an aftereffect rather than an afterimage because your eye was not stationary during adaptation to the tilted grating.)

ment of orientation sensitivity may be influenced by visual experience, just as ocular dominance is influenced by visual experience.

To test this hypothesis, kittens have been raised in visual environments consisting of stripes of only one orientation. For example, animals can be raised in an environment consisting of only vertical stripes. After the animals mature, recordings are made from single neurons in striate cortex.

If the orientation of the visual world plays a role in visual development, then it is expected that a kitten raised in a vertical environment will display a disproportionate number of cortical cells selective for vertical stimuli. Although the experimental results are somewhat controversial, it does appear that the orientation of the visual environment plays a role in visual development (Blakemore and Cooper, 1970; Stryker and Sherk, 1975; Stryker et al, 1978). Animals raised in an environment consisting of only one orientation have a disproportionately large number of cortical cells sensitive to this orientation, and they have disproportionately few neurons sensitive to other orientations.

If a patient presents with a substantial amount of astigmatism, it is possible that this astigmatism was present during the critical period (Mohindra et al, 1978). Consequently, the patient's visual system may have developed with one meridian more in focus than other meridians. On the basis of the experimental results discussed earlier, the expectation is that these patients will manifest better vision in certain meridians than in other meridians.

Consider the following hypothetical case of a 14-year-old child who received his first prescription at the age of 10 years:

| | | |
|---|---|---|
| OD | pl = −4.00 × 180 | 20/25 |
| OS | pl = −4.00 × 180 | 20/25 |

This type of refractive error, uncorrected, results in vertical gratings being clear and horizontal gratings being blurred.

If visual resolution is determined for this patient when fully corrected, using both vertical and horizontal gratings, it is found that resolution is better for vertical gratings than for horizontal gratings. This patient manifests **meridional amblyopia** (Mitchell et al, 1973).

Meridional amblyopia occurs when a child progresses through the critical period with one visual meridian clear and the other out of focus. Presumably, the clear meridian wins out in a competition for cortical cells, dominates more cortical cells, and manifests better visual resolution. The blurred meridian loses this competition, drives disproportionately few cortical cells, and manifests relatively poor resolution.

Meridional amblyopia is commonly seen in clinical practice. Patients with high degrees of astigmatism, when first corrected, often have slightly reduced visual acuity. (Over time, the acuity of these patients tends to reach normal levels.) Certain optotypes are especially difficult for these patients to resolve. The specific optotypes that are difficult to resolve depend on the meridian affected. For instance, a patient with a high degree of compound myopic, with-the-rule astigmatism has difficulty resolving horizontal gratings. Consequently, this patient finds it difficult to resolve optotypes such as **E** or **F,** which have substantial horizontal components.

Infants tend to be born with astigmatism. One study showed that half of neonates had astigmatism of between 0.75 and 2.00 D (Howland et al, 1983). The axis of the astigmatism of neonates may depend on the child's race. While Caucasian neonates are likely to show against-the-rule astigmatism, Chinese children are more likely to have with-the-rule astigmatism (Thorn et al, 1987). The amount of the astigmatism generally decreases over the first 5 to 6 years of life (Gwiazda et al, 1984).

It is unlikely that the low to moderate amounts of astigmatism that are commonly present at birth lead to meridional amblyopia (Gwiazda et al, 1985). Consequently, it is generally not advisable to optically correct low to moderate amounts of astigmatism in infants. The correction of astigmatism in young, school-age children (children 4 to 7 years of age) is controversial. It is possible that such a correction could interfere with the normal ocular growth that leads to reductions in astigmatism. However, significant amounts of astigmatism, especially against-the-rule astigmatism, may produce asthenopia (eye strain) that could discourage a child from reading. Based on these various considerations, it is probably best to consider prescribing lenses for young, school-age children if the astigmatism shows no signs of abating and is at least 2.00 D.

## PERCEPTUAL CONSEQUENCES OF BILATERAL VISUAL DEPRIVATION

As we have learned, early monocular visual deprivation leads to profound changes in striate cortex physiology with resultant amblyopia and loss of stereopsis. What is the effect of bilateral visual deprivation that occurs early in life and continues until maturity? Another way to phrase this question is as follows:

what would a person whose otherwise healthy eyes were occluded from birth see when the occlusion was removed as an adult? There are a few such cases reported in the literature.

An interesting case is the patient S.B. who developed corneal opacities early in life and had has vision surgically restored with a corneal transplant at the age of 52 (Gregory, 1974). (The opacities did not entirely occlude S.B.'s vision. He had rudimentary vision through his corneal opacities.) Following the corneal transplant, this patient learned simple visual tasks, such as recognizing letters; however, his vision was profoundly disturbed. Objects would appear different when viewed from different perspectives, and his motion and depth perception were not well developed. Consider the following quote from Gregory (1974):

> He would look at a lamp post, walk round it, stand studying it from a different aspect, and wonder why it looked different and yet the same. . . . He found traffic frightening, and would not attempt to cross even a comparatively small street by himself (p. 111).

This patient had not learned to see an object as being the same object regardless of the perspective from which it is viewed and had difficulty interpreting motion and depth, apparently due to deprivation during the critical period. This case is interesting because it demonstrates the effects that deprivation can have on higher level visual functions (e.g., form recognition, motion perception) that presumably involve higher cortical areas (see Chap. 15).

## DEVELOPMENT OF REFRACTIVE ERRORS

### Myopia: Nature Versus Nurture

The origin of myopia has been the subject of intense speculation and investigation for at least a century. For many years, there has been a vigorous debate between the advocates of two seemingly opposing theories. The advocates of the *nature* theory contend that myopia is an inherited condition. Supporters of a *nurture* theory believe that environmental factors (e.g., prolonged near work) cause myopia. Recent research suggests that both nature and nurture play a role in the development of myopia.

Strong support for a hereditary origin of myopia comes from studies on identical (monozygotic) twins. Such twins, when mature, tend to have highly correlated refractive errors (Teikari et al, 1988). Other evidence for the heritability of myopia includes the finding that myopic parents are more likely to have myopic children than are parents who are not myopic (Gwiazda et al, 1993).

Most growth of the eyeball occurs during the first 6 years of life. However, myopia is relatively uncommon when children enter school (2 percent of 6-year-old children are myopic), but increases in frequency throughout the school years (15 percent of 15-year-old children are myopic) (Mutti et al, 1996).This observation has lead to the suspicion that environmental factors, such as prolonged near work, may cause myopia. While prolonged near work appears to be associated with myopia, such correlation does not prove that the near work causes myopia. (Children grow taller during their school years, but attending school does not cause children to grow.) Much of contemporary research in myopia has been aimed at determining if near work causes myopia in certain individuals or is merely associated with the development of myopia.

Support for an environmental role in the development of myopia received much impetus from the finding that suturing an animal's eyelid closed at birth, or optically blurring the retinal image early in life, leads to the development of axial myopia (Wiesel and Raviola, 1977; Raviola and Wiesel, 1978; Siegwart and Norton, 1993). These results not only demonstrate that environmental factors may play a role in the development of myopia, but also suggest that a focused retinal image may be required for normal ocular growth leading to emmetropia.

Additional support for the role of environmental factors in the development of refractive errors, including myopia, comes from an experiment in which infant monkeys were raised wearing either minus lenses or plus lenses over one of their eyes (Hung et al, 1995). An eye raised with a minus lens apparently compensates for this defocus by maturing to a longer axial length than it would have otherwise. Consequently, when the minus lens is removed, the mature eye is myopic. Likewise, an eye that wears a plus lens during development matures to a shorter axial length than it would have otherwise and is hyperopic when the lens is removed. This and similar experiments demonstrate that the development of emmetropia (emmetropization) is an active process (Wildsoet and Wallman, 1995).

A fairly unambiguous conclusion from the recent work on the development of myopia is that a clear retinal image promotes emmetropization. One theory of myopia development is that certain children do not fully accommodate to near objects, leading to chronic near blur (Gwiazda et al, 1993). To compensate for this blur, it has been suggested that the eye's axial length increases, causing myopia. It has long been suspected that plus lenses at near, in the form of bifocals or progressive lenses, may lead to a clearer retinal image and forestall the development of myopia (Wallman and McFadden 1995). Further research is required to determine if this hypothesis is correct.

### *Development of Refractive Errors in Humans*

It is important to know the course of development of refractive errors (in humans) from birth through maturity so that the clinician can be aware of what is normal when he or she examines a child. Unfortunately, studies of the development of refractive errors in humans have led to inconsistent results due to the various techniques used to determine the refractive error (i.e., cycloplegia versus noncycloplegia, retinoscopy versus photorefraction). In general, these studies suggest that typical healthy humans are born with or develop a slight amount of hyperopia (less than 2.50 D) during the first year of life (Slataper, 1950; Dobson et al, 1981; Mohindra and Held, 1981). The amount of hyperopia in a typical child tends to decrease throughout childhood (Howland and Sayles, 1987).

The correction of refractive errors in children is controversial because the prescription of corrective lenses could potentially interfere with emmetropization. For instance, the prescription of minus lenses for myopia *may* lead to near defocus, thereby promoting the development of additional amounts of myopia (Hung et al, 1995). For this reason, lenses should be prescribed only after careful consideration of both the benefits that may accrue from the correction (e.g., clear vision, reduced asthenopia) and the potential interference with the emmetropization process that may result.

## DEVELOPMENT OF GRATING ACUITY

The resolution acuity of a 1-month-old infant, as measured with spatial gratings, is on the order of 20/600, and reaches adult levels by about 4 to 5 years of age (Teller, 1997). Grating acuity in infants (and other nonverbal patients) has been assessed using several different procedures that do not require the cooperation of the patient. These procedures are discussed next.

### *Optokinetic Nystagmus*

A moving grating produces an (involuntary) nystagmus, referred to as optokinetic nystagmus (OKN). This nystagmus consists of a slow following movement (smooth pursuit) followed by fast compensatory eye movement (saccade). OKN can be produced by positioning a rotating drum that displays a grating along the patient's visual axis (Fig. 17–8).

Optokinetic nystagmus is presumably dependent on the ability to resolve the grating. If the grating cannot be resolved, the OKN response is presumably

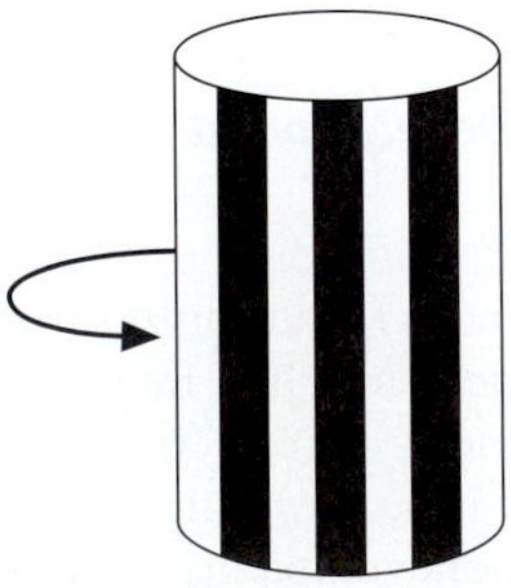

**FIGURE 17–8.** A drum with stripes is rotated to elicit an optokinetic nystagmus response.

not elicited. OKN has been used to assess visual capabilities in uncooperative patients including infants, malingerers, hysterics, and the mentally retarded.

Some caution is necessary when interpreting OKN results. It is not established that OKN relies on the same pathways as does conscious visual perception (Van Sluyters et al, 1990). Therefore, it is conceivable that a patient could have impaired vision yet show a normal OKN response.

### *Preferential Looking*

When given a choice, infants prefer to view a patterned stimulus rather than a nonpatterned stimulus. For example, when presented with the stimulus configurations in Figure 17–9A, an infant will choose to view the patterned stimulus on the right. Because the stimuli are of the same average luminance, it is the pattern itself that attracts the attention of the child. This is referred to as preferential looking (Teller, 1979; Teller and Movshon, 1986).

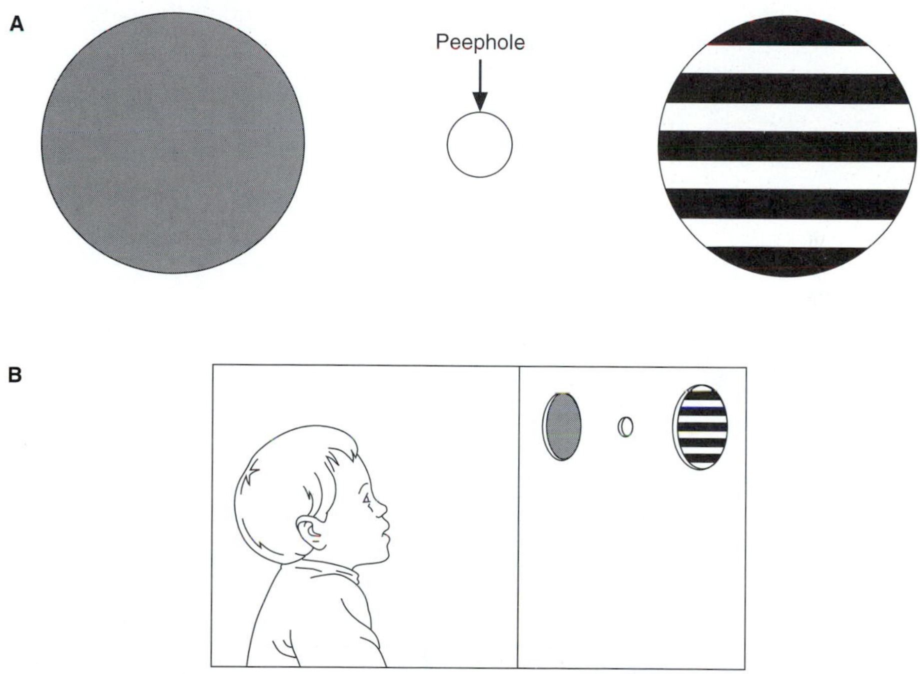


**FIGURE 17–9. A.** Stimulus arrangement viewed by an infant during forced choice preferential viewing. The examiner observes the infant's eyes through the peephole and guesses which side of the panel contains the grating. (The other side of the panel consists of uniform gray equal in luminance to the grating.) **B.** An infant participating in preferential viewing. The examiner is located behind the stimulus display and views the child's eyes through the peephole.

Preferential looking can be used to determine an infant's grating acuity. The infant typically sits on a parent's lap and views stimuli as illustrated in Figure 17–9. The examiner is located behind the stimulus display and views the infant's eyes through a peephole. By observing the infant's direction of gaze, the examiner guesses which side the pattern is on. As the examiner *must* guess which side the pattern is on, this is a forced choice procedure and is referred to as **forced-choice preferential looking (FPL).** The positions of the patterned and nonpatterned stimuli are randomly interchanged; therefore, the examiner does not know which side the pattern is on. Consequently, the examiner must rely on observation of the child's gaze to determine the location of the pattern.

Several trials are conducted at each of a large number of spatial frequencies. The results are plotted in the form of a psychometric function, similar to that given in Figure 17–10. The percentage correct for the highest spatial frequencies is 50 percent, which represents chance performance for a two-alternative forced choice (2AFC) procedure (i.e., the infant cannot resolve the spatial frequency gratings). As the spatial frequency decreases, the percentage correct increases. As discussed in Chapter 11, threshold is represented by the point midway between chance performance and 100 percent performance. For

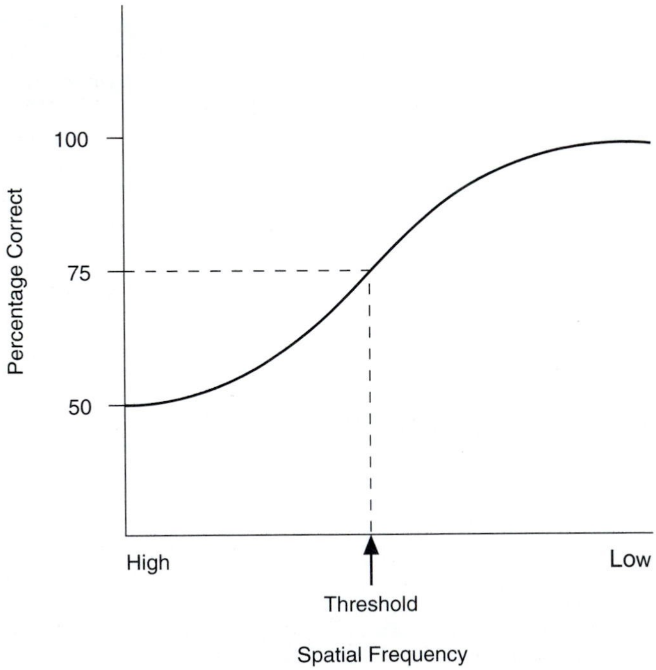


**FIGURE 17–10.** Psychometric function for a two-alternative forced choice preferential viewing task.

a 2AFC procedure, this is 75 percent correct. The spatial frequency that elicits 75 percent correct performance represents the infant's grating acuity.

While the information provided by FPL is valuable for research purposes, the procedure is time consuming; therefore, it is of limited usefulness in standard clinical practice. A technically less stringent variation of preferential looking, which is clinically practicable, involves the use of Teller acuity cards (McDonald et al, 1985). These rigid, rectangular, hand-held, gray cards have a peephole in the center, and a grating with a luminance that is equal to the gray card to one side of the peephole. If the infant looks at the grating, it is assumed he or she can resolve it. Presenting the grating one or two times is usually sufficient to determine if a grating can be resolved. (The location of the grating can be switched by flipping the card over.) To determine the infant's acuity, the clinician simply presents gratings of increasing frequency until the infant does not consistently tend to the location of the grating.

Teller acuity cards elicit results that are similar to those obtained with the more stringent FPL method, but their relatively low test-retest reliability limits their effectiveness is diagnosing subtle reductions is acuity that may be associated with clinically significant amblyopia (Dobson, 1993; Teller 1997). As indicated in Figure 17–11, studies with these cards suggest that healthy 1-month-old infants have acuities of about 20/600 (1 cycle/degree) (Mayer et al, 1995). Resolution acuity improves rapidly during the first year of life, with 1-year-old children manifesting acuities of about 20/100 (6 cycles/degree). This is followed by

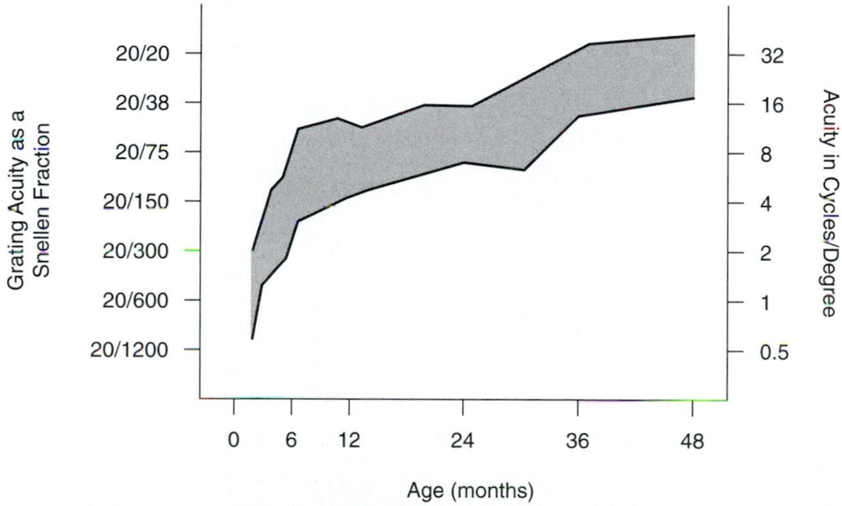


**FIGURE 17–11.** Visual acuity as a function of age as determined with Teller Acuity Cards.The shaded area shows the 95 percent prediction limits. (*Adapted from Mayer DL et al. Monocular acuity norms for the Teller Acuity Cards between ages one month and four years.* Invest Ophthalmol Vis Sci. *1995;36:671–685.*)

a slower improvement in acuity: adult levels of 20/20 acuity are not reached until 3 to 5 years of age, a finding that is consistent with common clinical experience. Immaturities in the retina, particularly the foveal cones, apparently account for the poor acuity of infants during the first year of life (Abramov et al, 1982; Brown et al, 1987; Banks et al, 1988).

### *Visually Evoked Potentials*

Visually evoked potentials (VEPs) have been used to assess the visual acuity of infants. The procedure for determining visual acuity with VEPs is discussed in Chapter 16.

Visually evoked potentials yield results that are somewhat different than those obtained with forced preferential looking (FPL) (Norcia and Tyler, 1985; Teller and Movshon, 1986). Whereas FPL suggests that adult levels of resolution acuity are reached between 3 and 5 years of age, VEPs show adult levels at 6 to 8 months. The different results obtained with FPL and VEPs may be related to the greater cognitive demands associated with FPL (Dobson and Teller, 1978).

## *DEVELOPMENT OF OTHER VISUAL ATTRIBUTES*

### *Contrast Sensitivity*

Figure 17–12 illustrates contrast sensitivity functions (CSFs) for 1, 2, and 3-month-old infants that were obtained with a preferential viewing procedure. The CSF shifts to the right and upwards as infants mature, revealing increased contrast sensitivity for most spatial frequencies and improved visual acuity (Banks and Salapatek, 1978; Movshon and Kiorpes, 1988). The peak of the CSF is probably at the adult location (~4 cycles/degree) at about 6 months (Teller, 1997). Limitations in spatial vision that are present during the first year of life are primarily due to immaturities of the retina rather than the central visual pathways (i.e., the cortex) (Hawken et al, 1997).

### *Hyperacuity*

Although hyperacuity is classified as a form of visual acuity, it is subserved by different mechanisms than grating acuity, leading to the suspicion that the time course for maturation of the two forms of acuity may be different (see Chap. 7). Studies (using preferential looking) of the development of vernier acuity, a form of hyperacuity, suggest that vernier acuity, like grating acuity, matures rapidly during the first year or so and then matures more slowly, reaching adult levels at slightly older ages than grating acuity (Manny and Klein, 1984; 1985; Kiorpes, 1992). Since vernier acuity is thought to depend on cortical processing, it is not surprising that it reaches adult levels late in life, paralleling the slow maturation of the cortex (Ciuffreda et al, 1991; Levi, 1992).

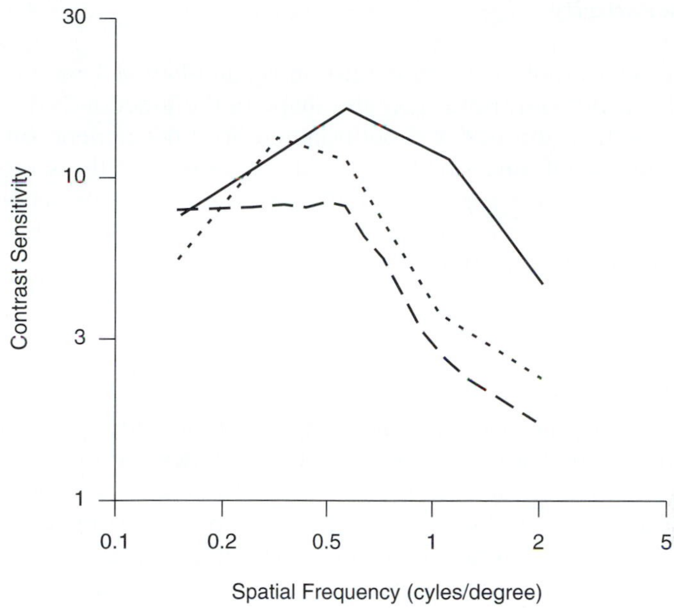


**FIGURE 17–12.** Contrast sensitivity functions shift upwards and to the right as an infant matures. The dashed, dotted, and solid curves are CSFs for infants of 1, 2, and 3 months of age, respectively. (*Adapted from Banks M, Salapatek, P. Acuity and contrast sensitivity in 1-, 2-, and 3-month-old human infants.* Invest Ophthalmol Vis Sci. *1978;17:361–365.*)

## *Stereopsis*

Preferential looking studies of stereopsis are designed to determine if infants respond to stimuli that produce retinal disparity (see Chap. 10). Interestingly, these studies reveal that while few infants manifest stereopsis prior to 3 months of age, it has a rapid onset between 3 and 6 months (Birch et al, 1982; Teller, 1982). Stereoacuity matures rapidly thereafter reaching 1 minute of arc by 6 months (Held et al, 1980; Held, 1993).

## *Temporal Vision: Critical Flicker Fusion Frequency*

Whereas spatial vision (i.e., grating and vernier acuity) does not reach adult levels until 3 to 5 years of age, the critical flicker fusion frequency is 40 Hz at 1 month of age and reaches adult levels of about 55 Hz by 3 months (Regal, 1981). The retinal and cortical immaturities that limit grating and vernier acuity, respectively, in young infants apparently have little effect on temporal resolution.

### *Scotopic Sensitivity*

The form of the scotopic sensitivity function is adult-like at 1 month (Powers et al, 1981). This is not surprising since the shape of the function is determined by the absorption characteristics of rhodopsin and does not depend on postreceptoral processing of information. The absolute sensitivity of the scotopic system (i.e., the sensitivity for a stimulus of 507 nm presented under conditions that maximize scotopic sensitivity) apparently reaches adult levels by about 6 months of age (Hansen and Fulton, 1993).

### *Color Vision*

Preferential viewing has been used to examine both red–green and blue–yellow color discrimination. These studies reveal that rudimentary red–green discrimination arises during the second month of life (Adams et al, 1990; Allen et al, 1993). Discrimination is worst for small stimuli, probably due to poor spatial summation secondary to retinal immaturities (Packer et al, 1984). Adult levels of red–green chromatic discrimination are apparently obtained by the end of the first year of life (Morrone et al, 1993; Kelly et al, 1997). Visually evoked potentials suggest that the photopic spectral sensitivity function is adult-like in young infants (Bieber et al, 1995).

The emergence of blue–yellow color discrimination is less well understood. Certain studies have found crude blue–yellow discrimination in 2-month-old infants, while other studies suggest a slower time course for the development of this aspect of color vision (Teller et al, 1978; Varner et al, 1985).

### *Summary of Visual Development*

Figure 17–13 summarizes the development of various visual attributes in infants and children. While vision is rudimentary at birth, substantial improvements occur early in life, with certain attributes such as the CFF and the forms of the scotopic, photopic, and contrast sensitivity functions showing adult-like characteristics within the first 6 months. Other attributes, including stereopsis and color vision, emerge within the first 3 months of life and probably approach adult levels within the first year or so. Grating and vernier acuity rapidly improve during the first year, but then slowly mature until the child is 3 to 5 years old.

The different rates of maturation for the various visual functions (i.e., grating acuity, hyperacuity, etc.) are consistent with the notion that each of these visual functions has a different critical period (Harwerth et al, 1987; Levi and Carkeet, 1993). For instance, the critical period for the development of scotopic sensitivity may terminate at a much younger age than the critical period for the development of hyperacuity.

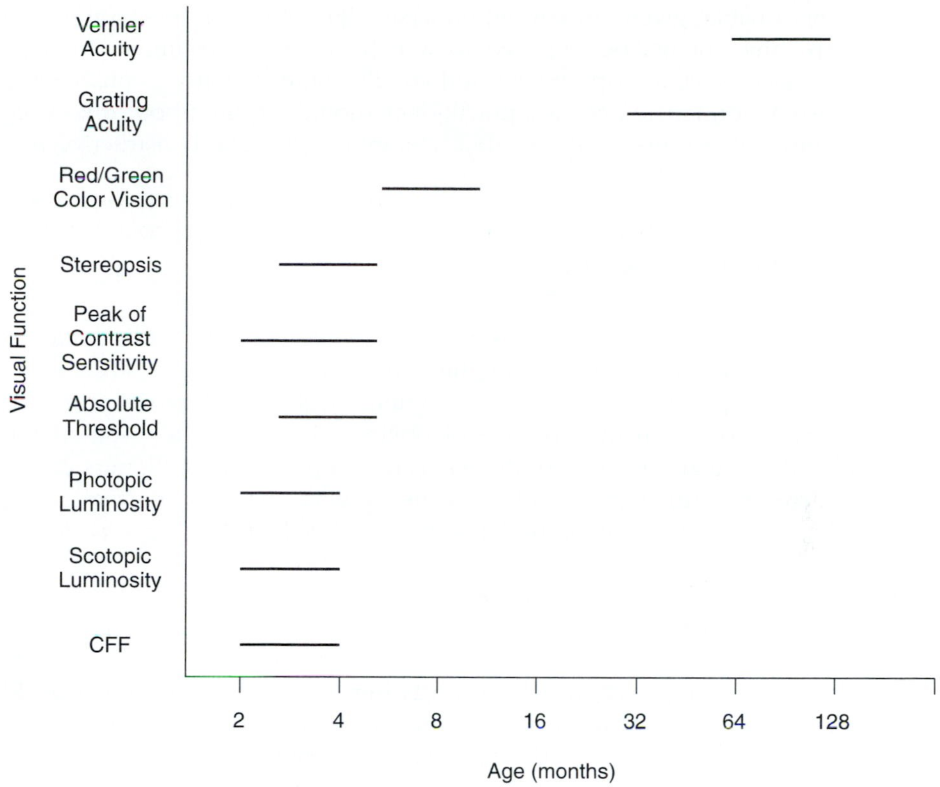


**FIGURE 17–13.** Time frame for development of various visual attributes. (*Adapted from Levi DM. Amblyopia: A developmental disorder of spatial vision.* Optom Vis Sci. *1992:69(12s):123.*)

## *VISUAL DEVELOPMENT: CLINICAL CONSIDERATIONS*

If the developing visual system does not receive normal visual input, it does not develop properly. Conditions such as anisometropia, strabismus, cataracts, and ptosis all may produce visual deprivation that can lead to permanent visual loss in the form of amblyopia. Because the visual system becomes hard-wired early in life, it is important that these conditions be diagnosed and treated at the earliest possible time. This necessitates eye exams early in life.

It is unfortunate that some practitioners continue to inform concerned parents that their children must be of school age before they can be examined. Objective clinical tests can readily be used to assess the ocular status of nonverbal infants and toddlers. Retinoscopy, the cover test, ophthalmoscopy, and other procedures can reveal the presence of conditions that, if treated in a timely manner, are preventable causes of severe visual loss.

It is reasonable, given our current understanding of visual development, to recommend that infants be exposed to a rich visual environment. Visually complex objects, such as crib mobiles and visually interactive toys, enhance the infant's visual world. The eye care practitioner should inquire about the visual environment that parents create for their children, and make constructive recommendations.

## VISION IN THE LATER YEARS

With respect to vision, it has been said that, "things start out badly [infants], then they get better; then, after a long time, they get worse again" (Teller and Movshon, 1986, p. 1483). As the visual system ages, it undergoes profound changes. These occur in the absence of obvious disease. As a result of improved health care and increased life expectancy, eye care practitioners examine an increasing number of elderly patients who manifest normal aging changes in their vision. Some of these are discussed in the following sections.

### Contrast Sensitivity

Figure 17–14 shows typical contrast sensitivity functions (CSFs) for a 60-year-old individual and a 20-year-old individual. Note that contrast sensitivity for the 60-year-old person is reduced at moderate and high spatial frequencies.

Several factors contribute to this reduction in contrast sensitivity. Primary among these factors is the reduction in retinal illumination produced by senile miosis. A 60-year-old individual behaves as if a neutral density filter that transmits only 33 percent of the incident light (OD = 0.48) has been placed in front of his or her eyes (Weale, 1963).

Other factors may lead to the reduction in contrast sensitivity. Increased light scatter secondary to nuclear sclerosis is clearly a factor. The aging of neural elements, both retinal and more central, may also play a contributing role.

**Senile Miosis.** The pupil becomes smaller with age, leading to a condition referred to as senile miosis. A typical 20-year-old individual has a pupil diameter of about 5.3 mm, whereas a 60-year-old person has a pupil diameter of about 3.2 mm (Owsley et al, 1983). Due the reduction in pupil area, a 60-year-old individual receives one third of the retinal illumination that a 20-year-old individual receives. This reduction in retinal illumination has profound consequences for visual function, leading to diminished increment and contrast sensitivity and impaired color discrimination.

There are, however, some advantages to a small pupil. A small pupil behaves like a pinhole, thereby increasing the patient's depth of field. Therefore, patients with senile miosis often report less reliance on their spectacles, particularly under high illumination that mitigates the loss of light due to reduced pupillary area.

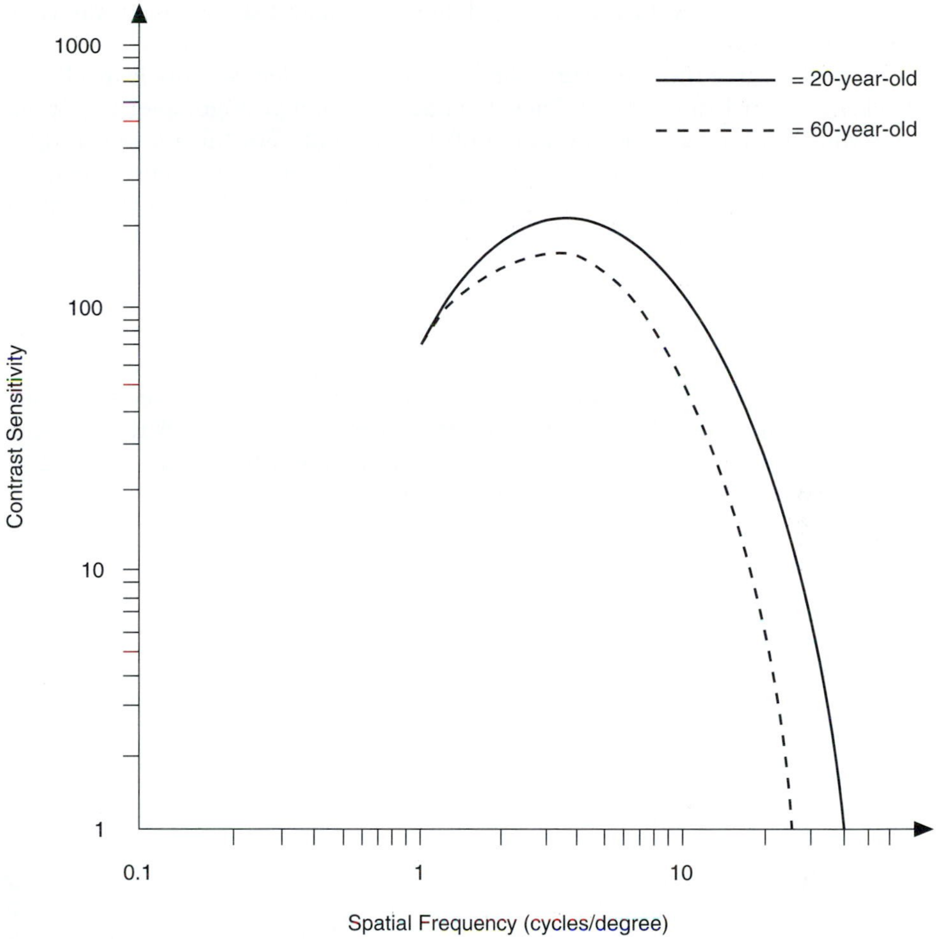


**FIGURE 17–14.** Contrast sensitivity functions for a 20-year-old and a 60-year-old. (*Adapted from Owsley C, Sekular R, Siemsen D. Contrast sensitivity throughout adulthood.* Vision Res. *1983;23:689–699.*)

***Nuclear Sclerosis.*** The crystalline lens of a young adult is colorless. In comparison, the typical elderly patient's lens appears yellow. The yellowing of the nucleus of the crystalline lens, which is readily observed during slit lamp biomicroscopy, is referred to as nuclear sclerosis.

The yellow appearance indicates increased absorption of blue light by the aging lens. One can think of the young lens as absorbing ultraviolet light, but not blue light. As the lens ages, however, it accumulates damage due to the absorption of this high energy ultraviolet light, leading to the absorption of increasing amounts of blue light and its yellow appearance. This increased absorption results in a reduction in retinal illumination and slight changes in color perception (Weale, 1992).

It is likely that the same (or a similar) process that leads to nuclear sclerosis also leads to nuclear cataracts. These cataracts occur at younger ages in populations with substantial exposure to ultraviolet radiation. For this reason, and because ultraviolet radiation may accelerate the development of certain retinal diseases (e.g., age-related macular degeneration), it is important to recommend that patients wear lenses with ultraviolet filters when outdoors (Weale, 1983).

### *Resolution Acuity*

The age-related reduction in high spatial frequency sensitivity is seen clinically as a reduction in visual acuity (Owsley et al, 1983). Figure 17–15 shows visual acuity as a function of age. The same factors that contribute to the overall reduction in the CSF contribute to this reduction in visual acuity.

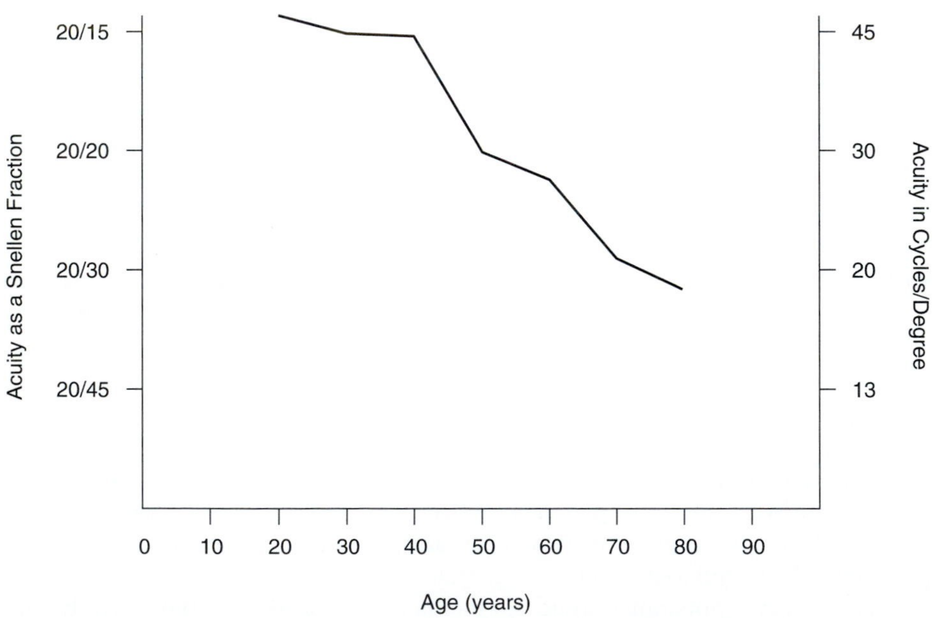


**FIGURE 17–15.** Effect of normal aging on visual acuity. (*Adapted from Pitts DG. The effects of aging on selected visual functions: Dark adaptation, visual acuity, stereopsis, and brightness contrast. In: Sekular R, Kline DW, Dismukes K, eds.* Aging in Human Visual Functions. *New York: Liss; 1982.*)

### *Increment Sensitivity*

Increment sensitivity decreases with increasing age. Senile miosis, yellowing of the crystalline lens, and neural factors all appear to play a role in this age-related reduction in sensitivity (Weale, 1992).

Age-related reductions in increment sensitivity occur across the retina, leading to a sinking of the hill of vision (see Fig. 3–23). This age-related reduction in sensitivity must be taken into account when performing and interpreting visual fields.

### *Useful Field of View*

Elderly people are more likely to be involved in automobile accidents than are younger people (Ball and Owsley, 1991). Why is this the case? Age-related declines in visual acuity and other traditional measures of visual function do not appear to explain this finding and cannot be effectively (or fairly) used to predict which elderly drivers are at risk of involvement in an automobile accident (Shinar and Schieber, 1991). An attention-based measure of visual function—the *useful field of vision*—provides a foundation for such predictions (Ball et al, 1993).

In traditional visual field testing, increment thresholds are determined across the visual field (see Chap. 3). This test is exceedingly important for the diagnosis of many ocular and neurologic conditions. Additionally, it provides important information regarding a patient's lateral and vertical extent of vision that can be used in counseling the patient regarding his or her visual limitations. However, traditional visual fields do not characterize the usefulness of the patient's field of vision. That is, a patient may have a normal visual field, yet not be able to effectively process, or use, information presented within this field of vision.

The useful field of vision has been assessed by determining how well patients can divide their attention between two stimuli. The task is to *identify* a centrally (foveally) fixated target while also *identifying* a target presented in the peripheral visual field. In essence, the useful field of vision is a measure of visual attention within the visual field.

There are data suggesting that the size (extent) of the useful field of vision can predict which elderly drivers are more likely to be involved in automobile accidents (Ball et al, 1993). Those subjects with small useful fields of vision are more likely to be involved in accidents. This is a promising example of the manner in which psychophysical testing can be used to assess visual function as it relates to day-to-day activities.

### *Color Vision*

Color discrimination is commonly affected by normal aging processes (Weale, 1992). Reduction in retinal illumination and yellowing of the crystalline lens contribute to changes in color discrimination. These changes are often manifested as a shift toward a tritan (blue–yellow) defect.

### *Temporal and Motion Aspects of Vision*

Although not exhaustively studied, it appears that sensitivity to temporal modulation decreases with age for all temporal frequencies (Mayer at al, 1988; Casson et al, 1993). The ability to detect motion, as measured by minimum displacement thresholds, has also been demonstrated to diminish with age (Wood and Bullimore, 1995). It is not yet known if these changes in temporal and motion thresholds are optical or neural in origin (Lachenmayr et al, 1994; Spear et al, 1994).

### *Presbyopia*

The ability to accommodate decreases with age (Fig. 17–16) (Donders, 1864). When this reduction in accommodation produces symptoms such as blur and eyestrain when reading, it is referred to as presbyopia. Symptoms are usually first noticed when patients are in their mid-40s. Presbyopia is one of the primary reasons patients seek eye care.

Although somewhat controversial, it appears that one factor in the development of presbyopia is a decrease in elasticity of the lens capsule (Weale, 1992).

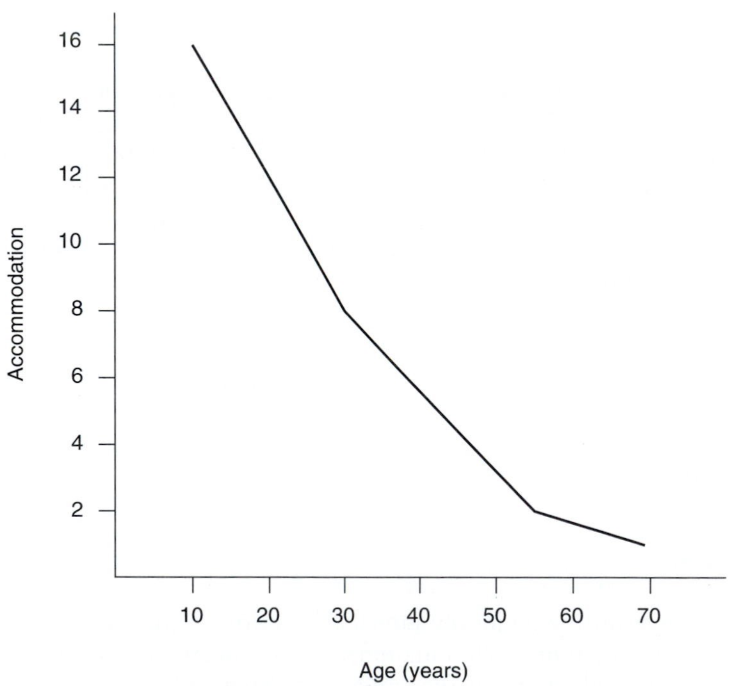


**FIGURE 17–16.** Accommodation as a function of age.

In younger patients, the capsule is very elastic. When the ciliary muscle constricts in younger people, it releases tension on the lens zonules and capsule, allowing the supple lens to bulge anteriorly (see Fig. 2–2). This increases the dioptric power of the eye. The bulging forward of the anterior lens surface depends on an elastic lens capsule. Consequently, as the lens capsule ages and becomes less elastic, accommodation is impaired. Presbyopia is treated with convex (plus) lenses. These lenses compensate for the loss of near dioptric power.

### *Astigmatism*

The aging crystalline lens shows increasing dioptric power in the horizontal meridian relative to the vertical meridian. Clinically, this manifests as a gradual shift from with-the-rule to against-the-rule astigmatism as we age (Morgan and Rosenbloom, 1993). Changes in the crystalline lens apparently account for this observation.

### *Summary of Vision in the Later Years: Clinical Considerations*

As the population ages, eye care practitioners will see increasing numbers of elderly patients. These patients should be educated with respect to expected changes in their visual capabilities and the manner in which these changes can influence their daily activities. Eye care practitioners should make practical recommendations that enable patients to enhance their visual environment.

One factor all too often overlooked by patient and doctor alike is the proper use of light. In this chapter, we have stressed that reduction in retinal illumination is a primary factor in reducing visual function in elderly patients. It cannot be overemphasized that elderly patients need sufficient light in order to maximize their visual capabilities. Patients should be questioned with respect to the lighting conditions they use for various tasks. On the basis of the patient's visual status, work status, and hobbies, specific practical recommendations should be made.

# Self-Assessment Questions

1. An infant has a high spatial frequency cutoff of 4 cycles/degree. Express the visual acuity as a Snellen function.

2. At the age of 20, a patient's pupillary diameter is 7 mm. At age 70, this same patient's pupillary diameter is 2 mm. **A.** Calculate the percentage reduction in the amount of light reaching this patient's retina. **B.** What is the optical density of a neutral density filter which, when placed in front of the 20-year-old eye, will reduce the light level to that experienced by the 70-year-old eye?

3. A 4-year-old who has never worn spectacles has the following refraction and corrected acuities:

| | | |
|---|---|---|
| OD | plano | 20/20 |
| OS | +3.00 DS | 20/200 |

   **A.** Given that all other ocular findings are unremarkable, what is your diagnosis? **B.** Would you expect this patient's stereoacuity to be normal? **C.** Provide a treatment plan for the patient.

4. A 30-year-old patient presents with a dense cataract in the left eye. The patient claims this cataract has been present for the past 15 years. Following cataract extraction, the best corrected acuity in the left eye is 20/1000. Assuming that the left eye is healthy and has never suffered trauma, and that there are no postsurgical complications, provide an explanation for this reduction in acuity.

5. A 10-year-old child undergoes strabismus surgery to correct a congenital constant right eye esotropia. The child has received no previous treatment and the presurgical acuity in the deviated eye is 20/1000. **A.** Do you expect the child to regain normal or near-normal acuity in the right eye following surgery? **B.** What degree of stereopsis is expected following the surgery?

# A Answers to Self-Assessment Questions

## *CHAPTER 3. DUPLEX NATURE OF THE RETINA*

**1.** A. Photophobia, squinting, poor daytime vision, reduced visual acuity (≈ 20/200), nystagmus, poor fixation.
B. Long-pass sunglasses (red) are helpful because long wavelength light is least effective at bleaching rhodopsin.

**2.** Locate these wavelengths on the photopic and scotopic spectral sensitivity functions. The 507 and 555-nm stimuli are equally bright under photopic conditions only when the 507-nm stimulus has more energy. (This is because the photopic system is less sensitive to 507 nm than to 555 nm.) If the intensities of these two equally bright stimuli are decreased by equal amounts, the 507-nm stimulus continues to contain more energy. Under scotopic conditions, the 507-nm stimulus appears brighter because it has more energy and because the scotopic system is more sensitive to 507 nm than to 555 nm.

**3.** The scotopic visual system is most sensitive to 507 nm because this wavelength is most effective at bleaching rhodopsin.

**4.** A. Red, because threshold detection of 610 nm, after 20 minutes of dark adaptation, is mediated by the cones.
B. The 465-nm stimulus has no color after 20 minutes of dark adaptation because it is detected by the scotopic system.

**5.** A. About 4 log units (photochromatic interval).
B. About 0.5 log unit (photochromatic interval).

**6.** A. After 1.5 minutes, 50 percent of the photopigment has regenerated and 50 percent remains bleached. Over the next 1.5 minutes, 50 percent of the remaining photopigment recovers. Consequently, the total amount of cone photopigment that recovers after 3 minutes is 50 percent plus 25 percent, or 75 percent.

B. The rod–cone break occurs at about 35 minutes. The half-life for rhodopsin regeneration is 5 minutes. Therefore, after 5 minutes, 50 percent has regenerated. And after 10 minutes, 75 percent has regenerated. Carrying out this calculation to 35 minutes shows that at this time 99.22 percent of the rhodopsin has regenerated.

**7.** A. Although the cones are more sensitive after 11 minutes of dark adaptation, the rods are capable of detecting the stimulus if it is sufficiently intense. According to Figure 3–8B, the stimulus would need to be on the order of 6 relative log units to be detected by the rods. (Note that after 5 minutes of dark adaptation, the rods could not detect the stimulus because their threshold approaches infinity.)

B. The cones plateau at about 3.75 relative log units. They maintain this same threshold at 20 minutes (and beyond).

C. The difference between the cone and rod plateaus is about 3 log units.

**8.** A. The 507-nm patch is brighter because it results in more quantal absorptions by rhodopsin.

B. Both patches have the same brightness because they bleach the same number of rhodopsin molecules.

## CHAPTER 4. PHOTOMETRY

**1.** Formula:

(number of watts) (visual efficiency) (680 lumens/watt) = number of lumens

Solve for number of watts:

$$(\text{number of watts})\ (0.62)\ (680\ \text{lumens/W}) = 1000\ \text{lumens}$$
$$\text{number of watts} = 2.37\ \text{W}$$

**2.** Use the formula from Problem 4–1 to calculate the number of lumens for each wavelength. Abney's law allows the addition of these amounts to determine the total number of lumens.

# A

| | | |
|---|---|---|
| 500 nm: | (10 W) (0.35) (680 lumens/W) = 2380 lumens | |
| 550 nm: | (5 W) (1.00) (680 lumens/W) = 3400 lumens | |
| 650 nm: | (20 W) (0.10) (680 lumens/W) = 1360 lumens | |
| | Total = 7140 lumens | |

**3.** Observe $V'(\lambda)$. There are 680 scotopic lumens/W at 555 nm. The number of scotopic lumens per watt at other wavelengths is determined by a proportionality factor.

| | |
|---|---|
| 500 nm: | (10 W) (1.0/0.4) (680 scotopic lumens/W) = 17,000 scotopic lumens |
| 550 nm: | (5 W) (0.50/0.40) (680 scotopic lumens/W) = 4250 scotopic lumens |
| 650 nm: | (20 W) (0) (680 scotopic lumens/W) = 0 scotopic lumens |
| | Total = 21,250 scotopic lumens |

**4.** Seventy foot-candles fall on a probe that measures 3 × 3 cm. The area of this probe is 0.0097 ft$^2$. Therefore,

$$(70\ \text{lumens/ft}^2)\ (0.0097\ \text{ft}^2) = 0.67\ \text{lumens}$$

**5.** Place a filter with the transmission characteristics of the $V(\lambda)$ function in front of the probe. The device would then need to be calibrated.

**6.** $E = I/d^2$

$E = 100$ lumens/(2ft)$^2$ = 25 lumen/ft$^2$ or 25 foot-candles

Convert to lux:

$$(25\ \text{foot-candles})\ (10\ \text{lux/foot-candle}) = 250\ \text{lux}$$

**7.**

$$E_1 = E_2$$
$$I_1/d_1^{\,2} = I_2/d_2^{\,2}$$
$$50\ \text{cd}/(1\ \text{ft})^2 = X/(3\ \text{ft})^2$$
$$X = 450\ \text{cd}$$

**8.** $E = (I/d^2)\cos\theta$

As lux is metric, convert distance to meters:

$$2\ \text{ft} = 0.6096\ \text{m}$$

# A

Substitute:

$$100 = I/(0.6096)^2 (\cos 60)$$
$$I = 74.32 \text{ cd}$$

**9.**
$$OD = \log (1/T)$$
$$OD = \log (1/0.25)$$
$$OD = 0.60$$

**10.** Combined OD = 0.50 + 1.0 = 1.5

$$OD = \log(1/T)$$
$$1.5 = \log(1/T)$$
$$10^{1.5} = 1/T$$
$$31.62 = 1/T$$
$$T = 0.032$$
$$\text{Percent transmitted} = (100)(0.032) = 3.2\%$$
$$\text{Percent absorbed} = 100 - 3.2 = 96.8\%$$

**11.**
$$L = rE$$
$$50 = 0.7E$$
$$E = 71.43 \text{ foot-candles}$$

**12.** (25 cd) ($4\pi$ lumens/cd) = 314 lumens

**13.** $L = rE$

Convert 100 lumens/m² to foot-candles:

$$(100 \text{ lumens/m}^2)\left(\frac{1 \text{ foot-candle}}{10 \text{ lumens/m}^2}\right) = 10 \text{ foot-candles}$$

$$L = rE$$
$$5 = r(10)$$
$$r = 0.5$$

# A

## CHAPTER 5. COLOR VISION

1. The observer will behave as a monochromat because he or she continues to have only one photopigment. (If, however, the observer compares perceptions with the red sunglasses to perceptions without the red sunglasses, he or she will behave as a dichromat.)

2. A. About 500 nm.
   B. About 0.64.
   C. A nonspectral purple.

3. A. About 595 nm.
   B. About 0.50.
   C. About 480 nm.

4. Illuminant $D_{65}$, because it has a higher color temperature, appears more blue than illuminant A. That is, relative to illuminant $D_{65}$, illuminant A appears reddish yellow. This is consistent with the location of illuminant $D_{65}$ in the "blue corner" of the CIE diagram; illuminant A is located relatively closer to the red–yellow region of this diagram.

5. A. Trichromacy of vision.
   B. Paints, when mixed together, produce a subtractive color mixture. This subtractive mixture is less bright than any of the original paints. Consequently, mixing of paints produces a dim color. This can be alleviated by brightly illuminating the picture. Alternatively, access to more than three primaries allows the artist to optimize brightness, as well as to match hues.

6. A red filter (or almost any colored filter) would be useful. The metameric match, which the camouflaged clothing produces with the background, holds up only under normal viewing conditions. When viewed with a colored filter, which results in a subtractive color mixture, the metameric match no longer holds.

7. The invariant hues presumably represent those wavelengths that perfectly balance one of the opponent color channels. For example, 578 nm perfectly balances the red–green channel and stimulates only the yellow

channel. As the stimulus intensity increases, the red–green channel remains "neutralized," and there is no change in hue.

## CHAPTER 6. ANOMALIES OF COLOR VISION

**1.** A. Typically, yes.
B. The number on the plate is not seen by a color-defective patient because it is a metameric match with the background. The red filter forms a subtractive mixture with the plate and eliminates the metamerism, enabling the color-defective patient to see the number. Another way to think of this is that a combined filter and retinal photopigment absorption spectrum is displaced from that of the photopigment alone. Consequently, the original metameric match no longer holds.

**2.** A. No.
B. Top mixture field appears red and the bottom test field appears black.
C. The red filter transmits only the longer wavelengths that emerge from the anomaloscope (subtractive mixture). Consequently, for the top mixture field, only red is transmitted. For the bottom test field, little or no light is transmitted.

**3.** A. Yes.
B. Both the mixture and test field appear green.
C. Exposure of the eye to a red light produces a disproportionate bleaching of erythrolabe. The result is that subsequently viewed objects appear relatively more green. This is true for the mixture and test fields which initially appeared yellow. They remain metamers, but now appear green.

**4.** A. 670 nm is matched by a very dim yellow test field, whereas 546 nm is matched by a relatively bright test field.
B. The scotopic spectral sensitivity curve peaks at 510 nm; consequently, 546 nm is brighter than 670 nm.

# A

## CHAPTER 7. SPATIAL VISION

**1.** A. The visual acuity is 20/15. First, calculate the minimum angle of resolution (MAR):

$$15/20 = 0.75' \text{ arc}$$

Therefore, the size of the threshold detail is 0.75′ arc. This means each bar of the grating subtends 0.75′ arc (see Fig. 7–18). If each bar subtends 0.75′ arc, then a cycle of a grating (a dark and bright bar together) subtends 1.50′ arc. Convert this to cycles/degree:

$$\left(\frac{1 \text{ cycle}}{1.5 \text{ arc}}\right)\left(\frac{60' \text{ arc}}{1 \text{ degree}}\right) = 40 \text{ cycles/degree}$$

B. 7.5 cycles/degree.
C. 4.0 cycles/degree.

**2.** A. The contrast sensitivity function cutoff is 5 cycles/degree. If the grating has 5 cycles in one degree, then each cycle must subtend one fifth of a degree. Each cycle of a grating consists of both a bright and dark bar. The bars themselves represent the detail of the grating (see Fig. 7–18). Therefore, the detail is one half of one cycle of the grating, or (1/2)(1/5 degree) = 1/10 degree. This is the MAR in degrees. We must convert this MAR to minutes of arc:

$$\left(\frac{1}{10} \text{ degree}\right)\left(\frac{60' \text{ arc}}{1 \text{ degree}}\right) = 6' \text{ arc}$$

The MAR is 6′ arc. Because the acuity measurement is at 20 ft, the Snellen fraction is 20/120 (120/20 = 6′ arc). An alternative solution involves recalling that a 20/20 acuity corresponds to 30 cycles/degree. Five cycles/degree represents a MAR six times as large (30/5 = 6) as does an acuity of 20/20. Therefore, the Snellen fraction corresponding to 5 cycles/degree is 20/120.
B. 20/30.
C. 20/10.

# A

**3.** The visual acuity is 20/100.

A. By definition, the threshold letter subtends 5′ arc overall at 100 ft. The tangent relationship is used to calculate the letter's physical size. First, convert 5′ arc to degrees:

$$(5' \text{ arc})\left(\frac{1 \text{ degree}}{60' \text{ arc}}\right) = 0.0833 \text{ degree}$$

Next, convert 100 ft to millimeters:

$$(100 \text{ ft})\left(\frac{12 \text{ in}}{1 \text{ ft}}\right)\left(\frac{25.4 \text{ mm}}{1 \text{ in}}\right) = 30{,}480 \text{ mm}$$

Tangent relationship:

$$\tan(0.0833 \text{ degree}) = \frac{\text{overall letter size}}{30{,}480 \text{ mm}}$$

$$\text{overall letter size} = 44.31 \text{ mm}$$

B. The detail of the letter is one fifth this overall size or

$$(1/5)(44.31 \text{ mm}) = 8.86 \text{ mm}$$

**4.** For 20/80, the MAR is 4′ arc (i.e., 80/20 = 4). To maintain a MAR of 4′ arc, the fraction would need to be 10/40.

**5.** A. The patient's high-frequency cutoff is 30 cycles/degree. This measurement represents a MAR of 1′ arc. This MAR does not change with distance. The size of the stimulus (grating bars or acuity letters) required to produce this MAR will change, but the MAR remains constant. Consequently, the patient's high-frequency cutoff will be 30 cycles/degree at both 20 and 10 ft.

B. As there is 30 cycles/degree, each cycie must subtend 1/30th of a degree. A single bar is one half of a cycle (see Fig. 7–18). Therefore, each bar subtends (1/2)(1/30 degree) = 1/60 degree. We can use the tangent relationship to calculate the size of a bar. First, we must convert the distance to millimeters:

$$(20 \text{ ft})\left(\frac{12 \text{ in}}{1 \text{ ft}}\right)\left(\frac{25.4 \text{ mm}}{1 \text{ in}}\right) = 6096 \text{ mm}$$

Tangent relationship:

$$\tan\left(\frac{1}{60}\right) = \frac{\text{bar width}}{6096\ \text{mm}}$$

$$\text{bar width} = 1.77\ \text{mm}$$

C. The angle is the same as in B, but the distance is now 10 ft. Convert 10 ft to millimeters and substitute as follows:

$$\tan\left(\frac{1}{60}\right) = \frac{\text{bar width}}{3048}$$

$$\text{bar width} = 0.89\ \text{mm}$$

This means that to obtain 30 cycles/degree, the bars used at 10 ft are one half the size as those used at 20 ft. The key is to recognize that the angle of resolution remains constant.

**6.** A. The measured acuity is expected to be less than 20/20.
B. The overhead lights decrease the contrast of the letters of the projected chart. This results in a reduction in the contrast sensitivity function's high-frequency cutoff leading to a reduction in measured visual acuity.

## ***CHAPTER 8.*** ***TEMPORAL ASPECTS OF VISION***

**1.** 20 Hz = 20 cycles/s. Each cycle is 1/20th of a second or 0.05 second. One half of a cycle is the on-phase; its duration is (1/2)(0.05) = 0.025 second. Convert to milliseconds:

$$(0.025\ \text{s})\ (1000\ \text{ms/s}) = 25\ \text{milliseconds}$$

**2.** A total cycle is 40 milliseconds, or 1 cycle/40 ms. Convert to hertz:

$$(1\ \text{cycle}/40\ \text{ms})\ (1000\ \text{ms/s}) = 25\ \text{cycles/s or } 25\ \text{Hz}$$

**3.** The percentage modulation, $(A/l_{ave})(100)$, remains constant at low frequencies as $l_{ave}$ is increased. Because the amplitude ($A$) remains a constant fraction of the background illumination ($I_{ave}$), Weber's law is followed (see Chap. 11).

## *CHAPTER 9. MOTION PERCEPTION*

**1.** Cortical activity can be measured in alert human subjects with functional magnetic resonance imaging (fMRI) or positron emission tomography (PET). As described in Chapter 15, the subject views a moving object while cortical activity is measured. The level of cortical activity is then measured when the same object is stationary. The difference in activity between the moving and stationary conditions is presumably greatest in those cortical areas that are involved in motion perception.

## *CHAPTER 10. DEPTH PERCEPTION*

**1.** Since monovision contact lenses interfere with stereopsis, we need to consider the importance of stereopsis for flying an airplane. Many of a pilot's visual tasks are performed at far distances. At these far distances, stereopsis is of little or no value because objects would need to be separated by great linear distances to produce a threshold disparity. For comparatively close tasks, such as a visual landing, stereopsis may play a role.

## *CHAPTER 11. PSYCHOPHYSICAL METHODOLOGY*

**1.** A. Perfect performance = 100%.
Chance performance = 33%.

$$\text{Midpoint} = \frac{(100\% - 33\%)}{2} + 33\% = 66.5\%.$$

# A

B. Perfect performance = 100%.
Chance performance = 20%.

$$\text{Midpoint} = \frac{(100\% - 20\%)}{2} + 20\% = 60\%.$$

**2.** Forced choice methodology is preferable because different criteria may be used for the detection of stable and flickering gratings.

## *CHAPTER 12. FUNCTIONAL RETINAL PHYSIOLOGY*

**1.** Gratings are optimal stimuli for ganglion cells, which are "designed" to detect contrast. The various spatial frequencies may be coded by ganglion cells with various receptive field dimensions. That is, low spatial frequencies may be coded by peripheral ganglion cells with large receptive fields, and high frequencies may be coded by foveal ganglion cells with small receptive fields.

**2.** The receptive fields of foveal ganglion cells are smaller than those of peripheral ganglion cells. These smaller foveal receptive fields manifest less spatial summation, but better spatial resolution, than the larger peripheral receptive fields.

**3.** The antagonistic surround of ganglion cells is less apparent under dark adaptation. This allows greater spatial summation with a resultant increase in sensitivity (and reduction in resolution) (Barlow et al, 1957).

## *CHAPTER 13. PARALLEL PROCESSING*

**1.** Cats respond to movement but may ignore stationary objects. This presumably reflects a highly developed "where" system and a less well developed "what" system.

# A

2. The color detection function is expected to manifest reduced sensitivity relative to the flicker detection function.

3. Visual acuity targets are high spatial frequency targets. If glaucoma initally affects the magno pathway, which codes low spatial frequencies, it is unlikely to result in reduced visual acuity. (As it progresses, glaucoma results in reduced acuity, perhaps due to damage to the parvo system.)

4. This procedure assumes that magno neurons code luminance and that all magno neurons have the same spectral sensitivity. The first assumption is controversial. The second assumption is not correct; not all magno neurons demonstrate the same spectral sensitivity (Cavanagh, 1991).

## *CHAPTER 14. THE STRIATE CORTEX*

1. Injection of a radioactive tracer into the optic nerve of one eye at various stages of development would provide such information.

2. *Left cell:* A red light falling on the cell's receptive field center, surrounded by a green annulus on the surround, would elicit maximum excitation. *Right cell:* A green light falling on the cell's receptive field center, surrounded by a red annulus falling on the surround, would elict maximum excitation.

3. See Chapters 12, 13, and 14.

## *CHAPTER 15. INFORMATION STREAMS AND EXTRASTRIATE PROCESSING*

1. If the tilt aftereffect is mediated by binocular cortical neurons, it should be transferrable from one eye to the other eye. That is, if a subject stares at lines tilted slightly counterclockwise with his or her left eye, vertical lines subsequently viewed with the right eye should appear tilted clockwise. If

# A

an effect does not show interocular transfer, it is probably mediated by monocular neurons located lower in the visual system (e.g., dLGN). (As discussed in Chapter 17, the tilt aftereffect does show interocular transfer.)

## CHAPTER 16. GROSS ELECTRICAL POTENTIALS

1. Visually evoked potential (VEP). If the VEP is normal, the visual pathways are intact up through at least primary visual cortex.
2. A patient with a lesion in the higher visual centers could manifest a normal electrooculogram, electroretinogram, and visually evoked potential because these tests sample the visual system at lower levels.
3. The evoked potential is primarily a foveal response. A version of gaze will result in a reduced potential.
4. The pattern electroretinogram (PERG) tests retinal function, whereas the VEP tests cortical function. Amblyopia affects the cortex, not the retina. Consequently, the VEP is abnormal, and the PERG is normal.

## CHAPTER 17. DEVELOPMENT AND MATURATION OF VISION

1. Each cycle = 1/4 degree
   Each half-cycle = 0.5/4 degree
   Convert to minutes of arc:

$$\left(\frac{0.5}{4}\text{ degree}\right)\left(\frac{60'\text{ arc}}{\text{degree}}\right) = 7.5'$$

   Convert to a Snellen fraction:

$$\text{visual acuity} = 20/150$$

(See Chap. 7 for a detailed discussion of these calculations.)

# A

**2.** A. Twenty-year-old patient:

$$r = 3.5 \text{ mm}$$
$$A_1 = \pi r^2$$
$$A_1 = \pi\,(3.5)^2$$
$$A_1 = 12.15\pi$$

Seventy-year-old patient:

$$r = 1 \text{ mm}$$
$$A_2 = \pi r^2$$
$$A_2 = \pi\,(1)^2$$
$$A_2 = \pi$$

Percentage reduction:

$$(A_1 - A_2)/A_1 = (12.25\,\pi - \pi)/12.25\pi = 92\%$$

B. $OD = \log(1/T)$

$$T = \pi/12.25\pi$$
$$T = 0.0816$$
$$OD = \log(1/T)$$
$$OD = 1.09$$

**3.** A. Anisometropic amblyopia of the left eye.

B. No. The expected reduction in binocular cortical neurons results in reduced stereoacuity.

C. i. Fully correct the refractive error.

ii. Encourage use of left eye by part-time patching of the right eye.

iii. Prescribe orthoptics which require the simultaneous use of both eyes.

iv. Carefully monitor the patient's progress.

**4.** As there are no indications of pathology, the left eye may be amblyopic; however, a cataract that develops at 15 years of age does not produce amblyopia. Perhaps the cataract was present earlier in life, during the critical period, but was cosmetically noticeable at age 15.

**5.** A. No. The child is past the critical period.

B. Very poor stereopsis. No binocular cortical cells have developed.

# References


Abney WW. *Researches in Color Vision and the Trichromatic Theory.* London: Longmans, Green; 1913.

Abramov I, Gordon J, Hendrickson A, et al. The retina of the newborn human infant. *Science.* 1982;217:265–267.

Adams AJ. Impact of new and emerging instrumentation on optometry. *Optom Vis Sci.* 1993;70:272–278.

Adams AJ, Bodis-Wollner I, Enoch JM, et al. Normal and abnormal mechanisms of vision: Visual disorders and visual deprivation. In: Spillman L, Werner JS, eds. *Visual Perception: The Neurophysiological Foundations.* New York: Academic Press; 1990:381–416.

Adams AJ, Haegerstrom-Portnoy G. Color deficiency. In: Amos JF, ed. *Diagnosis and Management in Vision Care.* Boston: Butterworths; 1987.

Adams AJ, Rodic R, Husted R, Stamper R. Spectral sensitivity and color discrimination changes in glaucoma and glaucoma-suspect patients. *Invest Ophthalmol Vis Sci.* 1982;23:516–524.

Adams RJ, Maurer D, Cashin HA. The influence of stimulus size on newborn's discrimination of chromatic from achromatic stimuli. *Vision Res.* 1990;30:2023–2030.

Adelson EH, Movshon JA. Phenomenal coherence of moving visual patterns. *Nature.* 1982;300:523– 525.

Aguilar M, Stiles WS. Saturation of the rod mechanism of the retina at high levels of stimulation. *Opt Acta.* 1954;1:59–65.

Ahissar M, Hochstein S. Task difficulty and the specificity of perceptual learning. *Nature.* 1997;387:401–406.

Albright JD. Direction and orientation selectivity of neurons in visual area MT of the macaque. *J Neurophysiol.* 1984;52:1106–1130.

Allen D, Banks MS, Norcia AM. Does chromatic sensitivity develop more slowly than luminance sensitivity? *Vision Res.* 1993;33:2553–2562.

Alpern M, Moeller J. The red and green cone visual pigments of deuteranomalous trichromacy. *J Physiol.* 1977;266:647–675.

Alpern M, Torii S. The luminosity curve of the protanomalous fovea. *J Gen Physiol.* 1968a;52:717–737.

Alpern M, Torii S. The luminosity curve of the deuteranomalous fovea. *J Gen Physiol.* 1968b;52:738–749.

Alpern M, Wake T. Cone pigment in human deutan colour vision defects. *J Physiol.* 1977;266:595–612.

Apple DJ, Rabb MF. *Ocular Pathology: Clinical Applications and Self Assessment.* St. Louis: Mosby-Year Book; 1991.

Applegate RA, Bonds AB. Induced movement of receptor alignment toward a new pupillary aperture. *Invest Ophthalmol Vis Sci.* 1981;21:869–873.

Arden GB, Barrada A. Analysis of the electrooculograms of a series of normal subjects. *Br J Ophthalmol.* 1962;46:468–481.

Arden GB, Barrada A, Kelsey JH. New clinical test of retinal function based upon the standing potential of the eye. *Br J Ophthalmol.* 1962;46:449–467.

Armington JC. *The Electroretinogram.* New York: Academic Press; 1974.

Bailey IL, Lovie JE. New design principles of visual acuity letter charts. *Am J Optom Physiol Opt.* 1976;53:740–745.

Ball K, Owsley C. Identifying correlates of accident involvement in older drivers. *Hum Factors.* 1991;33:583–595.

Ball K, Owsley C, Sloane ME, et al. Visual attention problems as a predictor of vehicle crashes in older adults. *Invest Ophthalmol Vis Sci.* 1993;34:3110–3123.

Ball KK, Sekuler R. A specific and enduring improvement in visual motion discrimination. *Science.* 1982;218:697–698.

Banks MS, Aslin RN, Letson RD. Sensitive period for the development of human binocular vision. *Science.* 1975;190:675–677.

Banks M, Bennett P. Optical and photoreceptor immaturaties limit the spatial and chromatic vision of human neonates. *J Opt Soc Am A.* 1988;5:2059–2079.

Banks M, Salapatek P. Acuity and contrast sensitivity in 1-, 2-, and 3-month-old human infants. *Invest Ophthalmol Vis Sci.* 1978;17:361–365.

Barlow HB. Retinal noise and absolute threshold. *J Opt Soc Am.* 1956;46:634–639.

Barlow HB. Temporal and spatial summation in human vision at different background intensities. *J Physiol.* 1958;141:337–350.

Barlow HB. Optic nerve impulses and Weber's law. *Cold Spring Harb Symp Quant Biol.* 1965;30:539–546.

Barlow HB, Blakemore C, Pettigrew JP. The neural mechanisms of binocular depth discrimination. *J Physiol.* 1967;193:327–342.

Barlow HB, Fitzhugh R, Kuffler SW. Change in organization in the receptive fields of the cat's retina during dark adaptation. *J Physiol.* 1957;137:338–354.

Barmack NH. Dynamic visual acuity as an index of eye movement control. *Vision Res.* 1970;10:1377–1391.

Barnes S, Werblin F. Gated currents generate single spike activity in amacrine cells of tiger salamander retina. *Proc Natl Acad Sci USA.* 1986;83:1509–1512.

Bartley SH. Subjective brightness in relation to flash rate and the light/dark ratio. *J Exp Psychol.* 1938;23:313–319.

Bartley SH. *Vision: A Study of Its Basis.* New York: Hafner; 1963.

Barton JJS, Sharpe JA, Raymond JE. Directional defects in pursuit and motion perception in humans with unilateral cerebral lesions. *Brain.* 1996;119:1535–1550.

Baylor DA, Nunn BS, Schnapf JL. The photocurrent, noise and spectral sensitivity of rods of the monkey *Macaca fascicularis. J Physiol.* 1984;357:575–607.

Beard BL, Levi DM, Reich LN. Perceptual learning in parafoveal vision. *Vision Res.* 1995;35:1679–1690.

Bearse MA, Sutter EE, Sim D, et al. Glaucomatous dysfunction revealed in higher order components of the electroretinogram. In: *Vision Science and Its Applications, 1996 OSA Technical Digest Series, Vol. 1,* Washington, D.C.: Optical Society of America; 1996:104–107.

Berson EL. Electrical phenomena in the retina. In: Hart MH, ed. *Adler's Physiology of the Eye,* 9th ed. St. Louis: Mosby-Year Book; 1992:641–707.

Bieber M, Volbrecht V, Werner J. Spectral efficiency measured by heterochromatic flicker photometry is similar in human infants and adults. *Vision Res.* 1995;35:1385–1392.

Birch E, Gwiazda J, Held R. Stereoacuity development for crossed and uncrossed disparities in human infants. *Vision Res.* 1982;22:507–513.

Birch EE, Stager DR. Monocular acuity and stereopsis in infantile esotropia. *Invest Ophthalmol Vis Sci.* 1985;26:1624–1630.

Birch J. *Diagnosis of Defective Colour Vision.* Oxford: Oxford University Press; 1993.

Bisiach E, Rusconi ML. Breakdown of perceptual awareness in unilateral neglect. *Cortex.* 1990;26:643–649.

Blakemore C, Campbell FW. On the existence of neurones in the human visual system selectively sensitive to the orientation and size of retinal images. *J Physiol.* 1969;203: 237–260.

Blakemore C, Cooper CF. Development of the brain depends on the visual environment. *Nature.* 1970;228:477–478.

Blakemore CB, Van Sluyters RC. Reversal of the physiological effects of monocular deprivation in kittens: Further evidence for a sensitive period. *J Physiol.* 1974;237:195–216.

Bodis-Wollner I, Atkin A, Raab E, Wolkstein M. Visual association cortex and vision in man: Pattern-evoked occipital potentials in a blind boy. *Science.* 1977;198:629–630.

Bodis-Wollner I, Camisa JM. Contrast sensitivity measurement in clinical diagnosis. In: Lessel S, Van Dalen JTW, eds. *Neuroophthalmology 1980.* Amsterdam: Excerpta Medica; 1980;1:373–401.

Bosworth CF, Sample PA, Weinreb RN. Motion perception thresholds in areas of glaucomatous visual field loss. *Vision Res.* 1997;37:355–364.

Bowmaker JK, Dartnall HJA, Lythgoe JN, Mollon JD. The visual pigments of rods and cones in the rhesus monkey, *Macaca mulatta. J Physiol.* 1978;274:329–348.

Boynton RM. Implications of the minimally distinct border. *J Opt Soc Am.* 1973;63:1037–1043.

Boynton RM. *Human Color Vision.* New York: Holt, Rinehart, and Winston; 1979.

Bradley A, Freeman RD. Contrast sensitivity in anisometropic amblyopia. *Invest Ophthalmol Vis Sci.* 1981;21:467–476.

Brannan JR, Williams MC. The effects of age and reading ability on flicker threshold. *Clin Vision Sci.* 1988;3:137–142.

Breitmeyer BG. *Visual Masking.* New York: Oxford University Press; 1984.

Breitmeyer BG. Parallel processing in human vision: History, review, and critique. In: Brannon H, ed. *Applications of Parallel Processing in Vision.* Amsterdam: Elsevier; 1992:37–38.

Brenner E, Van Damme WJM. Judging distance from ocular convergence. *Vision Res.* 1998;38:493–498.

Broca A, Sulzer D. La sensation lumineuse en fonction du temps. *J Physiol Pathol Gen.* 1902;4:632–640.

Broca A, Sulzer D. La sensation lumineuse en fonction du temps. *J Physiol Pathol Gen.* 1904;6:55–68.

Brown A, Dobson V, Maier J. Visual acuity of human infants at scotopic, mesopic and photopic luminances. *Vision Res.* 1987;27:1845–1858.

Brown KT, Wiesel JW. Localization of origins of electroretinogram components by intraretinal recording in the intact cat eye. *J Physiol.* 1961;158:257–280.

Bullimore MA, Wood JM, Swenson K. Motion perception in glaucoma. *Invest Ophthalmol Vis Sci.* 1993;34:3526–3533.

Burr DC, Morrone MC, Ross J. Selective suppression of the magnocellular visual pathway during saccadic eye movements. *Nature*. 1994:371:511–513.

Campbell FW, Maffei L. Electrophysiological evidence for the existence of orientation and size detectors in the human visual system. *J Physiol*. 1970;207:635–652.

Campbell FW, Robson JG. Application of Fourier analysis to the visibility of gratings. *J Physiol*. 1968;197:551–566.

Carr RE, Siegel JM. *Visual Electrodiagnostic Testing: A Practical Guide for the Clinician*. Baltimore: Williams and Wilkins; 1982.

Casson EJ, Johnson CA, Nelson-Quigg JM. Temporal modulation perimetry: The effects of aging and eccentricity on sensitivity in normals. *Invest Ophthalmol Vis Sci*. 1993; 34:3096–3102.

Cavanagh P. Vision at equiluminance. In: Kulikowski JJ, Walsh V, Murray IJ, eds. *Limits of Vision*. Boca Raton, FL: CRC Press; 1991:234–250.

Cavanagh P. When colours move. *Nature*. 1996;379:26.

Cavanagh P, MacLeod DIA, Anstis SM. Equiluminance: Spatial and temporal factors and the contribution of blue-sensitive cones. *J Opt Soc Am [A]*. 1987;4:1428–1438.

Chapanis A. Spectral saturation and its relation to color-vision defects. *J Exp Psychol*. 1944;34:24–44.

Ciuffreda KJ, Levi DM, Selenow A. *Amblyopia*. Boston: Butterworth-Heinemann; 1991.

Ciuffreda KJ, Tannen B. *Eye Movement Basics for the Clinician*. St. Louis: Mosby; 1995.

Corbetta M, Miezin FM, Dobmeyer S, et al. Attentional modulation of neural processing of shape, color, and velocity in humans. *Science*. 1990;248:1556–1559.

Cornsweet T. *Visual Perception*. New York: Academic Press; 1970.

Crawford MLJ, von Noorden GK. Optically induced concomitant strabismus in monkeys. *Invest Ophthalmol Vis Sci*. 1980;19:1105–1109.

Cropper SJ, Derrington AM. Rapid colour-specific detection of motion in human vision. *Nature*. 1996;379:72–74.

Curcio CA, Allen KA. Topography of ganglion cells in human retina. *J Comp Neurol*. 1990;300:5–25.

Damasio A, Yamada T, Damasio H, et al. Central achromatopsia: Behavioral anatomic and physiologic aspects. *Neurology*. 1980;30:1064–1071.

deLange H. Research into the dynamic nature of the human fovea cortex systems with intermittent and modulated light: II. Phase shift in brightness and delay in color perception. *J Opt Soc Am*. 1958;48:784–789.

DeMonasterio FM, Gouras P. Functional properties of ganglion cells of the rhesus monkey retina. *J Physiol*. 1975;251:167–195.

Derrington AM, Krauskopf J, Lennie P. Chromatic mechanisms in lateral geniculate nucleus of macaque. *J Physiol*. 1984;357:241–265.

Desimone R, Duncan J. Neural mechanisms of selective visual attention. *Ann Rev Neurosci*. 1995;18:193–222.

DeValois RL, Abramov I, Jacobs GH. Analysis of response patterns of LGN cells. *J Opt Soc Am*. 1966;56:966–977.

DeValois RL, Albrecht DG, Thorell LG. Spatial frequency selectivity of cells in macaque visual cortex. *Vision Res*. 1982;22:545–549.

DeValois RL, Morgan HC, Polson MC, et al. Psychophysical studies on monkey vision. I. Macaque luminosity and color vision tests. *Vision Res*. 1974;14:53–67.

DeVries HL. The quantum character of light and its bearing upon threshold of vision, the differential sensitivity and visual acuity of the eye. *Physica*. 1943;10:553–564.

DeYoe EA, Van Essen DC. Concurrent processing streams in monkey visual cortex. *Trends Neurosci*. 1988;11:219–226.

Dobson V. Visual acuity testing in infants: From laboratory to clinic. In: Simons K, ed. *Early Visual Development: Normal and Abnormal*. New York: Oxford University Press; 1993:318–334.

Dobson V, Fulton AB, Manning K, et al. Cycloplegic refractions of premature infants. *Am J Ophthalmol*. 1981;91:490–495.

Dobson V, Teller D. Visual acuity in human infants: A review and comparison of behavioral and electrophysiological studies. *Vision Res*. 1978;18:1469–1483.

Donders FC. *On the Anomalies of Accommodation and Refraction of the Eye*. London: New Sydenham Society; 1864.

Dowling JE. Chemistry of visual adaptation in the rat. *Science*. 1960;188:114–118.

Dowling JE. *The Retina: An Approachable Part of the Brain*. Cambridge, MA: Harvard University Press; 1987

Dowling JE, Boycott BB. Organization of the primate retina: electron microscopy. *Proc R Soc Lond Biol Sci*. 1966;166:80–111.

Dreher B, Fukada Y, Rodieck RW. Identification, classification and anatomical segregation of cells with X-like and Y-like properties in the lateral geniculate nucleus of old-world primates. *J Physiol*. 1976;258:433–452.

Einthoven W, Jolly WA. The form and magnitude of the electrical response of the eye to stimulation by light at various intensities. *Q J Exp Physiol*. 1908;1:373–416.

Engel S, Zhang X, Wandell B. Colour tuning in human visual cortex measured with functional magnetic resonance imaging. *Nature*. 1997;388:68–71.

Enoch JM, Birch DG. Inferred positive phototropic activity in human photoreceptors. *Philos Trans R Soc Lond Biol Sci*. 1981;291:293–303.

Enoch JM, Fry GA. Characteristics of a model retinal receptor studied at microwave frequencies. *J Opt Soc Am*. 1958;48:899–911.

Enroth-Cugell C, Robson JG. The contrast sensitivity of retinal ganglion cells of the cat. *J Physiol*. 1966;187:517–552.

Fain GL, Mathews, HR. Calcium and the mechanism of light adaptation in vertebrate photoreceptors. *Vis Neurosci*. 1990;10:981–989.

Famiglietti EV, Kolb H. Structural basis for ON- and OFF-center responses in retinal ganglion cells. *Science*. 1976;194:193–195.

Fechner GT. *Elemente der Psychophysik*. Leipzig: Breitkopf und Hartel; 1860.

Ferry ES. Persistence of vision. *Am J Sci*. 1892;44:192–207.

Fiorentini A, Berardi N. Perceptual learning specific for orientation and spatial frequency. *Nature*. 1980;287:43–44.

Flom MC, Weymouth FW, Kahneman D. Visual resolution and contour interaction. *J Opt Soc Am*. 1963;53:1026–1032.

Fuster JM, Jervey JP. Inferotemporal neurons distinguish and retain behaviorally relevant features of visual stimuli. *Science*. 1981;212:952–955.

Gallant JL, Braun J, Van Essen DC. Selectivity for polar, hyperbolic, and cartesian gratings in macaque visual cortex. *Science*. 1993;259:100–103.

Gilbert CD. Laminar differences in receptive field properties of cells in cat primary visual cortex. *J Physiol*. 1977;268:391–421.

Gouras P, Carr RE. Cone activity in the light-induced DC response of monkey retina. *Invest Ophthalmol*. 1965;4:318–321.

Gouras P, Du J, Yamamoto S, Kjeldbye H. Anatomy and physiology of photoreceptor transplants in degenerate C3H mouse retina. *Invest Ophthalmol Vis Sci*. 1993;34:1096.

Granit R, Harper P. Comparative studies on the peripheral and central retina: II. Synaptic reaction in the eye. *Am J Physiol.* 1930;95:211–228.

Grassman H. On the theory of compound colors. *Philos Mag.* 1854;7:254–264.

Gregory RL. *Concepts and Mechanisms of Perception.* London: Duckworth; 1974.

Gregory RL. *Eye and Brain.* 3rd ed. New York: McGraw-Hill; 1978.

Gross CG. Inferotemporal cortex and vision. *Prog Physiol Psychol.* 1973;5:77–115.

Gwiazda J, Mohindra I, Brill S, Held R. Infant astigmatism and meridional amblyopia. *Vision Res.* 1985;25:1269–1276.

Gwiazda J, Scheiman M, Mohindra I, Held R. Astigmatism in infants: Changes in axis and amount from birth to six years. *Invest Ophthalmol Vis Sci.* 1984;25:88–92.

Gwiazda J, Thorn F, Bauer J, et al. Emmetropization and the progression of manifest refraction in children followed from infancy to puberty. *Clin Vision Sci.* 1993;8:337–344.

Haegerstrom-Portnoy G. The vision of rod monochromats. *Optom Vis Sci.* 1991;68(12s): 21.

Halliday AM, McDonald WI, Mushin J. Delayed visual responses in optic neuritis. *Lancet.* 1972;1:982–985.

Hansen RM, Fulton AB. Development of scotopic retinal sensitivity. In: Simons K, ed. *Early Visual Development: Normal and Abnormal.* New York: Oxford Press; 1993:130–142.

Harwerth RS, Smith EL, Duncan GC, et al. Multiple sensitive periods in the development of the primate visual system. *Science.* 1987;232:235–238.

Hawken MJ, Blakemore C, Morley JW. Development of contrast sensitivity and temporal-frequency selectivity in primate lateral geniculate nucleus. *Exp Brain Res.* 1997;114:86–98.

Heath GG. Color vision. In: Wick R, Hirsch MJ, eds. *Children's Vision.* Philadelphia: Chilton; 1963.

Hecht S. Rods, cones and the chemical basis of vision. *Physiol Rev.* 1937;17:239–290.

Hecht S, Haig L, Chase AM. The influence of light adaptation on subsequent dark adaptation of the eye. *J Gen Physiol.* 1937;20:831–850.

Hecht S, Shlaer S, Pirenne MH. Energy, quanta, and vision. *J Gen Physiol.* 1942; 25:819–840.

Held R. What can rates of development tell us about underlying mechanisms? In: Granrud C, ed. *Visual Perception and Cognition in Infancy.* Hillsdale: Erlbaum; 1993:75–89.

Held R, Birch EE, Gwiazda J. Stereoacuity of human infants. *Proc Natl Acad Sci USA.* 1980;77:5572–5574.

Hering E. *Outlines of a Theory of Light Sense* (translated by Hurvich LM, Jameson D). Cambridge, MA: Harvard University Press; 1964 (originally published 1920).

Hess RF, Carney LG. Vision through an abnormal cornea. *Invest Ophthalmol Vis Sci.* 1979;18:470–483.

Hess RF, Woo G. Vision through cataracts. *Invest Ophthalmol Vis Sci.* 1978;17:428–435.

Higgins KE, Moskowitz–Cook A, Knoblauch K. Color vision testing: An alternative "source" of illuminant C. In: Verriest G, ed. *Modern Problems in Ophthalmology.* Basel: Karger; 1978;19:113–121.

Hitchcock PF, Hickey TL. Ocular dominance columns: Evidence for their presence in humans. *Brain Res.* 1980;182:176–179.

Hoffman KP, Stone J. Conduction velocity of afferents to cat visual cortex: A correlation with cortical receptive field properties. *Brain Res.* 1971;32:460–466.

Holopigian K, Blake R, Greenwald MJ. Selective losses in binocular vision in anisometropic amblyopes. *Vision Res.* 1986;26:621–630.

Hood DC, Holopigian K, Greenstein V, et al. A comparison of visual field loss to multifocal ERG changes in patients with RP. In: *Vision Science and Its Applications, 1997 OSA Technical Digest Series, Vol. 1,* Washington, D.C.: Optical Society of America; 1997:272–275.

Howland HC, Braddick O, Atkinson J, Howland B. Optics of photorefraction: Orthogonal and isotropic methods. *J Opt Soc Am.* 1983; 73:1701–1708.

Howland HC, Sayles N. A photorefractive characterization of focusing ability of infants and young children. *Invest Ophthalmol Vis Sci.* 1987;28:1005–1015.

Hsia Y, Graham CH. Spectral luminosity curves for protanopic, deuteranopic and normal subjects. *Proc Natl Acad Sci USA.* 1957;43:1011–1019.

Hubel DH. *Eye, Brain, and Vision.* New York: Scientific American Library; 1988.

Hubel DH, Wiesel TN. Receptive fields of single neurons in the cat's striate cortex. *J Physiol.* 1959;148:574–591.

Hubel DH, Wiesel TN. Receptive fields, binocular interaction and functional architecture in the cat's visual cortex. *J Physiol.* 1962;160:106–154.

Hubel DH, Wiesel TN. Receptive fields and functional architecture in two non-striate visual areas (18 and 19) of the cat. *J Physiol.* 1965a;28:229–289.

Hubel DH, Wiesel TN. Binocular interaction in striate cortex of kittens reared with artificial squint. *J Neurophysiol.* 1965b;28:1041–1059.

Hubel DH, Wiesel TN. Receptive fields and functional architecture of monkey striate cortex. *J Physiol.* 1968;195:215–243.

Hubel DH, Wiesel TN. Sequence regularity and geometry of orientation columns in the monkey striate cortex. *J Comp Neurol.* 1974;158:267–294.

Hubel DH, Wiesel TN. Functional architecture of macaque monkey visual cortex. *Proc R Soc Lond Biol Sci.* 1977;198:1–59.

Hubel DH, Wiesel TN, Stryker MP. Anatomical demonstration of orientation columns in macaque monkey. *J Comp Neur.* 1978;177:361–380.

Hung L-F, Crawford MLJ, Smith EL. Spectacle lenses alter eye growth and the refractive status of young monkeys. *Nature Med.* 1995;1:761–765.

Hurvich LM. *Color Vision.* Sunderland, MA: Sinauer Associates; 1981.

Ingling CR, Martinez-Uriegas E. Simple opponent receptive fields are asymmetrical: G-cone centers predominate. *J Opt Soc Am.* 1983;73:1527–1532.

Ishai A, Sagi D. Common mechanisms of visual imagery and perception. *Science.* 1995; 268:1772–1774.

Ittleson WH, Kilpatrick FP. Experiments in perception. *Sci Am.* 1951;185:50–55.

Johnson CA. Early losses of visual function in glaucoma. *Am J Optom Physiol Opt.* 1995;72:359–370.

Johnson CA, Casson EJ, Adams AJ, et al. Progression of glaucomatous visual field loss over five years: A comparison of white-on-white and blue-on-yellow perimetry. *Invest Ophthalmol Vis Sci.* 1992;33:1384.

Johnson EP, Riggs LA, Schick AML. Photopic retinal potentials evoked by phased alterations of a barred pattern. In: Burian HM, Jacobson JH, eds. *Clinical Electroretinography, Proceedings of the Third International Symposium.* Oxford: Pergamon; 1966:75–91.

Judd DB. *Color in Business, Science, and Industry.* New York: Wiley; 1952.

Judd DB, Wyszecki G. *Color in Business, Science, and Industry.* New York: Wiley; 1963.

Kaiser PK, Comerford JP, Bodinger DM. Saturation of spectral lights. *J Opt Soc Am.* 1976;66:818–826.

Kalmus H. The familial distribution of congenital tritanopia with some remarks on some similar conditions. *Ann Hum Genet.* 1955;20:39–56.

Kaufman L, Rock I. The moon illusion. I. *Science.* 1962;136:953–961.

Kelly DH. Visual responses to time-dependent stimuli. 1. Amplitude sensitivity measures. *J Opt Soc Am.* 1961;51:422–429.

Kelly DH. Spatiotemporal variation of chromatic and achromatic contrast thresholds. *J Opt Soc Am.* 1983;73:742–750.

Kelly JP, Borchert K, Teller DY. The development of chromatic and achromatic contrast sensitivity in infancy as tested with the sweep VEP. *Vision Res.* 1997;37:2057–2072.

King-Smith PE, Carden D. Luminance and opponent-color contributions to visual detection and adaptation and to temporal and spatial integration. *J Opt Soc Am.* 1976;66:709–717.

Kiorpes L. Development of vernier acuity and grating acuity in normally reared monkeys. *Vis Neurosci.* 1992;9:243–251.

Knowles A. The biochemical aspects of vision. In: Barlow HB, Mollon JD, eds. *The Senses.* Cambridge: Cambridge University Press; 1982;82–101.

Kolb B, Whishaw IQ. *Fundamentals of Human Neuropsychology.* San Francisco: Freeman; 1980.

Köllner H. *Die Störungen des Farbensinnes. ihre klinische Bedeutung und ihre Diagnose.* Berlin: Karger; 1912.

Korte A. Kinematoskopische Untersuchungen. *Z Psychol.* 1915;72:193–206.

Kosslyn SM, Oschner KN. In search of occipital activation during visual mental imagery. *Trends Neurosci.* 1994;17:290–292.

Krauskopf J, Mollon JD. The independence of the temporal integration properties of individual chromatic mechanisms in the human eye. *J Physiol.* 1971;219:611–623.

Krill AE. Congenital color defects. In: Krill AR, Archer DB, eds. *Krill's Hereditary Retinal and Choroidal Diseases. Vol. II. Clinical Characteristics.* Hagerstown, MD: Harper and Row; 1977.

Kuffler SW. Discharge patterns and functional organization of mammalian retina. *J Neurophysiol.* 1953;16:37–68.

Lachenmayr BJ, Kojetinsky S, Ostermaier N, et al. The different effects of aging on normal sensitivity in flicker and light-sense perimetry. *Invest Ophthal Vis Sci.* 1994;35:2741–2748.

Lamb T. Transduction in vertebrate photoreceptors: The roles of cyclic GMP and calcium. *Trends Neurosci.* 1986;May:224–228.

Land EH. The retinex. *Sci Am.* 1964;52:247–264.

Lee BB, Martin PR, Valberg A. The physiological basis of heterochromatic flicker photometry demonstrated in the ganglion cells of the macaque retina. *J Physiol.* 1988;404:323–347.

Lee BB, Pokorny J, Smith VC, et al. Luminance and chromatic modulation sensitivity of macaque ganglion cells and human observers. *J Opt Soc Am [A].* 1990;7:2223–2236.

LeGrand Y. *Light Color and Vision.* London: Chapman and Hall; 1968.

Lennie P. Recent developments in the physiology of color vision. *Trends Neurosci.* 1984;7:243–248.

Lennie P, Krauskopf J, Sclar G. Chromatic mechanisms in striate cortex of macaque. *J Neurosci.* 1990;2:649–669.

Lennie P, Trevarthen C, Van Essen D, Wässle H. Parallel processing of visual information. In: Spillman L, Werner JS, eds. *Visual Perception: The Neurophysiological Foundations.* New York: Academic Press; 1990:103–128.

Leopold DA, Logothetis NK. Activity changes in early visual cortex reflect monkeys' percepts during binocular rivlary. *Nature.* 1996;379:549–553.

Lerman S. *Radiant Energy and the Eye.* New York: MacMillan; 1980.

Lettvin JY, Maturana HR, McCulloch WS, Pitts WH. What the frog's eye tells the frog's brain. *Proc Inst Radio Eng.* 1959;47:1940–1951.

Levi DM. Amblyopia: A developmental disorder of spatial vision. *Optom Vis Sci.* 1992;69 (12s):123.

Levi DM, Carkeet A. Amblyopia: A consequence of abnormal visual development. In: Simons K, ed. *Early Visual Development: Normal and Abnormal.* New York: Oxford Press; 1993:391–408.

Levi DM, Harwerth RS. Spatiotemporal interactions in anisometropic and strabismic amblyopia. *Invest Ophthalmol Vis Sci.* 1977;16:90–95.

Levi DM, Klein SA, Aitsebaomo AP. Vernier acuity, crowding, and cortical magnification. *Vision Res.* 1985;25:963–977.

Levi DM, Polat U, Ying-Sheng H. Improvement in vernier acuity in adults with amblyopia. *Invest Ophthal Vis Sci.* 1997;38:1493–1510.

Levine MW, Shefner JM. *Fundamentals of Sensation and Perception.* 2nd ed. Pacific Grove, CA: Brooks/Cole; 1991.

Liebman P. Microspectrophotometry of photoreceptors. In: Dartnall HJA, ed. *Handbook of Sensory Physiology VII/1.* New York: Springer–Verlag; 1972.

Lindberg KA, Fisher SK. An ultrastructural study of inter-plexiform cell synapses in human retina. *J Comp Neurol.* 1986;243:561–576.

Livingstone MS, Hubel DH. Psychophysical evidence for separate channels for the perception of form, color, movement, and depth. *J Neurosci.* 1987;7:3466–3468.

Livingstone MS, Hubel DH. Segregation of form, color, movement, and depth: Anatomy, physiology, and perception. *Science.* 1988;240:740–749.

Livingstone MS, Rosen GD, Drislane FW, Galaburda AM. Physiological and anatomical evidence for a magnocellular defect in developmental dyslexia. *Proc Natl Acad Sci USA.* 1991;88:7943–7947.

Logothetis NK. Physiological studies of motion inputs. In: Smith AT, Snowden RJ, eds. *Visual Detection of Motion.* New York: Academic Press; 1994:177–216.

Logothetis NK, Schiller PH, Charles ER, Hurlbert AC. Perceptual deficits and the activity of the color-opponent and broad-band pathways at isoluminance. *Science.* 1990;247: 214–217.

Lovegrove WJ, Garzia RP, Nicholson SB. Experimental evidence for a transient system deficit in specific reading disability. *J Am Optom Assoc.* 61;1990:137–146.

Lund JS, Henry GH, MacQueen CL, Harvey AR. Anatomical organization of the primary visual cortex (area 17) of the cat. A comparison with area 17 of the macaque monkey. *J Comp Neurol.* 1979;184:599–618.

MacAdam DL. *Sources of Color Vision.* Cambridge, MA: The MIT Press; 1970.

Maddess T, Henry GH. Performance of nonlinear visual units in ocular hypertension and glaucoma. *Clin Vision Sci.* 1992;7:371–383.

Maffei L, Fiorentini A. Electroretinographic responses to gratings before and after section of the optic nerve. *Science.* 1981;211:953–955.

Manny RE, Klein SA. The development of vernier acuity in infants. *Curr Eye Res.* 1984;3:453–462.

Manny RE, Klein SA. A three alternative tracking paradigm to measure vernier acuity of older infants. *Vision Res.* 1985;25:1245–1252.

Matin E. Saccadic suppression: A review and analysis. *Psychol Bull.* 1974;81:899–917.

Matin E, Clymer A, Matin L. Metacontrast and saccadic suppression. *Science.* 1972;178: 179–182.

Maunsell JHR. The brain's visual world: Representation of visual targets in cerebral cortex. *Science.* 1995;270:764–769.

Maunsell JHR, Nealey TA, DePriest DD. Magnocellular and parvocellular contributions to responses in the middle temporal visual area (MT) of the macaque monkey. *J Neurosci.* 1990;10:3323–3334.

Maunsell JHR, Newsome WT. Visual processing in monkey extrastriate cortex. *Ann Rev Neurosci.* 1987;10:363–401.

Maunsell JH, Van Essen DC. Functional properties of neurons in the middle temporal area of the macaque monkey. I. Selectivity for stimulus direction, speed, and orientation. *J Neurophysiol.* 1983;49:1127–1147.

Mayer DL, Beiser AS, Warner AF, et al. Monocular acuity norms for the Teller Acuity Cards between ages one month and four years. *Invest Ophthalmol Vis Sci.* 1995;36: 671–685.

Mayer MJ, Kim CBY, Svingos A, Glucs A. Foveal flicker sensitivity in healthy aging eyes: I: Compensating for pupil variation. *J Opt Soc Am A.* 1988;5:2201–2209.

Mayer MJ, Spiegler JJ, Ward B, et al. Mid-frequency loss of foveal flicker sensitivity in early stages of age-related maculopathy. *Invest Ophthalmol Vision Sci.* 1992;33: 3136–3142.

McDonald MA, Dobson V, Sebris SL, et al. The acuity card procedure: A rapid test of infant acuity. *Invest Ophthalmol Vis Sci.* 1985;26:1158–1162.

Merbs SL, Nathans J. Absorption spectra of human cone pigments. *Nature.* 1992;356: 433–435.

Merigan WH. Chromatic and achromatic vision of macaques: Role of the P pathway. *J Neurosci.* 1989;9:776–783.

Merigan WH, Maunsell JHR. Macaque vision after magnocellular lateral geniculate lesions. *Vis Neurosci.* 1990;5:347–352.

Merigan WH, Maunsell JHR. How parallel are the primate pathways? *Ann Rev Neurosci.* 1993;16:369–402.

Miller JW, Ludvigh E. The effect of relative motion on visual acuity. *Surv Ophthalmol.* 1962;7:83–116.

Millodot M. Image formation in the eye. In: Barlow HB, Mollon JD, eds. *The Senses.* Cambridge: Cambridge University Press; 1982:46–61.

Mishkin M, Ungerleider LG, Macko KA. Object vision and spatial vision: Two cortical pathways. *Trends Neurosci.* 1983;6:414–417.

Mitchell DE, Freeman RD, Millodot M, Haegerstrom G. Meridional amblyopia: Evidence for modification of the human visual system by early visual experience. *Vision Res.* 1973;13:535–558.

Mitchell DE, Reardon J, Muir DW. Interocular transfer of motion aftereffect in normal and stereo blind observers. *Exp Brain Res.* 1975;22:163–173.

Mohindra I, Held R. Refraction in human infants from birth to five years. *Doc Ophthalmol.* 1981;28:19–27.

Mohindra I, Held R, Gwiazda J, Brill S. Astigmatism in human infants. *Science.* 1978;202:329–331.

Mollon JD, Bowmaker, JK. The spatial arrangement of cones in the primate fovea. *Nature.* 1992;360:677–679.

Moran J, Desimone R. Selective attention gates visual processing in extrastriate cortex. *Science.* 1985;229:782–784.

Morgan MW, Rosenbloom AA. *Vision and Aging*. 2nd ed. Boston: Butterworth-Heinemann; 1993.

Morrone MC, Burr DC, Fiorentini A. Development of infant contrast sensitivity to chromatic stimuli. *Vision Res*. 1993;33:2535–2552.

Motter BC. Neural correlates of attentive selection for color or luminance in extrastriate area V4. *J Neurosci*. 1994;14:2178–2189.

Movshon JA, Adelson EH, Gizzi MS, Newsome WT. The analysis of moving visual patterns. In: Chagas C, Gattass R, Gross C, eds. *Pattern Recognition Mechanisms*. Vatican City: Pontifical Academy of Sciences; 1985:117–151.

Movshon JA, Eggers HM, Gizzi MS, et al. Effects of early unilateral blur on the macaque's visual system: III. Physiological observations. *J Neurosci*. 1987;7:1340–1351.

Movshon JA, Kiorpes L. Analysis of the development of spatial contrast sensitivity in monkey and human infants. *J Opt Soc Am A*. 1988;5:2166–2172.

Mutti DO, Zadnick K, Adams AJ. The nature versus nurture debate goes on. *Invest Ophthalmol Vis Sci*. 1996;37:952–957.

Nakayama K. Biological motion processing: A review. *Vision Res*. 1985;25:625–660.

Nakayama K, Tyler CW. Psychophysical isolation of movement sensitivity by removal of positional cues. *Vision Res*. 1981;21:427–433.

Nathans J. The genes for color vision. *Sci Am*. 1989;260(2):42–49.

Nathans J, Piantanida TP, Eddy RL, et al. Molecular genetics of inherited variation in human color vision. *Science*. 1986a;232:203–210.

Nathans J, Thomas D, Hogness DS. Molecular genetics of human color vision: the genes encoding blue, green, and red pigments. *Science*. 1986b;232:193–202.

Neitz J, Jacobs GH. Polymorphism of long-wavelength cone in normal human colour vision. *Nature*. 1986;323:623–625.

Neitz J, Neitz M. Color Vision Defects. In: Wright AF, Barrie, J, eds. *Molecular Genetics of Inherited Eye Disorders*. Harwood Academic Publishers; 1994:217–257.

Neitz J, Neitz M, Kainz PM. Visual pigment gene structure and the severity of color vision defects. *Science*. 1996;274:801–803.

Newman N. *Neuro-Ophthalmology: A Practical Text*. Norwalk, CT: Appleton & Lange; 1992.

Newsome WT, Paré EB. A selective impairment of motion perception following lesions of middle temporal visual area (MT). *J Neurosci*. 1988;8:2201–2211.

Newsome WT, Wurtz RH. Probing visual cortical function with discrete chemical lesions. *Trends Neurosci*. 1988;11:394–400.

Norcia AM, Tyler CW. Spatial frequency sweep VEP: Visual acuity in the first year of life. *Vision Res*. 1985;25:1399–1408.

Norcia AM, Tyler CW, Allen D. Electrophysiological assessment of contrast sensitivity in human infants. *Am J Optom Physiol Opt*. 1986;63:12–15.

Ogle KN. *Researches in Binocular Vision*. Philadelphia: Saunders; 1950.

Olson CR, Freeman RD. Profile of the sensitive period for monocular deprivation in kittens. *Exp Brain Res*. 1980;39:17–21.

Østerberg G. Topography of the layer of rods and cones in the human retina. *Acta Ophthalmol Suppl*. 1935;6:1–103.

Owsley C, Sekular R, Siemsen D. Contrast sensitivity throughout adulthood. *Vision Res*. 1983;23:689–699.

Packer O, Hartmann EE, Teller DY. Infant color vision: The effect of field size on Rayleigh discriminations. *Vision Res*. 1984;24:1247–1260.

Pelli PG, Robson JG, Wilkins AJ. The design of a new letter chart for measuring contrast sensitivity. *Clin Vision Sci*. 1988;2:187–199.

Pirenne MH. *Vision and The Eye*. London: Chapman and Hall; 1967.

Pitt FHG. *Characteristics of Dichromatic Vision with an Appendix on Anomalous Trichromatic Vision*. Great Britain Medical Report Series, no. 200; 1935.

Pitts DG. The human ultraviolet action spectrum. *Am J Optom Arch Am Acad Optom*. 1974;51:946–960.

Pitts DG. The effects of aging on selected visual functions: Dark adaptation, visual acuity, stereopsis and brightness contrast. In: Sekular R, Kline DW, Dismukes K, eds. *Aging in Human Visual Functions*. New York: Liss; 1982.

Pokorny J, Smith VC. Wavelength discrimination in the presence of chromatic fields. *J Opt Soc Am*. 1970;60:562–569.

Pokorny J, Smith VC, Verriest G, Pinckers AJLG. *Congenital and Acquired Color Vision Defects*. New York: Grune and Stratton; 1979.

Polyak SL. *The Retina*. Chicago: University of Chicago Press; 1941.

Porter TC. Contributions to the study of flicker, II. *Proc R Soc Lond*. 1902;70A:313–329.

Posner MI. Seeing the mind. *Science*. 1993;262:673–674.

Powers MK, Schneck M, Teller DY. Spectral sensitivity of human infants at absolute visual threshold. *Vision Res*. 1981;21:1005–1016.

Priest IG, Brickwedde FG. The minimum perceptible colorimetric purity as a function of dominant wavelength. *J Opt Soc Am*. 1938;28:133–139.

Pugh EN, Cobbs WH. Visual transduction in vertebrate rods and cones. *Vision Res*. 1986;26:1613–1643.

Purkinje J. *Opera Omnia Beobachtungen und Versuche zur Physiologie der Sinne*. Vol. 1. Prague: JG Calve; 1819.

Quigley HA, Addicks EM, Green WR. Optic nerve damage in human glaucoma. III. Quantitative correlation of nerve fiber loss and visual field defect in glaucoma, ischemic neuropathy, papilledema, and toxic neuropathy. *Arch Ophthalmol*. 1982;100: 135–146.

Quigley HA, Sanchez RM, Dunkelberger GR, et al. Chronic glaucoma selectivity damages large optic nerve fibers. *Invest Ophthalmol Vis Sci*. 1987;28: 913–920.

Rao SC, Rainer G, Miller EK. Integration of what and where in the primate prefrontal cortex. *Science*. 1997;276:821–824.

Ratliff F, Hartline HK, Miller WH. Spatial and temporal aspects of retinal inhibitory interaction. *J Opt Soc Am*. 1963;53:110–120.

Ratliff F, Riggs LA. Involuntary motions of the eye during monocular fixation. *J Exp Psychol*. 1950;40:687–701.

Raviola E, Wiesel TN. Effect of dark-rearing on experimental myopia in monkeys. *Invest Ophthalmol Vis Sci*. 1978;17:485–488.

Lord Rayleigh. Experiments on colour. *Nature*. 1881;25:64–66.

Rea MS. *Lighting Handbook: Reference and Application*. New York: Illuminating Engineering Society of North America; 1993.

Reeves BC, Wood JM, Hill AR. Vistech VCTS 6500 Charts—within and between session reliability. *Optom Vis Sci*. 1991;68:728–737.

Regal DM. Development of critical flicker fusion frequency in infants. *Vision Res*. 1981;21:549–555.

Regan D. *Human Brain Electrophysiology: Evoked Potentials and Evoked Magnetic Fields in Science and Medicine*. New York: Elsevier; 1989.

Riggs LA, Ratliff F, Cornsweet JC, Cornsweet TN. The disappearance of steadily fixated test objects. *J Opt Soc Am*. 1953;43:495–501.

Riggs LA, Wooten BR. Electrical measures and psychophysical data on human vision. In: Jameson D, Hurvich LM, eds. *Handbook of Sensory Physiology*. Vol. VII/4. *Visual Psychophysics*. New York: Springer-Verlag; 1972:690–731.

Rodenstock HB, Swick DA. Color discrimination for the color blind. *Aerospace Med.* 1974;145:1194–1197.

Rodieck RW. Which cells code for color? In: Valberg A, Lee BB, eds. *From Pigments to Perception: Advances in Understanding Visual Processes*. New York: Plenum; 1991:83–93.

Rodman HR, Albright TD. Single-unit analysis of pattern-motion selective properties in the middle temporal visual area (MT). *Exp Brain Res.* 1989;75:53–64.

Rolls ET, Tovée MJ. Sparseness of the neuronal representation of stimuli in the primate temporal cortex. *J Neurophysiol.* 1995;73:713–726.

Rose A. The sensitivity performance of the human eye on an absolute scale. *J Opt Soc Am.* 1948;38:196–208.

Rushton WAH. Rhodopsin measurement and dark adaptation in a subject deficient in cone vision. *J Physiol.* 1961;156:193–205.

Rushton WAH. A cone pigment in the protanope. *J Physiol.* 1963a;168:345–359.

Rushton WAH. Cone pigment kinetics in the protanope. *J Physiol.* 1963b;168:374–388.

Rushton WAH. The Ferrier lecture. Visual adaptation. *Proc R Soc Lond Biol Sci.* 1965a;162:20–46.

Rushton WAH. A foveal pigment in the deuteranope. *J Physiol.* 1965b;176:24–37.

Rushton WAH. Visual pigments and color blindness. *Sci Am.* 1975;232(3):64–74.

Salzman CD, Newsome WT. Neural mechanisms for forming a perceptual decision. *Science.* 1994;264:231–237.

Salzmann M. *The Anatomy and Physiology of the Human Eyeball in the Normal State* (translated by Brown EVC). Chicago: University of Chicago Press; 1912.

Schiller PH. The effects of V4 and middle temporal (MT) area lesions on visual performance in the rhesus monkey. *Vis Neurosci.* 1993;10:717–746.

Schiller PH, Finlay BL, Volman SF. Quantitative studies of single-cell properties in monkey striate cortex. I. Spatiotemporal organization of receptive fields. *J Neurophysiol.* 1976;39:1288–1319.

Schiller PH, Logothetis NK, Charles ER. Functions of the color-opponent and broad-band channels of the visual system. *Nature.* 1990a;343:68–70.

Schiller PH, Logothetis NK, Charles ER. Role of color-opponent and broad-band channels in vision. *Vis Neurosci.* 1990b;5:321–346.

Schiller PH, Malpeli JG. Functional specificity of lateral geniculate laminae of the rhesus monkey. *J Neurophysiol.* 1978;41:788–797.

Schnapf JL, Baylor DA. How photoreceptors respond to light. *Sci Am.* 1987;256(4):40–47.

Schnapf JL, Kraft TW, Baylor DA. Spectral sensitivity of human cone photoreceptors. *Nature.* 1987;325:439–441.

Schneck ME, Haegerstrom-Portnoy G. Color vision defect type and spatial vision in the optic neuritis trial. *Invest Ophthalmol Vis Sci.* 1997;38:2278–2289.

Schwartz SH. Reaction time distributions and their relationship to the transient/sustained nature of the neural discharge. *Vision Res.* 1992;32:2087–2092.

Schwartz SH. Colour and flicker thresholds for high frequency increments. *Ophthalmic Physiol Opt.* 1993;13:299–302.

Schwartz SH. Spectral sensitivity of dichromats: Role of postreceptoral processes. *Vision Res.* 1994;34:2983–2990.

Schwartz SH, Godwin LD. Masking of the achromatic system: Implications for saccadic suppression. *Vision Res.* 1996;36:1551–1559.

Shapley R. Visual sensitivity and parallel retinocortical pathways. *Annu Rev Psychol.* 1990;41:635–658.

Shevell SK. Saturation in human cones. *Vision Res.* 1977;17:427–434.

Shinar D, Schieber F. Visual requirements for safety and mobility of older drivers. *Hum Factors.* 1991;33:507–519.

Sekuler R, Blake, R. *Perception.* New York: McGraw-Hill; 1990.

Siegwart JT, Norton TT. Refractive and ocular changes in tree shrews raised with plus or minus lenses. *Invest Ophthalmol Vis Sci.* 1993;34:1208.

Silverman SE, Trick GL, Hart WM. Motion perception is abnormal in primary open-angle glaucoma and ocular hypertension. *Invest Ophthalmol Vis Sci.* 1990;31:722–729.

Slaghuis WL, Lovegrove WJ. Spatial-frequency-dependent visible persistence and specific reading disability. *Brain Cogn.* 1985;4:219–240.

Slataper FJ. Age norms of refraction and vision. *Arch Ophthalmol.* 1950;43:466–481.

Slaughter MM, Miller RF. The role of glutamate receptors in information processing in the distal retina. In: Gallego A, Gouras P, eds. *Neurocircuitry of the Retina, A Cajal Memorial.* New York: Elsevier; 1985:51–65.

Smith VC, Pokorny J. Spectral sensitivity of the foveal cone photopigments between 400 nm and 500 nm. *Vision Res.* 1975;15:161–171.

Sokol S. The visually evoked cortical potential in optic nerve and visual pathway disorders. In: Fishman GA, Sokol S, eds. *Electrophysiologic Testing in Disorders of the Retina, Optic Nerve, and Visual Pathway.* San Francisco: American Academy of Ophthalmology; 1990:105–141.

Spear PD, Moore RJ, Kim CBY, et al. Effects of aging on the primate visual system: Spatial and temporal processing by lateral geniculate neurons in young adult and old rhesus monkeys. *J Neurophysiol.* 1994;72:402–420.

Sperling HG, Harwerth RS. Red-green cone interactions in the increment-threshold spectral sensitivity of primates. *Science.* 1971;172:180–184.

Sperling HG, Jolliffe CL. Intensity-time relationships at threshold for spectral stimuli in human vision. *J Opt Soc Am.* 1965;55:191–199.

Steinman BA, Steinman SB, Lehmkuhle S. Visual attention mechanisms show a center-surround organization. *Vision Res.* 1995;35:1859–1869.

Steinman SB, Levi DM, McKee SP. Discrimination of time and velocity in the amblyopic visual system. *Clin Vision Sci.* 1988;2:265–276.

Steinman SB, Steinman BA. Vision and Attention. I: Current models of visual attention. *Optom Vis Sci.* 1998;75:146–155.

Stell WK, Ishida AT, Lightfoot DO. Structural basis for on- and off-center responses in retinal bipolar cells. *Science.* 1977;198:1269–1271.

Stevens SS. On the psychophysical law. *Psychol Rev.* 1957;64:153–181.

Stiles WS. The directional sensitivity of the retina and the spectral sensitivities of the rods and cones. *Proc R Soc Lond Biol Sci.* 1939;127:64–105.

Stiles WS. Further studies of visual mechanisms by the two-colour threshold method. In: *Collequio Sobre Problemas Opticos de la Vision.* Madrid; 1953:63–103.

Stone J, Dreher B, Levanthal A. Hierarchical and parallel mechanisms in the organization of visual cortex. *Brain Res Rev.* 1979;1:345–394.

Stoner GR, Albright TD. The interpretation of visual motion: Evidence for surface segmentation mechanisms. *Vision Res.* 1996;36:1291–1310.

Stryer L. Cyclic GMP cascade of vision. *Annu Rev Neurosci.* 1986;9:87–119.

Stryker MP, Sherk H. Modification of cortical orientation selectivity in the cat by restricted visual experience: A reexamination. *Science.* 1975;190:904–906.

Stryker MP, Sherk H, Levanthal AG, Hirsch HVB. Physiological consequences for the cat's visual cortex of effectively restricting early visual experience with oriented contours. *J Neurophysiol.* 1978;41:896–909.

Sutter E, Tren D. The field topography of ERG components in men-1. The photopic luminance response. *Vision Res.* 1992;32:435–446.

Svaetichin G. Spectral response curves from single cones. *Acta Physiol Scand.* 1956;39 (suppl 134):17–46.

Swanson WH, Ueno T, Smith VC, Pokorny J. Temporal modulation sensitivity and pulse-detection thresholds for chromatic and luminance perturbations. *J Opt Soc Am [A].* 1987;4:1992–2005.

Swets JA, Tanner WP Jr, Birdsall TG. Decision processes in perception. *Psychol Rev.* 1961;68:301–340.

Tanaka K, Saito H, Fukada Y, Moriya M. Coding visual images of objects in the inferotemporal cortex of the macaque monkey. *J Neurophysiol.* 1991;66:170–189.

Teikari JM, Kaprio J, Koskenvuo MK, et al. Heritability estimate for refractive errors: A population-based sample of adult twins. *Gen Epidemiol.* 1988;5:171–181.

Teller DY. The forced-choice preferential looking procedure: A psychophysical technique for use with human infants. *Infant Behav Dev.* 1979;2:135–153.

Teller DY. Scotopic vision, color vision, and stereopsis in infants. *Curr Eye Res.* 1982;2: 199–210.

Teller DY. First glances: The vision of infants. *Invest Ophthalmol Vis Sci.* 1997;38: 2183–2203.

Teller DY, Morse R, Borton R, Regal D. Visual acuity for vertical and diagonal gratings in human infants. *Vision Res.* 1974;14:1433–1439.

Teller DY, Movshon JA. Visual development. *Vision Res.* 1986;26:1483–1506.

Teller DY, Peeples DR, Sekel M. Discrimination of chromatic from white light by two-month-old human infants. *Vision Res.* 1978;18:41–48.

Thorn F, Held R, Fang L. Orthogonal astigmatic axes in Chinese and Caucasian infants. *Invest Ophthalmol Vis Sci.* 1987;28:191–194.

Tomita T. Electrical activity of vertebrate photoreceptors. *Q Rev Biophys.* 1970;3:179–222.

Tootell RBH, Reppas JB, Dale AM, et al. Visual motion aftereffect in human cortical area MT revealed by functional magnetic resonance imaging. *Nature.* 1995;375:139–141.

Tovée MJ. *An Introduction to the Visual System.* Cambridge: Cambridge; 1996.

Tovée MJ, Cohen-Tovée EM. The neural substrates of face processing: A review. *Cogn Neuropsychol.* 1993;10:505–528.

Trick GL. Retinal potentials in patients with primary open angle glaucoma: Physiological evidence for temporal frequency tuning defects. *Invest Ophthalmol Vis Sci.* 1985;26:1750–1758.

Trick GL, Steinman SB, Amyot, M. Motion perception deficits in glaucomatous optic neuropathy. *Vision Res.* 1995;35:2225–2233.

Troxler D. Ueber das verschwinden gegebener Gegenstande innerhalb unseres Gesichtskreises. In: Himly K, Schmidt JA, eds. *Ophthalmische Bibliothek.* Jena: Fromann; 1804;2:51–53.

Ts'o DY, Gilbert CD. The organization of chromatic and spatial interactions in the primate striate cortex. *J Neurosci.* 1988;8:1712–1727.

Tyler CW. Specific defects of flicker sensitivity in glaucoma and ocular hypertension. *Invest Ophthalmol Vis Sci.* 1981;20:204–212.

Tyler CW, Ernst W, Lyness AL. Photopic flicker sensitivity losses in simplex and multiplex retinitis pigmentosa. *Invest Ophthalmol Vis Sci.* 1984;25:1035–1042.

Ungerleider LG. Functional brain imaging studies of cortical mechanisms for memory. *Science*. 1995;270:769–775.

Vaegan, Taylor D. Critical period for deprivation amblyopia in children. *Trans Ophthalmol Soc UK*. 1980;99:432–439.

Van Essen DC, Andersen CH, Felleman DJ. Information processing in the primate visual system: An integrated systems perspective. *Science*. 1992;255:419–423.

Van Loo JA, Enoch JM. The scotopic Stiles–Crawford effect. *Vision Res*. 1975;15:1005–1009.

Van Sluyters RC, Atkinson J, Banks MS, et al. The development of vision and visual perception. In: Spillman L, Werner JS, eds. *Visual Perception: The Neurophysiological Foundations*. New York: Academic Press; 1990;349–379.

Varner D, Cook JE, Schneck ME, et al. Tritan discriminations by 1- and 2-month-old human infants. *Vision Res*. 1985;2:821–831.

Verriest G, Uvijls A. Central and peripheral increment thresholds for white and spectral lights on a white background in different kinds of congenitally defective colour vision. *Atti Fond Giorgio Ronchi*. 1977;32:213–254.

Wagner G, Boynton RM. Comparison of four methods of heterochromatic photometry. *J Opt Soc Am*. 1972;62:1508–1515.

Wald G. Human vision and spectrum. *Science*. 1945;101:653–658.

Wallman J, McFadden S. Monkey eyes grow into focus. *Nature Med*. 1996;1:737–739.

Walraven J, Enroth-Cugell C, Hood DC, et al. The control of visual sensitivity: Receptoral and post-receptoral processes. In: Spillman L, Werner JS, eds. *Visual Perception: The Neurophysiological Foundations*. New York: Academic Press; 1990:53–101.

Walraven J, Valeton JM. Visual adaptation and response saturation. In Van Doorn AJ, Van de Grind WA, Koenderink JJ, eds. *Limits in Perception*. Utrecht: VNU Science Press; 1984.

Wandell BA. *Foundations of Vision*. Sunderland: Sinauer; 1995.

Wasserman GS, Kong KL. Illusory correlation of brightness enhancement and transients in the nervous system. *Science*. 1974;184:911–913.

Watson JD, Myers R, Frackowiak RSJ, et al. Area V5 of the human brain: Evidence from a combined study using positron emission tomography and magnetic resonance imaging. *Cereb Cortex*. 1993;3:79–94.

Weale RA. *The Aging Eye*. London: Lewis; 1963.

Weale RA. Senile cataract: The case against light. *Ophthalmology*. 1983;90:420–423.

Weale RA. *The Senescence of Human Vision*. New York: Oxford University Press; 1992.

Weiskrantz L. *Blindsight. A Case Study and Implications*. Oxford: Oxford University Press; 1986.

Werblin FS, Dowling JE. Organization of the retina of the mudpuppy, *Necturus maculosus*. II. Intracellular recording. *J Neurophysiol*. 1969;32:339–355.

Westheimer G. The spatial sense of the eye (Proctor lecture). *Invest Ophthalmol Vis Sci*. 1979;18:893–912.

Wiesel TN, Hubel DH. Single-cell responses in striate cortex of kittens deprived of vision in one eye. *J Neurophysiol*. 1963;26:1003–1017.

Wiesel TN, Hubel DH. Spatial and chromatic interactions in the lateral geniculate body of the rhesus monkey. *J Neurophysiol*. 1966;29:1115–1156.

Wiesel TN, Raviola E. Myopia and eye enlargement after neonatal lid fusion in monkeys. *Nature*. 1977;266:66–68.

Wildsoet C, Wallman J. Choroidal and scleral mechanisms of compensation for spectacle lenses in chicks. *Vision Res*. 1995;35:1175–1194.

Williams DR. Seeing through the photoreceptor mosaic. *Trends Neurosci.* 1986;9:193–198.

Wong-Riley MTT. Changes in the visual system of monocularly sutured or enucleated cats demonstrable with cytochrome oxidase histochemistry. *Brain Res.* 1979;171:11–28.

Woo G, Hess R. Contrast sensitivity function and soft contact lenses. *Int Contact Lens Clin.* 1979;6:171–176.

Wood JM, Bullimore MA. Changes in the lower displacement limit for motion with age. *Ophthalmic Physiol Opt.* 1995;15:31–36.

Wright WD. The sensitivity of the eye to small colour differences. *Proc Physiol Soc Lond.* 1941;53:93–112.

Wright WD. *Researches on Normal and Defective Color Vision.* London: Henry Kimpton; 1946.

Wright WD. The characteristics of tritanopia. *J Opt Soc Am.* 1952;42:509–520.

Wyszecki G, Stiles WS. *Color Science: Concepts and Methods, Quantitative Data and Formulae.* 2nd ed. New York: Wiley; 1982.

Young MP, Scannell JW. Analysis and modelling of the mammalian cerebral cortex. In: Othmer HG, Main RK, Murray JD, eds. *Experimental and Theoretical Advances in Biological Pattern Formation.* New York: Plenum Press; 1993:369–384.

Young RW. Visual cells. *Sci Am.* 1970;223(4):80–91.

Young RW. The renewal of rod and cone outer segments in the rhesus monkey. *J Cell Biol.* 1971;49:303–318.

Young RW. Visual cells, daily rhythms, and vision research. *Vision Res.* 1978;18:573–578.

Young T. On the theory of light and colours. *Philos Trans.* 1802;92:21–71.

Zaidi Q. Simultaneous estimation of illuminance and object colors. *Invest Ophthalmol Vis Sci.* 1997;38(suppl):S476.

Zeki SM. The distribution of wavelength and orientation selective cells in different areas of the monkey visual cortex. *Proc R Soc Lond Biol Sci.* 1983;217:449–470.

Zeki S. *A Vision of the Brain.* Oxford: Blackwell Scientific; 1993.

Zihl J, von Cramon D, Mai N. Selective disturbance of movement vision after bilateral brain damage. *Brain.* 1983;106:313–340.

# Index